Life in Crisis

Life in Crisis

*The Ethical Journey
of Doctors Without Borders*

———

Peter Redfield

UNIVERSITY OF CALIFORNIA PRESS

Berkeley   Los Angeles   London

University of California Press, one of the most distinguished university presses in the United States, enriches lives around the world by advancing scholarship in the humanities, social sciences, and natural sciences. Its activities are supported by the UC Press Foundation and by philanthropic contributions from individuals and institutions. For more information, visit www.ucpress.edu.

University of California Press
Berkeley and Los Angeles, California

University of California Press, Ltd.
London, England

Library of Congress Cataloging-in-Publication Data

Redfield, Peter, 1965-
    Life in crisis : the ethical journey of Doctors without Borders /
Peter Redfield.
        p. ; cm.
    Ethical journey of Doctors without Borders
    Parts of the chapters were published previously.
    Includes bibliographical references and index.
    ISBN 978-0-520-27484-6 (cloth : alk. paper) — ISBN 978-0-520-27485-3
(pbk. : alk. paper)
    I. Title.   II. Title: Ethical journey of Doctors without Borders.
    [DNLM: 1. Médecins sans frontières (Association)   2. Voluntary
Health Agencies—ethics.   3. Altruism.   4. Anthropology, Cultural.
5. Disaster Medicine—ethics.   6. Health Policy.   7. Internationality.
WA 1]
    362.1—dc23   2012034935

Manufactured in the United States of America

21   20   19   18   17   16   15   14   13   12
10   9   8   7   6   5   4   3   2   1

For Zoë, in the name of Sofia

CONTENTS

FIGURES

ACKNOWLEDGMENTS

For all its urgent subject matter, this book has been distinctly slow in coming. My list of debts is therefore long and my ability to enumerate them grossly inadequate. Whatever is valuable in this work owes much to the generosity and forbearance of those who consulted, hosted, counseled, questioned, and otherwise lived adjacent to it.

First and foremost I thank the many current and former members of MSF (expatriate and national staff alike) who spoke with me, whether in offices or at mission sites, amid hectic days or in moments of off-duty respite. Most will remain nameless here, but this project would have languished without their honest engagement. Some contributed tolerantly and repeatedly over many years, others briefly but to fortuitous effect. A few figures merit particular mention. In the New York office first Kris Torgeson and then Kevin Phelan offered unflagging support, providing contacts, updates, and publications, while Nicolas de Torrenté shared commentary and a copy of his thesis. In Paris Stéphan Oberreit went far beyond duty in offering orientation, astute observations, and advice. In Brussels and Amsterdam Ed Rackley likewise played a key initial role, followed by years of periodic commentary. During the last phase of writing in Cape Town, Eric Goemaere kindly made time for reading the section on AIDS and discussing the South African case. And at the final hour Hernan del Valle and Olga Overbeek in Amsterdam helped locate a cover photo.

I owe a particular debt to several old friends in Uganda, particularly Jaco Homsy, Rachel King, Jono Mermin, and Becky Bunnell. They and their extended households hosted me on several occasions, matching generosity with invaluable advice. Beyond MSF I thank members of the Centers for Disease Control (CDC), the Aids Support Organization (TASO), and Traditional and Modern Health Practitioners Together against AIDS (THETA), who also welcomed me amid their daily work.

My research enjoyed support from a National Endowment for the Humanities Summer Stipend and a National Endowment for the Humanities Fellowship, as well as from several sources at UNC Chapel Hill, including the University Research Council, the Odum IRSS Latane fund, the Spray-Randleigh Fellowship fund, and a Junior Faculty Development Grant. I also benefited from a semester in residence at the Institute for Arts and Humanities at UNC and composed the bulk of the manuscript as a Weatherhead Fellow at the School for Advanced Research in Santa Fe.

It was my good fortune to craft much of this text at sites of privilege in beautiful surroundings. Writing about suffering in places like Santa Fe and Cape Town posed troubling contradictions, but it also served as a reminder to view life through its range of possibility and not just troubling episodes of despair. My cohort of fellows at SAR—Tutu Alicante, Omri Elisha, Joe Gone, Tiya Miles, Malena Mörling, Monica Smith, James Snead, and Angela Stuesse—proved as inspiring as the scenery. Thanks also to the wonderful staff, especially Rebecca Allahyari, James Brooks, Catherine Cocks, John Kantner, Nancy Owen Lewis, and Leslie Shipman. Members of the Advanced Seminar on Humanitarianism held at SAR likewise contributed greatly to my thinking at a critical stage; warm thanks go to Jonathan Benthall, Lawrence Cohen, Harri Englund, Didier Fassin, Ilana Feldman, Sandra Hyde, Liisa Malkki, Mariella Pandolfi, Miriam Ticktin, and especially my co-conspirator, Erica Bornstein.

Over the past decade I have shared parts of the manuscript and related work in many venues, including departments of anthropology at the University of Chicago, Cornell University, Duke University, the New School, Stellenbosch University, Université de Montréal, the University of Cape Town, the University of Copenhagen, the University of New Mexico, the University of Oslo, and the University of Sussex, as well as centers for African studies at Emory University and Cambridge University, the Department of Geography at UNC, the School for Advanced Research, departments of social medicine at Harvard University and McGill University, the Institute for Public Knowledge at NYU, and the Max Planck Institute for Social Anthropology. Elements of it featured in several workshops at the Social Science Research Council, as well as in workshops held at Amherst College, Cambridge University, Columbia University, Eindhoven Technical University, the Georgia Institute of Technology, Rice University, Université de Lille, the University of Michigan, and the University of Virginia. I thank all of these institutions, and even more the audience members who provided invaluable observations and suggestions.

Closer to home I owe a debt to present and former colleagues in the Anthropology Department at the University of North Carolina, who for many years have provided an open and collegial setting in which to work and think. Special thanks to Judy Farquhar, who served as my initial mentor and left distinctive comments on my early writing on this topic, and to the members of the shifting medical anthropology collective, who have provided many fruitful insights. Between Chapel Hill and Duke, Anne Allison, Rudi Colloredo-Mansfeld, Marisol de la Cadena, Bob Daniels, Arturo Escobar, Terry Evens, Dottie Holland, Matt Hull, Scott Kirsch, Fred Klaits, Bill Lachicotte, Paul Leslie, Cathy Lutz, Chris Nelson, Charlie Piot, Michele Rivkin-Fish, Barry Saunders, Mark Sorensen, Orin Starn, Brad Weiss, and Amy Weil all bear special mention, as does Diane Nelson, who thankfully never forgets how to laugh. A number of students contributed to this work while pursuing their own. Sara Ackerman, Juan Ricardo Aparicio, Laurel Bradley, Ashley Carse, Thom Chivens, Jason Cross, Amelia Fiske, Euryung Jun, Lili Lai, Louisa Lombard, Karie Morgan, Dawn Peebles, Dana Powell, Eduardo Restrepo, and Lindsey Wallace all provided useful intervention, whether or not they recall it themselves. Particular thanks go to Laura Wagner and Saydia Kamal, insightful scholars of humanitarianism in their own right, and Johanna Rankin, who included directly relevant questions in her thesis research.

Old friends likewise contributed to this endeavor. Daniel Labovitz and Laura Boylan hosted me in New York several times, with lavish helpings of conversation and wry medical insight. Catherine Benoît first directed me to some key nodes in Paris, while Alex Miles and Anne-Marie Bruleaux let me squat in their empty apartment. Other friends old and new provided intellectual welcome, discussion, and inspiration; they include Michael Barnett, Dominic Boyer, Alice Bullard, Carlo Caduff, Craig Calhoun, Jennifer Cole, Stephen Collier, Stefan Ecks, Jim Faubion, Paco Ferrándiz, Bruce Grant, Jeremy Greene, Gabrielle Hecht, Seth Holmes, Guillaume Lachenal, Andy Lakoff, Fletcher Linder, Pierre Minn, Hiro Miyazaki, Vinh-Kim Nguyen, Rich and Sally Price, Paul Rabinow, Tobias Rees, Annelise Riles, Steven Robins, Richard Rottenburg, and Eric San Juan, as well as Wenzel Geissler and Ruth Prince. Renée Fox and Didier Fassin offered generous early encouragement, while Dan Bortolotti, Julie Laplante, and Darryl Stellmach kindly shared resources from their own work on MSF.

At the University of California Press I thank Stan Holwitz for his forbearance when my "short, quick" book turned long and slow, as well as Reed Malcolm, who proved equally patient and supportive when he inherited it. Two reviewers and a member of the Press's editorial review board provided exceptionally thoughtful commentary. Miriam Ticktin merits extra appreciation for her attention to the manuscript, as does Rich Price, for expeditious and candid feedback. Stacy Eisenstark and Mari Coates deftly steered the text into production, and Jan Spauschus provided judicious copyediting.

As always, I thank most deeply those closest to my own trajectory. My parents,

Charles and Margaret Redfield, have long and quietly embodied an ethical life. My brothers, Marc and Tim, have reliably, year after year, offered provocation in different directions. I could not ask for a more steadfast companion than Silvia Tomášková, bold enough to care and never failing to ask uncomfortable questions. Our daughter, Zoë, has grown up alongside this work. Although it belongs to that dull genre that she once memorably summarized as "the theory is . . . ," I hope someday she may receive a small return for what she has lent to it: a daily reminder of the importance not just of life, but of living.

ADDITIONAL ACKNOWLEDGMENTS:

A portion of chap. 1 was published in "Doctors, Borders and Life in Crisis," *Cultural Anthropology* 20 (3 [2005]). Parts of chap. 2 appeared in "Secular Humanitarianism and Sacred Life," in *What Matters? Ethnographies of Value in a (Not So) Secular Age,* ed. C. Bender and A. Taves (New York: Columbia University Press, 2012). Elements of chap. 3 were published in "Vital Mobility and the Humanitarian Kit," in *Biosecurity Interventions: Global Health and Security in Question,* ed. A. Lakoff and S. Collier (New York: Columbia University Press, 2008), and in "Cleaning Up the Cold War: Global Humanitarianism and the Infrastructure of Crisis Response," in *Entangled Geographies: Empire and Technopolitics in the Global Cold War,* ed. G. Hecht (Cambridge, MA: MIT Press, 2011). Sections of chap. 4 appeared in "A Less Modest Witness: Collective Advocacy and Motivated Truth in a Medical Humanitarian Movement," *American Ethnologist* 33 (1 [Feb. 2006]), and in "The Impossible Problem of Neutrality," in *Forces of Compassion: Humanitarianism between Ethics and Politics,* ed. E. Bornstein and P. Redfield (Santa Fe, NM: School for Advanced Research Press, 2011). Much of chap. 5 featured in "The Unbearable Lightness of Expats: Double Binds of Humanitarian Mobility," *Cultural Anthropology* 27 (2 [May 2012]). Elements of chap. 6 were published in "Sacrifice, Triage and Global Humanitarianism," in *Humanitarianism in Question: Politics, Power, Ethics,* ed. M. Barnett and T. Weiss (Ithaca, NY: Cornell University Press, 2008). A small part of chap. 7 was published in "Doctors Without Borders and the Moral Economy of Pharmaceuticals," in *Human Rights in Crisis,* ed. A. Bullard (Aldershot, UK: Ashgate Press, 2008). Chap. 8 draws partly on "The Verge of Crisis: Doctors Without Borders in Uganda," in *Contemporary States of Emergency: The Politics of Military and Humanitarian Interventions,* ed. D. Fassin and M. Pandolfi (New York: Zone Books, 2010). Previously published material reprinted with permission.

Introduction

Help us save a life today.
MSF FUNDRAISING BROCHURE, 2008

The prospect of "saving lives" now serves as a common point of moral reference. Variations on the theme figure prominently in fundraising appeals, suggesting that donations to aid organizations can transmute into rescue. Politicians and corporations, with varying degrees of sincerity, seek to validate their actions through an accounting of potential protection or harm. As a moral precept the preservation of human life offers the allure of simplicity: whatever else holds in the complexity of human affairs, surely helping others live should be a good thing.

Beyond rhetorical appeals to virtue, what would it mean to build a framework for action around an ethic of life, understood medically and cast on a global scale? The following pages pursue this question through the story of a particular organization, one founded with precisely such an aim in mind. The group's name— Médecins Sans Frontières, or Doctors Without Borders—reflects both its fundamental orientation to health and its distinctly universal ambition.[1] To the extent that its acronym, MSF, has become a staple reference in international aid, the group has realized its geographic aspiration. Its general goals and modes of engagement are far from unique; many other nongovernmental organizations practice humanitarian medicine. Nonetheless, MSF's historical trajectory and restless, critical ethos render it a particularly telling case. Over four decades the group has sought to save lives and push limits, reflecting upon and sometimes reconsidering its actions without abandoning its fundamental commitment to combat suffering. In settings where action itself stands for virtue (in the sense that "doing something" displays good character), MSF's engagement offers the abiding appeal of immediacy. When lives appear to be at stake, urgent medical care acquires an aura of moral purity. What more essential response, after all, could there be? Nonethe-

1

less, the actual practice of such intervention often proves complex and its implications fraught. Which threats are the most pressing? How long should a given response continue? When might aid projects metastasize, growing to choke their host like a cancer? MSF's evolving series of attempts to provide succor reflect the shifting dreams of the contemporary aid world; they also reveal the lines of tension running through its vision.

During Europe's first fling with the Enlightenment, there emerged a literary genre known as the bildungsroman. Recounting the uncertain passage of callow youth to the ripeness of mature wisdom, works like Goethe's *Wilhelm Meister's Apprenticeship* captured the mood of self-realization for a humanist age in which one's calling and place in the world emerged through personal experience rather than divine revelation. Although the sureness of genre may evaporate under careful scrutiny—like the larger terms of *humanism* and *enlightenment* themselves— I take such novels of self-formation as my guide for presenting the story of a particular organization. This literary form provided a vision of the human as a barometer for moral development, one that emerged in concert with both the nation-state and international law.[2] Voltaire's early incisive satire *Candide* thus offers a historically apt reference when considering relations between humanitarian action and the burden of misplaced hopes it often bears, a point I pursue in the final chapter. MSF's journey has yielded a wealth of experience, if not the comfort of certain wisdom.

What follows, then, is a bildungsroman of sorts, the story of the sentimental education of a collective enterprise, one conducted in the name of human virtue and common decency. I have ordered it as a series of overlapping histories interspersed with observations and analytic discussion. My approach is largely descriptive, since I retain faith in the suggestive power of specific detail. I also emphasize ethics rather than immediately asserting a political framing. Humanitarian action certainly entails politics, and always has political effects. But the specific motive here remains doing what is right in the most immediate sense, or at any rate doing what is least wrong. Unlike doctors openly dedicated to a certain ideology—Cuba's famous medical brigades, for example—the members of MSF share no sure vision of a public good beyond a commitment to the value of life.[3] Rather than evaluating this ethical field in formal terms (deontological, consequentialist, or virtue-based in one philosophical typology), I simply follow my chosen group's passage through the world of practice. At times MSF claims categorical duties; at others it measures impacts or defines character. Often it worries whether it has lost its way.

As for my own formation, I had several motives for this project. One was simple curiosity; having heard about MSF for years from friends who had encountered or worked with the group, I wanted to know more. My biography no doubt played a role as well, given that I grew up amid humanitarian sensibilities. But the most immediate impetus came from entering professional life as a university professor at a time when calls to relevance resounded. These calls came from strikingly different quarters: administrators bent on instilling business principles into the academy; older faculty who came of age in the 1960s; younger students who combined a thinner sense of history with an intense desire to "do good." The collective emphasis on action over contemplation convinced me that it would be worthwhile to examine intervention itself in some ethnographic and historical detail. Humanitarianism, particularly in its medical form, offered a highly concrete example of instrumental action, even as it broached significant ethical and political questions. MSF, as I soon discovered, dated from the very epoch that had shaped understandings of engagement in the university around me. It was an outgrowth of oppositional idealism that had transformed into a key example of the sort of nongovernmental organization now prominent in international affairs. Telling its story, therefore, seemed apt at this generational juncture.

As I continued to pursue this line of research my convictions about it only grew. In the pall that fell over the United States after September 11, 2001, topics that had once appeared comfortably distant acquired sharper relief in public discourse. Refugee camps, the Geneva Conventions, states of legal exception—indeed the very sense of emergency and crisis itself—became more immediate and imaginable concerns. Accumulating background knowledge in bits and pieces, I realized how little I had previously known about the thin fabric of institutions that govern international relations, or the larger histories of war and disaster. My progress was embarrassingly slow, particularly by the frantic standards of emergency projects. I had other duties and responsibilities, and the sensibilities of an academic rather than those of a journalist. As the years slipped by, world crises, not to mention project staff I encountered, came and went. By a humanitarian timeline my material receded into the dimmer reaches of history, and I was always belated as well as a bystander. However, this very inadequacy provided the rare luxury of a longer view.[4]

The research tradition known as ethnography in anthropology developed in villages, that is to say, in face-to-face settings imbued with a cyclical, usually agrarian rhythm. As anthropologists have expanded their vision to a more mobile world, they have also struggled to adapt their methodological inheritance. Many studies now proclaim themselves to be "multi-sited," patched together between places and times rather than layered in place. The following is certainly one such, shaped from encounters on three continents as well as the floating space of electronic exchange. I make no claims to have solved this methodological puzzle in any general sense, only to have muddled though in pursuit of a particular problem. No single person could know all of a global, shifting organization in any depth. However, elements of an organization prove easy to trace and follow, and if one does that repeatedly, they grow familiar. Thus I visited MSF offices in New

York, Paris, Amsterdam, Brussels, and Geneva to interview, observe, and become accustomed to their general ambiance. I likewise traveled over several years to field projects in different corners of Uganda, a country I chose largely on the basis of access and my connections, as well as its location within the central hub of humanitarian activity in sub-Saharan Africa.

As I am not an African specialist by training, let alone an expert across plural worlds, my understanding of particular settings remains regretfully foreshortened. At the same time, this book is less about Uganda than about encounters that took place within its borders. To reach these different settings I lived a version of the expat life, passing through multiple localities at different points in time. Friends also introduced me to other moments in the aid world beyond MSF. Although only glimpses of this larger background appear here, it helped situate my understanding of the particular projects I describe. The wider lives of those who encounter humanitarian action as its intended beneficiaries also exceed these pages. I have sought to include traces of their reactions, but in the limiting tradition of the bildungsroman this work remains focused on its protagonist, MSF.[5]

While researching this book I interviewed well over a hundred individuals, some repeatedly, and encountered hundreds more. Although I recorded a few of my more formal office visits, much of the time I simply took notes, and the further into the field I went—bouncing over dirt tracks and scribbling in a small pocket notebook—the more telegraphic they became. When it was difficult or inappropriate to write at a moment of encounter, I reconstituted events as best I could afterward. The majority of the conversations recounted here took place in English (the lingua franca of the aid world), others in French, and some in a mixture of the two, sometimes including occasional words from other languages. Many of the English conversations were with nonnative speakers of varying backgrounds and facility, people who speak "international English" rather than the literary version. Since this project focuses on the content of their statements rather than the form, I have massaged some quotations to fit convention. All translation involves compromise; I have favored clarity and style over verbatim transcription.

Anthropologists have a tradition of masking their sources when they write, both to protect those involved and to emphasize a perspective that approaches humans through collectivities. In keeping with this convention I name only those individuals who have already entered the public record, identifying others by their social roles or the use of a pseudonym. Given the range of backgrounds involved it is not always easy to find an appropriate alternative designation, let alone one that captures all the qualities of the original. In those cases I at least hope my substitutions do not detract from the authority of the speakers.

An organization like Médecins Sans Frontières generates a phenomenal amount of self-representation, from glossy brochures and electronic postings to a larger and more fragmentary array of internal memos, studies, essays, conferences, and other exchanges. During the course of this project I gathered a considerable archive of these items, including many issues of the house journals of MSF sections in Paris, Brussels, and Amsterdam. Much of this material lies in a gray area between public and private, moving closer to the light as the urgent moment of its creation fades. The few items that appeared particularly sensitive I have avoided citing, often finding alternatives already in circulation, since this work seeks to portray a general form, not to compromise individuals or reanalyze a particular intervention. A number of highly articulate and thoughtful studies have emerged within humanitarianism, including a striking number by sometime members of MSF. I have treated these as both primary and secondary literature in the historical sense, often finding source material and interpretive guidance within the same text.

MSF prides itself on maintaining a culture of internal argument and critical reflection. I owe this admirable tradition an incalculable debt, both for generating rich, diverse material and for granting me access to it. At the same time, that culture creates challenges of its own. Early on in this project an astute colleague warned me that the group's constant self-questioning might have the side effect of inoculating it against external criticism. Certainly few topics have escaped disputation within MSF over the years, and most of what I recount here will therefore be familiar to anyone with experience in the organization, or indeed the aid world, where critical consideration is no novelty. On occasion MSF appears to suffer from a common academic affliction—assuming that because an issue has generated passionate discussion, it is therefore resolved.

The group's self-questioning does exhibit certain limits. At an academic conference at an American university I heard a prominent African scholar ask representatives of MSF why they did not just let people die. Both his blunt provocation and subsequent elaboration highlighted the political stakes involved, suggesting that saving lives interfered with longer-term resolutions of human agony. It also uncovered an uncomfortable fault line of moral sentiment. MSF might quite ably discuss the dilemmas of aid, its shortcomings, limits, and negative side effects. But to willingly abandon the living—to sacrifice them for a potential future—remains unthinkable for a humanitarian organization. Even critics of humanitarianism rarely embrace openly antihumanitarian alternatives, such as the conscious exchange of living individuals or populations for future political gain. Progressive calls for social change now largely expect transformation to unfold without a guillotine. At this historical moment, then, it is not easy to stand completely outside the humanitarian frame of value, even if confronted with graphic evidence of its widespread and cynical violation. When writing about MSF, both hagiography and certain critique grow too comfortable.

Anthropologists tend to emphasize human dignity more than sheer survival and frequently worry about difference and self-determination. Predisposed to longer-term presence and invested in local knowledge, they challenge biomedical assumptions of universality on the one hand and emphasize larger patterns of political economy on the other. Even the work of Paul Farmer and his associates in Partners in Health—probably the closest corollary to MSF with anthropological roots—adopts a different strategic approach, making long-term collaborative investments in place and openly claiming ideals of social justice. Nonetheless, when facing acute episodes of human suffering, anthropologists also tend to measure moral failure in destruction and death. When disaster strikes they often display humanitarian impulses and expectations, desiring action and imagining a global response.

Like most potential readers of this book, I too care about the lives of others. However skeptical about salvation projects, I remain reluctant to denounce them out of hand. Calling for the dramatic transformation of human affairs offers little comfort if its fulfillment remains forever deferred. Rather, I would simply extend a question—whose salvation?—beyond the stark line dividing life and death, and back into an ever messy world. To the extent this study remains implicated in the broader humanitarian vision, then, it cannot resort to full-throated registers of critique. Acknowledging a degree of implication and shared values can never match the rhetorical fulfillment of denunciation. In recompense, however, it might recognize the imperfect conditions of our actual present, through which any concern for life and suffering must pass.

The following chapters expand on intertwined themes of life and crisis, offering background on MSF as an organization as well as on the values that animate it. Across them I trace a series of elements in MSF's evolving history of global ambition: the development of both independent fundraising and a mobile infrastructure for providing global care; the emergence of a signature practice of witnessing violations and suffering; and the complex interplay of human and financial resources across borders. I also present limits to its action: the troubling logic of choice inherent to open, mobile engagement; the reiterative expansion of projects beyond emergency care into crises that unfold more slowly, most significantly the provision of HIV/AIDS treatment; and the underlying uncertainty a setting like Uganda inspires in contrast to the moral clarity of emergency. Finally I take up the question of results and the problem of action without optimism.

In its collective experience MSF knows it can't save the world. Nonetheless, it operates within a wider field of expectations, inspiring hope and discontent well beyond its action. That is both its greatest quality and its greatest danger: to stand for virtue in what appears like a post-utopian age.

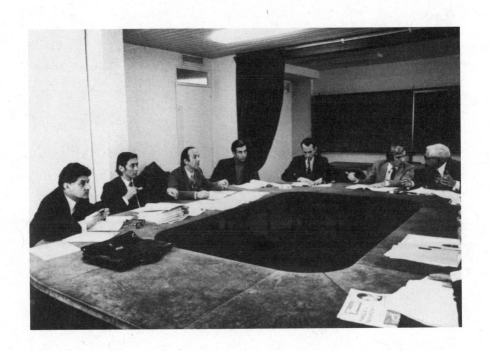

PART ONE

Terms of Engagement

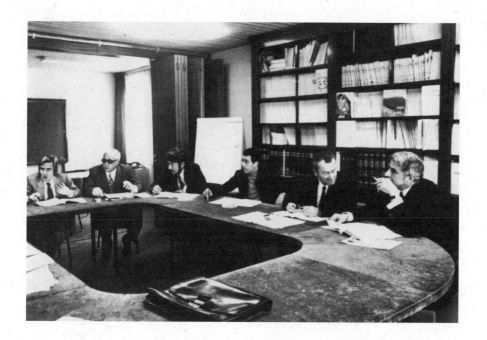

A Time of Crisis

*Our action is to help people in situations of crisis. And ours is not a contented
action.*

MSF, NOBEL PEACE PRIZE ACCEPTANCE SPEECH, 1999

THE NOBEL DREAM

On October 15, 1999, the Norwegian Nobel committee announced the last Peace
Prize of the twentieth century. It would go, the committee proclaimed with cus-
tomary fanfare, to the organization Médecins Sans Frontières. Known in English
as Doctors Without Borders and in the acronym-friendly aid world as MSF, this
group was, strictly speaking, focused on medical humanitarianism rather than
peace. Nonetheless, the committee noted the distinctive independence MSF
brought to disaster settings. By intervening swiftly and calling public attention to
abuses of power, it suggested, MSF's action inspired at least a glimmer of a brighter
future. "In critical situations, marked by violence and brutality, the humanitarian
work of Médecins Sans Frontières enables the organization to create openings for
contacts between the opposed parties," read the citation. "At the same time, each
fearless and self-sacrificing helper shows each victim a human face, stands for
respect for that person's dignity, and is a source of hope for peace and reconciliation."[1] The award hardly came as a complete surprise. MSF fit a long lineage of
humanitarian laureates and had received nominations for a number of years.
Indeed, given that the founder of the Red Cross movement had shared the very
first prize in 1901, it seemed fitting to end the century on a parallel note. What
better way to frame a bloody, violent era than with variants on the red and white
symbols of medical care?

As usual with the annual Nobel ritual, a flurry of news reports, mostly laudatory, profiled the committee's choice. Since MSF originated in France, the French
press went into a particular paroxysm of celebration. To the annoyance of MSF's
current members, considerable attention was focused on Bernard Kouchner, one

of the group's founders who had subsequently become a significant European political figure. Many reports emphasized Kouchner's signature issue—the *doit d'ingérence,* or right to intervene on humanitarian grounds—a concept that his successors at MSF had increasingly disavowed even as variants materialized in international precedent.[2] Alongside gauzy allusions to peace and hints of civilizing redemption, the accounts predictably emphasized national pride: this was France's great gesture of civil society, its response to Britain's Amnesty International and Switzerland's Red Cross. At the same time, the reviews skirted more controversial moments in the group's history, including the still-raw wounds of Rwanda.[3] As congratulatory letters poured in, celebration, not controversy, was the order of the day. For its part MSF basked in the attention, worried about how to respond appropriately, and debated what to do with the prize money.

December saw an award ceremony in Oslo, where representatives of the organization frantically drafted a final version of their collective address and donned special T-shirts to silently protest the Russian bombing of the Chechen capital Grozny. The speech sought to outline MSF's humanitarian vision and concerns, drawing a sharp distinction between MSF's actions and those of a state. "Humanitarianism occurs where the political has failed or is in crisis," it proclaimed, rejecting humanitarian justifications for political agendas. MSF's action was a struggle, and its independence included a right to witness and speak out. The T-shirt protest and subsequent march to the Russian embassy sought to exemplify this at a moment of heightened exposure. Although the small gesture drew no immediate response, the BBC subsequently announced that the Russian government had extended an ultimatum in the conflict, expressing concern about civilian suffering. As for the prize itself, MSF decided to invest the funds in its new initiative to combat neglected diseases and its campaign for greater access to essential medicines worldwide.[4] The celebratory mood continued though the final midnight of the year, when a young doctor from the group officially dropped the ball in New York's Times Square, ushering in a new millennium.

For all its obvious and sanctimonious pomp, the Nobel moment marked a watershed for MSF. Once considered a youthful and ragtag oppositional movement, the organization had grown into a fixture of international relief efforts and garnered official approval. *Le monde,* France's most established daily, described the group's mythic trajectory out of Nigeria's Biafran uprising as "the challenges of a generation." Other reports cited Paris's own turmoil in 1968, while Montreal's English-language *Gazette,* decrying the "humanitarian occupation of Third World countries," offered a more biting formulation: "Medical hippies go mainstream." At the opposite end of the spectrum a cartoon in a French satirical publication showed a young doctor returning to his stuffy, bourgeois parents, who wondered why he couldn't have received the medical prize instead.[5] Nearing thirty, MSF had clearly come of age. What was less clear was whether or not the group would experience some sort of midlife crisis, growing complacent, as some of its adherents feared, or preserving the status quo, as some of its critics charged. Had humanitarian action—even in its outspoken and independent form—grown routine?

At the time of the Nobel announcement I was already curious about Médecins Sans Frontières. Like many people I was familiar with the group's fundraising efforts, having received its solicitations from time to time. I also knew people who had worked for them. The name intrigued me, since the phrase "without borders" had grown synonymous with global mobility. Moreover, the humanitarian focus on saving lives suggested a universal appeal: minimal morality through emergency care. At the same time, MSF practiced medicine. The group's members not only spoke, but also acted, mounting complex missions in diverse settings. Their collective work combined technology and morality with a practical form of anthropology, defining and contesting a sense of humanity worldwide. This was indeed an attempt at global medicine.

Memoirs aside, much of the writing about nongovernmental organizations I could find at the time dealt with the topic from a methodological or theoretical remove. Some analysts surveyed a range of groups to create comparative models. Others positioned the recent prominence of civil society and the NGO form within a larger framework of neoliberal reform and privatized welfare. I sought a view closer to the ground, one involving historical detail and the loose ends of experience, albeit one more systematic than an individual memoir. For an anthropologist of my generation and orientation, what people did mattered as much as what they said. I knew MSF was venturing into new areas, such as the above-mentioned pharmaceutical campaign, and a major effort to treat AIDS. Before addressing those developments, however, I wanted to grasp the group's traditional customs and habits. The first task of studying this NGO, then, would be to examine its call to arms and vision for action.

In the Nobel address, MSF defined its mission as helping "people in situations of crisis," quickly adding that this endeavor was not "contented."[6] Beyond a general principle of the alleviation of suffering, then, the group's version of humanitarianism clearly depended on a concept of crisis. The life that MSF sought to save was not an ordinary one, in the sense of being burdened by everyday complaints. Rather it was the life located in an exceptional state of risk. Indeed, a persistent sense of urgency infused all of MSF's rhetoric and work. Although the group may have devoted its prize money to a new initiative for pharmaceutical equity, the Nobel citation reflected MSF's central public image: an emergency room team, on call worldwide. As I soon discovered, the details beneath that image proved more complex: the group included volunteer nurses, engineers, and administrators alongside doctors, relied on an army of local employees to perform a considerable part of the actual labor, and had grown to conduct a diverse range of missions. Nonetheless, the emergency idiom captured the organization's essential ethos.

Both *crisis* and *emergency* are native terms for MSF. Whereas the first indicates a critical condition or conjuncture, often including social and political contexts, the second references a more specific set of problems requiring rapid medical response.[7] In this work I will largely adhere to MSF's functional distinction. Moreover, I suggest that the line that distinguishes emergency from the more fluid concept of crisis raises unsettling questions about the group's humanitarian rationale and purpose. While emergency missions may no longer be the norm, they still represent a self-consciously "classic" form of action within MSF. Not every member may dream of being "eight to a tent in the Congo," as one veteran put it to me in Kampala in 2003, but such dramatic conditions remain romantic points of reference for the collective, and a sense of urgency courses through most of the group's rhetoric. To quote another of its former adherents, MSF "couldn't survive without the word *emergency*." At the same time, the organization addresses a wider field of problems, not all of which fit into an ambulance. As I detail later, AIDS and pharmaceutical equity are certainly crises from MSF's perspective, but they are not exactly emergencies. Both terms, however, prioritize the present over the past and the future. Moreover, they suggest a state of rupture and through it an imperative need for action: something must be done and done quickly. In this sense disaster—not development—lies at the heart of the organization. "We are much more attached to the notion of crisis," the French section's communications director told me in 2003, describing the group's particular niche in the wider aid complex. "A community has developed in its own particular way, encounters a moment of crisis, so we help them face it and then move on."[8] In this formulation at least, humanitarianism has come to define itself through exception.

LIFE IN CRISIS

In the fall of 2000, MSF brought a traveling exhibit to several sites in greater New York and Los Angeles. Part of a special publicity campaign on behalf of displaced people entitled "A Refugee Camp in the Heart of the City," it featured a model camp that could be moved and displayed in any public venue.[9] At each stop the exhibit also served as a de facto reunion for former aid workers, who came together both to raise public awareness and to see old comrades and like-minded souls. Staff at MSF's New York office assured me it would make for an excellent entrée into their world. Thus on a beautiful September morning I found myself in Central Park, the light clear and bright as it filtered through the buildings. A small group of MSF veterans milled about before a temporary enclosure, white shirts emblazoned with a bright red insignia. Throughout the day, they issued identity cards to a growing stream of visitors, shepherding them through a circle of structures representing a simulated refugee camp: tents and prefabricated huts, a mobile clinic, and a mock latrine.

This was a year before New York itself would experience the immediacy of disaster and five years before Hurricane Katrina would strike New Orleans. The images of panicked, fleeing people appeared comfortably remote, a problem of elsewhere. The camp here was a model, after all, meant to convey the gist of the humanitarian labor involved in caring for displaced populations to those who had only encountered glimpses of such things on television. Led by aid workers, including some former refugees, the tours offered another experiential reminder of human suffering and need through a display of the materials used to respond to them. In the name of research, I went on several tours over the course of the day. Although each varied in detail and emphasis according to the background and personality of the person leading it, the general pattern remained. The first section of the exhibit illustrated basic needs: shelter in the form of simple tents adapted to different climates, water purification in the form of a giant bladder dispensing five gallons per person per day, food in the form of compact bars providing 2,100 calories, and finally hygiene in the form of a latrine (the "VIP version") that was equipped with both a folk painting about hand washing and an ingenious method of trapping flies. To one side hung a small poster about mental health and trauma and beyond lay the medical zone, featuring a model clinic, a weighing station and vaccination center, and finally a cholera exclusion area. The tour closed with a depiction of land mines and a photographic testimonial to the plight of refugees.

As the press release for the event noted, the core of the exhibit emphasized "basic elements" of refugee existence. Here was a panorama of survival, in all its measured essence. When confronted by emergency, people's lives shrank to elemental, species-level needs: a place to stay, some means of sustenance, and collective cleanliness. Without these they would suffer, fall ill, or even die. At moments of crisis, the exhibit made clear, life itself was on the line. Humanitarian concern, therefore, focused on providing temporary substitutes for immediate necessities. Longer-term issues, although recognized, remained on the sidelines.

The choice of a refugee camp for MSF's publicity campaign was far from arbitrary. Rather, it reflected the setting within which the group had emerged and subsequently developed much of its equipment, experience, customs, and mores. As a medical organization it focused primarily on health concerns. Although MSF might offer shelter, food, or water if conditions required, its real expertise lay in the clinical areas of camp life, assessing nutrition, offering basic treatment, and dispensing health advice. Even if the group's activities now extended well beyond camp settings, its sensibilities remained those of urgent care. Medicine here centered on patients with pressing needs and prioritized rapid treatment. Although the patients experienced common conditions, they remained individual in the sense that one could not simply be substituted for another.

The official press kit for the exhibit provided ample and graphic evidence of the refugee experience. Beyond images, testimonial accounts, and a fact sheet, it offered a sample emergency nutritional biscuit and a swatch of the plastic sheeting commonly used in camps. It also included one of MSF's simplest instruments—a thin paper strip that the attached publicity card dubbed "The Bracelet of Life." As the card explained, the strip could be used to measure the middle upper arm circumference of children below the age of five. When looped and pulled tight it gave a quick indication of nutritional health, expressed both as a numerical measure and a declining gradation of colors: green, yellow, orange, and red. Inexpensive, easily replaced, and simple to use, it was an elegant tool for triage and assessment during famine.[10] The bracelet appeared a fascinating triumph of design. It also rendered most acutely a central dilemma confronted by MSF and similar organizations. Life, on this strip of paper, became most visible at the red end of the spectrum. There, existence itself was on the line. By contrast, the green reading indicated the absence of just one form of stress, not a secure childhood. Existence might be safe from starvation, but the significant gap between distress and happiness remained a cipher.

At the close of the 1950s the political philosopher Hannah Arendt suggested the term *life* might have more than one meaning. She drew a distinction between the cyclical life shared by all species, in which birth and death occur in repetitive patterns, and the linear life narrated by humans as a directional story, in which birth and death mark beginning and end.[11] Citing Aristotle, she suggested that the gap between them reflected two Greek terms for life, *zoe* and *bios,* the respective roots of the contemporary English terms *zoology* and *biography.* Decades later other thinkers would take up Arendt's distinction and elaborate on the broader problem of life and politics. We will return to some of these elaborations shortly. For the moment, however, the key thing to note is that MSF's bracelet belongs more to the cyclical realm of existence than to the narrative realm of life beyond it. "Saving lives" surely addresses living in the sense of biological survival, but not always life in the sense of living well or, as the expression goes, "having a life."

Although measuring a state of *zoe* far more than *bios,* the Bracelet of Life still tells a story of sorts. MSF members often cite nutritional work as an example of gratifying humanitarian experience, since children who remain above a threshold of survival recover with satisfying regularity once carefully fed. But they also describe frustration, recalling instances when patients would return for a second visit, their bodies withered anew by the same conditions that brought them to therapy in the first place. MSF cannot offer a happy ending, only sporadic attention to cruelly thin arms and the potential for short-term gain in the shape of specially formulated foods. It may be better than nothing for the chosen few, certainly, but hardly an ideal basis for a full life. Even recent initiatives to widen the availability of therapeutic foods define themselves against present realities, not future utopias. Humanitarianism of this sort is a stopgap gesture, as MSF's Nobel address sought to stress. It remains troubling work precisely because it responds to failure without offering a comprehensive solution. Lives are sustained and prolonged, more than they are "saved" in any final sense. Survival, after all, is a perpetually temporary outcome.

The facts of survival often prove uncomfortable—even undignified—when viewed outside of urgent contexts. Of all the exhibits in the model refugee camp, the sanitation equipment evoked perhaps the strongest response, at least in a country known for lavish lavatories. This was exemplified by one reaction I witnessed and later described:

> Two young men join the same group that I do. Their appearance and behavior exude an air of cool indifference. A simple concrete block, molded to include the impressions of two feet and a hole for a wooden pole captures their attention, however. The purpose of this artifact begins to dawn on one of them even before our guide launches into describing the dynamics of a temporary pit latrine. "No way," the young man says loudly, staring at it in incredulity. Absorbing the rawness of physical need that it reflects he then steps backward, one hand raised in emphatic rejection. "No way!"[12]

In recounting this anecdote to academic audiences, I discovered they too could find latrines disturbing. The technical considerations of what to do with human waste, although an urgent problem in the case of a sudden influx of people in an emergency, fit poorly into discussions of the lives of political subjects. Moreover, they resonated awkwardly in portrayals of parts of the world frequently associated with suffering and material lack. A latrine was not—at this level of discussion, at least—"empowering." It required delicate positioning to be mentionable, let alone a point of focus.

Humanitarian organizations such as MSF do care deeply about something they call "dignity." They refer to it frequently as a fundamental aspect of humanity, gesturing to it as a rhetorical ideal and denouncing its absence in particular contexts. Life for them thus certainly involves more than survival. A spirit of urgency, however, fuels their actual interventions, which therefore continue to foreground immediate existence. Outbreaks of infectious diseases like cholera haunt crowded settings with poor hygiene, resulting in predictable deaths. Sanitation therefore remains a fundamental part of most aid projects with a public health focus. MSF's ideal might be the VIP latrine, enclosed and free of flies. But if necessary its members are prepared to construct an open pit, shifting its stations, digging and backfilling repeatedly until a better system can be constructed. Survival, in this sense, is ever primary. Dignity remains a secondary consideration, a deeper matter of human recognition that might endure temporary, superficial embarrassment.

The construction of modest artifacts like latrines might appear well removed from the grander terrain of politics. However, modern forms of government actually devote considerable attention to such details. A contemporary state faces implicit and explicit expectations regarding the welfare of its population. Beyond projects such as roads or canals, public works now involve a much broader range of oversight, planning, and regulation. Even most poor and weak governments produce statistics about the well-being of their respective populations, and if they do not, then others do it for them. Birth rates, death rates, infant mortality, life expectancy, and health expenditure all find their measure. So too do more complex statistical artifacts, such as the disability-adjusted life year (DALY), an effort to indicate relative disease burden and compare conditions by calculating "the loss of the equivalent of one year of full health."[13] Infrastructure grows painfully visible when absent, particularly health infrastructure and the availability of care for treatable maladies. Life, in the sense of *zoe*, biological existence, has become a subject for constant accounting. Moments of crisis are thus not only readily apparent but find articulation through a language of health. The frame of a refugee camp both circumscribes a displaced population and reanimates its political significance through an economy of needs.

MINIMAL BIOPOLITICS

To situate MSF's work within this larger field of expectations, I extend an element of theoretical framing. Shortly after the organization was founded, the French thinker Michel Foucault underlined the growing significance of life processes in politics. He introduced the term *biopower* to describe the manner in which facts of existence became the focus of specific operations of government in eighteenth- and nineteenth-century Europe. Birth rates, public hygiene, and the regulation of sexual acts emerged as potential affairs of state and soon became the preoccupation of new cadres of experts. As Foucault famously summarized the shift: "One might say that the ancient right to take life or let live was replaced by a power to foster life or disallow it to the point of death."[14] The tools of politics, in other words, would now include finer instruments than a sword. To govern, and not simply rule, any legitimate sovereign needed a growing cadre of experts.

To the extent that MSF provides for basic needs—supplying shelter, food, water, sanitation, and medicine, urging a population to practice better hygiene—its work involves contemporary functions of governing, if on a minimal, immediate scale. In Foucault's formulation the group is fostering life, and thereby participating in the form of politics that such an endeavor entails. At the same time, however, MSF does not seek anything like classical sovereignty and rejects conventional claims to power. Like most nongovernmental organizations, it operates to one side of politics, claiming ethical motivation and justification for its work. In MSF's case the group's members frame their humanitarian response to suffering as what the Nobel speech termed an "ethic of refusal." In this formulation, action responds to outrage and derives from indignation as much as pity. Unequivocal and antagonistic, such action rejects any justification for either cruelty or neglect. Its adherents view it as an exceptional undertaking, a rejoinder to political failure that resists both the assumptions of charity and the temptations of rule. The goal, as the Nobel speech summarizes it, is to "build spaces of normalcy in the midst of what is profoundly abnormal."[15]

In this respect the group echoes the classic appeal of a humanitarianism rooted in war: responding to a moment of suffering that appears both exceptional and gratuitous. For Henri Dunant, the devout prophet of the Red Cross movement, it was groaning men on the battlefield of Solferino as they expired from lack of water, loss of blood, or a scavenger's knife. For some founders of Médecins Sans Frontières it was emaciated children, caught in the dwindling rebel enclave during the wretched excesses of the Biafran revolt in Nigeria.[16] An immediacy of revulsion reverberates through this humanitarian stream, implicating both the suffering itself and the conditions that allowed it to occur. But this very immediacy also limits political range. The Red Cross effectively sought to civilize war, not end it. MSF may strive to enable individuals to "regain their rights and dignity as human beings," but it prescribes no particular path for doing so. In both instances the emphasis rests on exceptional suffering. The lives in question are those currently in danger, not the legacy of ancestors or the prospects of future generations. The present thus expands to fill time forward and backward.[17]

Recently, the Italian philosopher Giorgio Agamben has extended questions about life and politics to issues of sovereignty and legal exception. Modifying and redirecting Foucault's vision with a central element from that of German political theorist Carl Schmitt, Agamben suggests that the state of exception provides a key form for sovereign rule. As he writes, the exception constitutes a "no-man's-land between public law and political fact, and between the juridical order and life"—a productive limit intimately tied to civil war, insurrection, and resistance.[18] In keeping with Schmitt's dictum, it is precisely this limit that reveals sovereign power, since the one who designates the state of exception stands beyond law. Agamben returns to Arendt's distinction between Greek terms for life, and focuses on the lower threshold of human possibility: naked, formless existence. Tracing a lineage from Auschwitz back to ancient Roman law, he perceives a seed of violence buried deep within the very political tradition that sought to define civility: the designation of those living in exception, whose killing does not constitute a sacrifice. From this perspective, Agamben suggests, we should contemplate anew Walter Benjamin's famous dictum that "the 'state of emergency' in which we live is not the exception but the rule."[19]

Agamben's intervention resonated widely enough to provoke considerable commentary, both positive and negative. Within anthropology it contributed to an upsurge in interest in topics like citizenship and sovereignty. As I suggest throughout this work, such political categories fit imperfectly against the actual conduct of a transnational NGO. MSF focuses quite emphatically on life rather than death. Likewise it defines itself through ethics rather than politics and displays only a reluctant and partial variety of mobile government. Still, whatever the relative merits of Agamben's larger argument and the terms it favors, his intervention highlights a critical axis of concern for this study: the complex contemporary politics of exception and the ambiguities of survival. It is in that spirit that I reference these themes here. Questions of survival and exception indeed lie at the heart of contemporary humanitarian action, particularly in its emergency medical form.[20]

Recall that what MSF seeks to save is, most literally, life in crisis. Some crises are more urgent than others, and the most sudden and dramatic ones demand an emergency response. But in all cases the group perceives the recipients of its care to be people threatened by "times of difficulty, insecurity and suspense" in the phrasing of The Oxford English Dictionary. This sense of crisis is not that of ancient medicine (the turning point of a disease) nor the essential instability of capitalism outlined by Marxist economics and celebrated by technological optimists.[21] Rather it designates a more general but categorically exceptional condition of threat. To borrow another of MSF's now well-worn designations, crisis describes the experience of "populations in danger."[22] In responding to their needs the group displays a lavish commitment to health standards and geographic scope, together with a minimal assurance of continuity in place. Given that war exemplifies the political state of exception, to the extent that MSF views its own existence to be exceptional—a reflection of the needless suffering in the world—one might say that the organization is perpetually at war.

The bracelet example cited above suggests the limits within which MSF operates, as well as the tension between its ideals and the means at its disposal. A colored ribbon might indicate the line between life and death for small children and suggest something about the nutritional state of a population, but it hardly encompasses the causes of human suffering. Often, as I try to suggest in these pages, MSF's general project has proved a work of minimalism, finding and highlighting varied and repeated threats to survival. Although particular interventions can appear extravagant, they remain circumscribed and attenuated, a "minimal biopolitics," if you will. The label fits uncomfortably, as this is action conducted in the name of an ethical rather than political vision. Its larger aims remain diffuse and open. The group's rhetoric routinely denounces threats to human dignity and occasionally suggests life as a longer arc. It does so, however, by claiming an exceptional, humanitarian ground, at once overarching and rigorously specific. The humanity of "populations in danger" remains ever embodied, not an abstract figure. Nonetheless I retain the reference to biopolitics here, not only because of the equipment and expertise MSF deploys (along with its effects), but also because of the form of political conscience it reveals. By responding to perceived state failures, the group asserts a strikingly clear vision of what any functioning state should do: foster life.

Designating MSF's activity as minimal biopolitics suggests a simultaneously attenuated and affirmative variation on the theme of Foucault's biopower. Such action constitutes itself negatively, directly resisting the sovereign right to kill. Rather than seeking control it demands governance by others, even as it provides a limited form of medical care. Unlike the emerging nation-state or Agamben's transcendent sovereign, MSF never names an enemy who must die to save the population, nor does it designate any death as being beyond sacrifice. If rebellious in attitude, it resists the violence of revolution along with the responsibility of rule. The only aspect of sovereignty the group claims is the Schmittian capacity to define an exception, in the sense of independently determining who is in crisis. Responding to those in crisis, it cannot deploy the full panoply of experts and technologies now associated with wealthy states; its action remains limited as well as medically focused. Yet it also marks a baseline, a minimum for moral legitimacy. That is the extent of its politics. In effect MSF dreams of a warmly nurturing state, one that would not designate exceptions or differentiate between those who should live or die. It would extend this dream worldwide to include all populations, *sans frontières*. But the group's own action does little to achieve such a utopian vision, beyond highlighting its continuing absence. It seeks to remain a minimal and temporary response, not the basis for a new regime.

Judging from its self-conception, MSF remains singularly untroubled by contradiction. The sociologist Rénee Fox aptly describes its overall vision as a "nonideological ideology" loosely based on the French legacy of the Rights of Man but directed against both abstract idealism and the existing order.[23] As we will see in the next chapter, the term *ideology* may imply a greater degree of coherence than the historical record. The group has grown, shifted, and fragmented, has often been riven by dispute, and has at times reversed course. However, two constants remain: a deeply realist geopolitical perspective and a categorical moral conscience about suffering. Its perspective combines anti-utopian skepticism with a near-utopian sense of engagement, implying close links between reason, emotion, and action. If MSF perceives a significant health crisis in any setting, be it an emergency such as a cholera outbreak among displaced people or a policy issue such as ineffective national malaria protocols, it tries to respond. Significantly, this response almost never claims to represent a comprehensive solution or to conform to conventional utilitarian rationales of public health. The majority of its operational programs justify themselves through moral legitimacy rather than through cost effectiveness. By demonstrating what is possible, the MSF doctrine suggests, a technically efficient project can highlight the failures of political will behind inadequate health care and remove the excuse that "it can't be done." Nonetheless, members of MSF rarely suggest that their work will directly build a better social order or achieve a state of justice. The goal is to agitate, disrupt, and encourage others to alter the world by practicing humanitarian medicine "one person at a time."[24]

Before proceeding further with this analysis, I turn to from MSF's theory to its practice and the more complicated terrain of the field. When responding to an exceptional state—even an emergency—the group must first determine whether one exists, and if so, what manner of reaction it warrants. Just as the clarity of conflict fades amid the fog of experience, the certainty of crisis can likewise prove elusive.

A VIEW FROM THE LAND CRUISER

A few years after visiting the model camp, I find myself in the back of a white Toyota Land Cruiser, bumping down a dirt track in northern Uganda. The classic transport of international aid organizations, the vehicle carries with it a small store of supplies, a team of field workers, and a connection to a wider world. A large radio antenna sways with each rut in the road, and team members clutch cell phones, checking the fading signal as we travel away from our base and into the countryside. MSF's red and white logo adorns the sides of the vehicle as well as the flag fluttering from the antenna. Another decal shows a rifle inside a slashed circle, emphasizing the unarmed nature of our business. Fittingly enough, this is an exploratory foray of sorts. Over the preceding months, a resurgence of violence in the country's long-simmering war has driven a new wave of people from their homes. MSF responded by launching several projects in the region. Now that conditions have begun to stabilize in the regional center and a neighboring camp, MSF representatives are moving out to visit and evaluate more remote settlements. In this case we are following rumors of a poor water supply and a trail suggested by cases of bloody diarrhea. Although little fighting has been reported recently, security remains tight. The Ugandan military restricts travel to daylight hours, and MSF is relatively unusual in declining to travel in convoys. Nonetheless, members of the team monitor the airwaves, call in at regular intervals, and keep an eye on the horizon. A few burned-out buildings by the roadside break the monotony of tall grass and scraggly trees. Otherwise there are few visible scars of war.

Traveling with me are an Australian nurse who serves as team coordinator, a Japanese doctor, and two Ugandans, our driver and a logistics assistant. En route we notice a growing stream of people joining us on the road and stop to query a man riding a bicycle. He informs us that the camp ahead of us is scheduled for a food distribution today. By the time we arrive a large crowd has gathered in front of an administration building. Stacks of large white and brown burlap bags line the field, marked with "USA" in large letters and containing a corn-soy blend. At a table in front of the building our coordinator, Mary, meets with the camp leader and a representative of the United Nations World Food Program (WFP). After a few pleasantries they get down to business while assistants in blue smocks wait impassively for direction. The camp leader and WFP representative disagree over the current population. The leader claims that well over 27,000 people live there at present; he's done a survey himself with the head of each camp cell. The WFP representative appears unimpressed and sticks to the number he has received from the Ugandan district administrator, which is closer to 21,000. Mary argues with him, pushing for more service, as she's heard that people return from the distribution without food. The WFP representative remains impassive; to alter anything he would "need to have figures and truth." If there is a discrepancy it is the district's responsibility to furnish new official figures. An informal community survey does not count. Noting that he is an experienced administrator, he intimates that he must guard against any attempt inflate a settlement's numbers.[25] He asks the camp leader to sign that the food has been received in good condition and then returns to his large UN car. Originally from South Asia, he has been in this post for three weeks.

As the distribution begins, our team divides up to get the lay of the land. The doctor will visit the health clinic and the cemetery to gain a sense of health services and death rates. The logistics assistant will inspect the latrines and water supply. Our driver will go shopping to check prices at the local trader. Meanwhile Mary and I begin an impromptu, thoroughly informal nutritional evaluation. Unlike the planned assessment I witnessed earlier at another site, we make no attempts to impose order. As the crowd presses in we walk against its flow, and she simply takes the arm of any passing child, measuring the middle upper arm with the multicolored bracelet. I record the results on a clipboard, filling in small bubbles on a sheet according to the color. Most are a healthy green, but as we walk further we find infants whose measurements are orange and red. In those cases Mary gestures to the bracelet to explain: "Orange getting very sick; red very sick," she repeats loudly in English when relevant. She knows little of the local language and we have no interpreter, but those who have been to school should have had some English instruction and may understand. She tells the mothers to find the MSF car and ask for a small food supplement.

While measuring, Mary also takes note of any other obvious disorders. She sees plenty of scabies, several signs of ringworm, a harelip, and possible cerebral palsy. At times she sacrifices efficiency for attention to specific cases; a child arriving only with her sister poses a problem, since the mother would need to be present to receive food. Mary urges the sister to find the mother, while telling her that vaccination is very important. We continue down the road meeting and greeting all available babies, really looking for the most vulnerable. As well as measuring their arms, Mary presses their feet to check for edema related to malnutrition. She catches a little boy who tries to wriggle off while a larger child in a blue shirt stands and stares. She meets a former patient from MSF's clinic in the trading center, calling her by name, and the two chat briefly. Cattle move among the people and an overloaded bicycle totters and crashes, to the amusement of passersby. The crowd streams on and on, and yet these are only a few of the camp's many residents. At last we reach the meeting point and find our vehicle. The other team members arrive and give their reports.

The driver informs us that there is a small market in the camp, its modest supplies selling at a markup. Informal transport leaves to a larger settlement once a day, but the high fare renders it a luxury for most residents. The settlement has four wells, but the chairman of the water association charges people to use them. When people cannot pay or the lines are too long or the water runs out, then they walk to the water hole, which is free but contaminated. Action Aid apparently works with the WFP here and UNICEF supports the health center, but otherwise the camp has received little international and even less governmental assistance. The doctor adds that the health center sees 60–70 patients a day, more than a quarter suffering from malaria. There are also reports of vomiting and gastrointestinal problems; and he announces with some satisfaction, "We have found our bloody diarrhea place." He and the logistics assistance both concur that water supply is a serious problem here. We all walk to the water hole, which proves to be little more than a muddy roadside puddle. Nonetheless, we find a throng of people using plastic cups to fill their jerry cans. The team takes photographs to use as evidence and on the way back to the car discusses the possibility of intervening. Water and sanitation are clearly the priority; perhaps MSF might assist WFP with a supplemental feeding center or work in the clinic, but only if the evidence supports it.

We return to the site of the food distribution, which is still in progress. People stand patiently in line to receive maize, oil, beans, and salt. Several of the mothers Mary enjoined to see us show up for their child's supplementary ration. Others crowd around the car, some with requests or complaints, others silently watching. A woman from a neighboring camp has somehow managed to get food at this distribution and looks hopefully for a ride. The driver ignores her. MSF will only carry patients and allows no one to clamber up on the roof. Mary does offer one mother transport funds to bring her severely withered child to the clinic. The logistics assistant advises another former patient to go to the local clinic. Our limited supplies are quickly exhausted and we head for home.

On the way back the doctor rests in the corner of one seat, closing his eyes and listening to music on earphones. Mary and the two Ugandans (who happen to share the same name) strike up a bantering conversation. The somewhat disjoined exchange—between bounces and over the roar of the engine—goes something like this:

> *Jonathan 1:* Look! That bird there, you can't kill that one or there won't be rain. That's what our people say.
>
> *Jonathan 2:* But we lost all our culture, thanks to you whites.
>
> *Mary:* Hey, that wasn't me, that was nineteenth-century missionaries!
>
> *Jonathan 1* [flashing smile]: It's OK, I would choose to change.
>
> *Jonathan 2:* But there was no big killing then. People rarely died. [pause] Before we didn't eat salt; there are all these new things for our bodies.

The Jonathans go on to tell Mary that there are rumors about the supplies included in food distributions. People only eat yellow corn because they are desperate, and some believe that it is part of a family planning effort to decrease the number of Africans. At another camp there was a riot when the corn-soy mix arrived. People were hungry but refused the mix, saying it caused diarrhea. The WFP switched to whole grain and that was better. Still, distrust lingers like it does with AIDS, which some rumors here ascribe to a foreign experiment. The camp mood remains suspicious, they assure her almost jovially.

The two Jonathans laugh frequently during this journey and like to point out incongruities on the road, such as a priest riding a motorbike illegally without a license plate (many soldiers do as well, one of the Jonathans adds). Such signs of double standards and political corruption are clearly a favored topic of humor. Indeed, the previous evening the entire team had carried on a running commentary about an ambulance donated by the Japanese government to the district hospital. The ambulance, it appeared, now sat idle for want of fuel, while the hospital director's motorcycle never seemed to run out. At one point someone pointed out gleefully that since the doctor was a Japanese taxpayer, he should simply go over and repossess the ambulance! Like most such humor, the joke aired a deeper frustration: the immobility of the hospital vehicle was a sore point for MSF staff, international and Ugandan alike. Routine medical transport fell under the hospital's purview, not theirs. And yet in the absence of an official ambulance, they faced continual requests for rides, which organizational protocol for nonemergency situations and insurance concerns forbid.

Mary has heard much of this before and wants to talk to WFP about encouraging a labor program, providing incentives to build latrines and improve sanitation; otherwise everyone focuses on food. She is clearly disturbed by the conditions in the camp we have just visited and wants to advocate with MSF's higher administration to start a project there. Back in the field office, she and I tabulate the results from our bracelet screening. She calculates the figures generously, rounding up and including all borderline cases, as if seeking support for intervention. The results are indeed discouraging but not obviously dire. In any case this is just a preliminary, informal impression. A convincing case will require a good deal more evidence. Among the many displacement camps in Uganda—let alone worldwide—why should MSF select this one? A grandmother with a full nursing career behind her, Mary has ample perspective and growing skepticism about the larger aid industry. She has already worked for MSF in South Sudan, where, as she puts it, "There's a whole generation that thinks shopping comes from the sky." Her time in Uganda is winding down, and soon she will find herself back in suburban Australia. Yet already she knows that once there, its material affluence will disturb her anew. Health care waste, disposable equipment, an everyday detachment from what she now sees as the real world will all prove unavoidable. Even worse is the display of ravenous consumption that now frightens her in supermarkets. The previous evening she had summarized her last return as a grotesquerie of surplus. "South Sudan didn't even have a plastic bag blowing around," she said. "I went home for Christmas and was horrified. What to give the grandchildren? They have everything." Once summoned to mind, this vision of excess lingers in our conversation. It contrasts starkly with MSF's relatively spartan office, which in turn appears munificent compared to its surroundings. This morning on the way to the camp we had passed little traffic other than a cotton truck, and as Mary observes, you can't eat cotton. Looking at the measurement numbers again, she sighs. "Today," she remarks softly to herself, "makes you want to stay."

Viewed from a field site rather than a model camp, the clarity of MSF's action wavers, overwhelmed by a distraction of details. Even basic needs can prove complex to calculate and reveal an assortment of varied interests. The population of a camp becomes a point of political tension between its leader and the official representative of international aid. Hints of corruption appear in the shape of an idle ambulance or a missing license plate. The head of the local water association seeks to profit from controlling a basic resource. History appears in the form of offhand references to tradition and colonial rupture. Rumors circulate among camp residents, who prove to have strong opinions about what is and what is not edible. Moreover, "aid" involves many discrete activities, and organizations rarely work in isolation. Entrepreneurs and traders move along the same roads that carry state officials, soldiers, and relief workers. MSF's representatives fumble their way through this varied array, gathering information and dispensing advice, whether requested or not. They follow procedures but also improvise. They also have significant capacity on a local scale. In the above case, should MSF commit to the project, the team could easily alleviate the camp's water supply problem by building a system of pumps and storage bladders. Team members could set up a supplemental feeding center to treat small children at risk of starvation. They could staff the clinic and provide excellent medical care or support and train such personnel as are already there. But at the same time, they have limits. They recognize that their organization cannot provide such assistance to every camp in the country, let alone the world. And the longer they stay in place, the more they risk becoming a fixture and fueling dependency. Even as they contemplate intervention, they know their organization will eventually seek to get out. All in all, the question of whether and how to act looks considerably less certain on the ground.

AN EXPANSIVE HORIZON

So far I have focused on emergency response and MSF's classic venue in and around refugee camps. As mentioned, at the time the group received its Nobel prize, it was also embarking on two ambitious and interrelated ventures: a commitment to offer treatment for victims of AIDS and an effort to advocate for greater access to medicines worldwide and foster pharmaceutical research on unprofitable diseases. Both the new AIDS program and the Access Campaign would alter the organization's profile and test its assumptions and procedures. They also illustrate the elasticity of the concept of crisis and its increasing extension beyond medical understandings of emergency. The HIV virus or an inadequate drug supply could certainly threaten a population and create what appeared to be exceptional circumstances. But neither fit easily into a delimited timeframe or invited techniques of rapid, mobile response. Here the crisis affecting life proved patently chronic and even structural in its scope.

The inclusion of nonemergency work in MSF's portfolio was not itself novel, but rather an alternative path present from the outset. As the group grew, it stressed innovation and took on fresh concerns. Unlike the Red Cross, it had no specific mandate or legal status beyond its internal charter and articles of incorporation. Led by an ever-shifting array of personnel and deeply infused with an oppositional ethos, the group's organizational structure fostered never-ending experimentation and critique. Many initiatives would prove short-lived, fading with the departure of key visionaries or eclipsed by later events. But over time MSF came to sponsor missions far beyond classic emergency responses to war or natural disaster. Although emergencies continued to define the group's public profile and sensibility, its definition of what constituted a crisis expanded to include problems such specific diseases and disenfranchised populations, conditions unlikely to be resolved quickly, cleanly, or conclusively. The Belgian section of the organization, in particular, flirted with sponsoring development projects, and even the French took on what they euphemistically called "longer-term" missions. Initially skeptical of offering mental health care, the group as a whole increasingly included it into its operations and later followed the aid world trend of drawing attention to gender and sexually based violence. MSF's sense of humanitarian crisis proved readily expansive.

MSF's *Activity Reports* provide a sense of the group's broader practice, so to situate the field anecdote above I turn to the 2003–2004 edition. As usual the volume contains not only a country-by-country synopsis of all projects, but also a world map, organizational statistics, a number of reflective and critical essays on humanitarian issues, and a carefully selected array of black-and-white images featuring aid workers and afflicted populations. It reflects, in this regard, what the sociologist Craig Calhoun terms "the emergency imaginary."[26] As the essays in the report indicate, at the time MSF recognized a series of significant challenges. These included the rise of military humanitarianism, which the group blamed for the recent death of five staff members in Afghanistan; an increasing focus on cost recovery, which it suggested favored macroeconomic theory over human life; and the emerging disaster in Darfur, to which it responded with a massive operation and publicity blitz, if stopping short of calling the situation genocide. In addition, the report highlights regional issues related to HIV/AIDS in Africa, tuberculosis control in Asia, and the plight of recent immigrants in Europe.

Alongside these general concerns, the statistical record suggests both clear patterns of geographic concentration and a considerable variety of topical focus. MSF's projects stretch worldwide and go well beyond emergency response. In 2003–2004 the group maintained a presence in seventy-seven countries: it had thirty-two missions in Africa, twenty-one in Asia, thirteen in Europe and the Middle East, and eleven in the Americas. The prevalence of Africa grows even clearer in monetary terms. The continent accounted for nearly 70 percent of the organization's program expenditure that year and four of its five most expensive programs, led by the Democratic Republic of the Congo and Sudan. Of the twenty-two programs with expenditures over three million euro, only six lay outside Africa: in Afghanistan, Chechnya, Iraq, Myanmar, Cambodia, and Russia. Not all of these major programs, however, concentrated on immediate emergency relief. In post-conflict settings like Angola, MSF treated malaria patients while lobbying to change government protocols, and in Liberia and Burundi it had begun new initiatives aimed at combating sexual violence. In Kenya and Malawi it focused on AIDS, providing antiretroviral therapy. If not matching the scale of operations in the Congo or Sudan (each of which involved over two hundred foreign and several thousand local staff), in the aggregate, nonemergency programs constituted a majority. Outside Africa, missions tended to be smaller and the projects even more varied. For its efforts to combat AIDS and malaria in Thailand and Cambodia, MSF deployed only a tenth of the personnel it had in Sudan. In Nicaragua it targeted Chagas disease, and in Uzbekistan multidrug-resistant tuberculosis. In Burkina Faso and Guatemala it sponsored psychological counseling for street children.

Even this quick survey of MSF's worldwide activity underscores the extent to which the organization's sense of crisis extends well beyond the refugee camp. A similar expansion of concern is evident in the American section's annual list of top ten "underreported humanitarian stories." Released every year since 1998, these lists match entries for specific countries with general problems such as cholera, street children, AIDS, drug resistance, access to medicine, neglected diseases, and malnutrition. Such issues reflect MSF's advocacy priorities and its increasing involvement in efforts to alter health policy and even pharmaceutical research. Although stopping short of full political engagement—let alone utopian ideals—such efforts extend beyond the immediacy of charity that David Rieff identifies with Brecht's apt phrase, "a bed for the night."[27] If MSF's annual reports and lists constitute snapshots of an emergency imaginary, then they reveal contours that stretch into longer-term ambitions and structural problems of inequality. Reading several in a row only further clouds the clarity of crisis itself. Missions open and close, problems reappear, dire predictions sometimes do and sometimes do not come to pass. The larger ensemble of MSF offers an empirical chart of ethical turmoil related to humanitarian intervention.

There were many sites on MSF's map I could have chosen for my research, some more or less significant by one historical measure or other. I came to focus on Uganda largely through serendipity and old connections. But the choice proved ultimately fortuitous for thinking about crisis, precisely because the term floated uncertainly there, suspended between memories, relative states, and an array of potential problems. For someone of my middling generation, Uganda evoked the name of Idi Amin, who cast an oversized media shadow in the 1970s as the postcolonial cannibal king. His regime might have been long gone, but the country still bore scars, sometimes revealed by continuing conflict in the north. Although Uganda itself had subsequently achieved a measure of stability, it remained surrounded by conflict, in Sudan to the north, Rwanda to the south, and the Democratic Republic of the Congo (formerly Zaire) to the west. Uganda further served as an epicenter of health research in Africa, in part due to its early prominence in HIV/AIDS. An astonishing number of international organizations fielded teams there, their four-wheel-drive vehicles struggling through the dense traffic of mopeds and minibuses on Kampala's central roundabout. Uganda, then, appeared a crossroads of African aid, at the intersection of both space and time.

Most writing about contemporary humanitarianism—by practitioners, journalists and academics alike—focuses on dramatic episodes of extreme emergency and human tragedy. Major disasters like the Ethiopian famine and the Rwandan genocide inspire ample commentary, analysis, and recrimination after the fact. Their significance established, they then serve as landmarks for humanitarian chronology, orienting subsequent problems within a lineage of inhuman events. In this manner they constitute classic forms of crisis, moments that appear as decisive turning points, while collectively suggesting the limits of humanity amid extreme conditions. Nonetheless, a great deal of actual practice by humanitarian organizations responds to less spectacular forms of suffering and more ambiguous contexts, ones that might or might not represent states of emergency. As in popular portrayals of medicine, the spectacular overshadows the routine, suggesting a world of active remedies rather than tentative trials and passive waiting. At the same time, even routine medicine can acquire a virtuous glow when practiced in settings with a surplus of suffering. To treat poor people, especially poor people living in poor countries and afflicted by curable conditions, now exemplifies the moral essence of medicine.

A REAL DOCTOR

During lunchtime at an MSF project in Uganda, one of my companions told a story about a successful plastic surgeon in Southern California. With the national trauma of September 11, 2001, this man apparently underwent a moral epiphany. Recognizing there were more important things than wealth and artificial beauty, he abruptly quit his practice and signed on for a field project with MSF. For the first time, he declared, he "felt like a real doctor." After returning from his first mission he launched into lower-income work at home and continued to volunteer periodically for humanitarian missions abroad. The story sounded second or third hand, and its particularities may have been apocryphal. Nonetheless, the tale captured a core sentiment I encountered again and again, both among people involved in aid work and those dreaming about it. Humanitarian medicine—whatever its realities, frustrations, or technical details—was fundamentally authentic in a way that wealthy suburban practice was not.

Claude, a French physician, had assured me of as much just the previous evening. "In Africa you see real problems," he said authoritatively, "not like in France." We were sitting at the table in his residence, eating dinner after a long day at the AIDS clinic and reflecting on the state of the world. "There it is all much more psychosomatic or small things overblown," he continued scornfully. "In developed countries people enlarge small problems." Life in suburban Europe was too easy, he felt, and as a consequence most patients there had forgotten how lucky they were. Claude waved his fork at the lantern that flickered dimly on our table, his tone hovering between wonder to disgust: "There you just turn on a switch and have light."

A deep sense of moral authenticity pervades MSF and similar aid organizations. Part of it entails a romantic rejection of material comfort and the illusions it generates. As Claude noted, people in wealthy countries ignore the ordinary miracles in their lives, forgetting to wonder at electricity or running water. Moreover, constant surplus dulls their perspective about what a real disruption of life might be like. By contrast, people focused on survival are rich in such awareness and know a real problem when they see one. Their visits to the hospital are more likely to involve matters of life and death, desperation as much as hope. A medical focus only amplifies this sense of touching reality: why treat the pampered and mildly sick when others need urgent care? Practicing humanitarian medicine offers moral liberation to health professionals trained amid excess. "You feel like the essence of a doctor," an American surgeon told me at the outset of my research in New York. Facing a conventional career in the United States, including the need to pay back school loans, she looked back on her experience as a volunteer with wistfulness as another, and perhaps more honest, education. Faced with limited resources, she had learned to rely on her intellect, not equipment. She had also found herself called upon to do everything, not just one specialized task. "It's pure medicine," she concluded, "not defensive, anti-lawsuit, documentation- and court-driven medicine."

The romance of medical authenticity takes many forms in individual lives. But at a collective level it defines the very core of common purpose for many adherents of MSF. A veteran Dutch nurse I met on my first visit to the Amsterdam office confessed that he had actually first joined the group simply to see the world. Over time, however, he had gradually transformed into a true believer: "What is MSF about for me? That people don't die of stupid things . . . Kala azar [visceral leishmaniasis] in Sudan, example: a black-and-white disease with a simple treatment. Malaria, cholera, sleeping sickness. Not only wars, but also simple things; this is the essence of refugee health care. Whatever the political issues, if people flee they shouldn't die of malaria."

I would encounter the phrase "stupid things" many times, both in MSF and throughout the world of international health.[28] Whatever else humanitarianism might signify for medical professionals immersed in it, it stood for the possibility of bringing need and care more closely in line, treating the treatable, and rejecting other considerations that might interfere. In MSF's case the adjective *stupid* bluntly delineated a terrain for action, sites where a minimal biopolitics of care might achieve immediate effects.

The degree to which the group identifies with both the possibilities and limits of the medical profession becomes equally clear in moments when the prospect of clinical attention redefines the situation. As a prominent figure within the French section of the organization suggested to me, medical personnel can claim a privileged perspective when it comes to facts of life:

> Doctors can diagnose causes and states. They are the ones who can measure. In Rwanda it was clear we couldn't protect the population during genocide. We were told at a checkpoint, you can fetch the wounded and we'll kill them here. But afterward, in prisons, life expectancy was six months, while the wait for trial something like ten years. So you had death before trial. Now who can get into prisons? Those who work there and those who work in health. So medical personnel can perform a diagnostic of a situation. It's a different angle than that of "they're all *génocidaires*"

(which many were, of course). We can view each of them as individuals, talk of people and their life chances, pathologies, and so on. It's a way of medically objectifying the political situation of why people are not living. It's about human facts, and not questions of philosophy, law, and the like. The doctor can speak of the sick, of a precise person and not in generalities. It's always individual—not talk of [abstract] desirable things, but of life and death. Doctors can talk in mortality rates.[29]

Although not a doctor herself, she saw that professional legacy—particularly the clinical tradition of focusing on specific cases and the precision of health measures—playing a central role in the group's collective persona. Claiming medical authority permitted not only access, but also a means of speaking that could redefine a situation by objectifying it, placing the ethical focus on considerations of individual existence.

In this sense the organization's name ultimately proves revealing. The complicated material and rhetorical assemblage of Médecins Sans Frontières does translate into an enacted statement of sorts, loosely characterized as "doctors yes, borders no." Such a statement distorts even as it reveals: the group's operations involve far more than doctors, and the original name intended to imply liberation from boundaries, not their eradication. However, the claim "doctors yes, borders no" also reflects the core motivation for MSF's volunteers and supporters: the opportunity to participate in the moral essence of a medical career. What could seem more pure, more certain than responding to obvious need?

THE ALLURE OF SIMPLICITY

Crisis is seductive in its very conception. The term descends from a Greek root for "discrimination" or "decision" and implies a condition of instability or a moment of decisive change. Within crisis, time contracts and one inhabits the present as intimately as possible—the "immediate present."[30] Language likewise reduces to the imperative mood, with exclamation: Do something! In this respect, crisis is the purest environment for a technical expert, a context in which expertise can and clearly must engage with the immanence of problems. It is also the natural habitat of a moral witness, who acquires the capacity to give testimony by virtue of presence. One can both act and know by being somewhere at just the right moment.[31]

For MSF, emergency missions go straight to the heart of crisis. Within the temporary shelter of a refugee camp, the group can (in theory at least) reach those near the edge of existence and provide them with urgent care. The appeal is vivid and direct: obvious suffering, critical need, a world of "black-and-white" diseases with simple treatments. Amid a world of political failure, disillusion and disappointment, the time of emergency offers moral clarity. Facing obvious rupture and lives at risk, medical action appears a natural and noble response. Like legal refugees—who are not just displaced, but have crossed a border—emergencies stand apart from everyday life, delimited from other problems. In real refugee camps such a distinction proves far less clear. We should not forget the small, complicating facts that linger even in the direst circumstances: the little treasures still secreted by those who "lost everything" at an earlier point in their story; the traces of memories that outlive bodies; the babies born during wartime. Moreover, as lives continue they quickly reacquire their complexity. Studies conducted in refugee settings suggest the power of the camp to both retain and sharpen moral political narratives and foster transformations over time.[32] When examining experience in detail, displaced people are rarely reduced to a pure state of merely living. Nonetheless, it has grown increasingly easy to imagine them in precisely such terms. Emergency provides a broad template for the political framing of problems, even as states co-opt the rhetoric of humanitarian appeals.

Even if medicine enjoys no monopoly on *emergency,* it provides a critical frame for its contemporary definition. At present it is hard to conceive of the term, or associated ones like *accident,* without expecting a response. In a society that measures health through risk and produces first-aid kits for even small calamities, life-threatening events naturally demand medical attention. However, neither the hospital emergency room nor the civilian ambulance, let alone the vast complex of artifacts we now associate with them, is all that old. Indeed, the concept of medical emergency itself may only have crystalized during the First World War, when the crushing reality of that destruction brought a complex of associated concepts into alignment: accident, ambulance, asphyxia, reanimation, resuscitation, shock, sudden death, and trauma. The ambulance was an older instrument in warfare, named for the "flying" version of battlefield treatment pioneered by France's chief surgeon during the Napoleonic wars, Dominique Larrey. If operating under a different conception of medicine, Larrey nonetheless advocated for the paramount importance of timely response, establishing a template for urgent care. During the long end of the nineteenth century ambulance societies began to respond to everyday problems in the industrial landscape. Only in the later decades of the twentieth century did organizational forms from military medicine translate into systems of emergency services common to wealthy countries. An ethos of war entered civilian life, as it were, through rapid medical care.[33]

The advent of Médecins Sans Frontières marks the extension of such an emergency sensibility worldwide. The group is hardly alone in pursuing this goal, of course, but it embodies the fundamental principles of urgency and action and seeks to provide global response. At its most fundamental level of justification it operates under an ethic of crisis, pursuing the good during moments of exception. The organization further expresses an ethos of crisis with its imperative atmosphere and an aesthetic of crisis with its breathless imagery. Most significantly, it refocuses political and economic problems through a medical prism. When doing so it both participates in the tendency of the larger historical moment and struggles to distinguish its particular form of response within it.

Although some of its elements may be very old, the configuration of "humanitarian crisis" now common to international affairs appears more recent. Like the discourse of human rights, it emerged with new force in the 1970s.[34] While more utopian framings for political history eroded—notably class struggle and anticolonial liberation—suffering appeared as a new point of moral reference. The articulation of a private humanitarian conscience within international affairs promises simplicity and certainty. By recognizing suffering and finding it unconscionable, groups like MSF assert moral clarity amid the grayer realm of politics. "If someone's drowning, you save them," one adherent told me in Uganda, describing her own conversion to humanitarian work. If uncertain about the universality of human rights, she knew she cared about the dying. The stark line of existence offers lucidity.[35] Unlike utopian dreams it proves directly relevant, while providing a grounds for judgment as well as action. One can distinguish between positions and policies in terms of the effects they have on life and death, and—once properly equipped—respond to ameliorate them. MSF's version of humanitarianism frames its work in an anti-heroic mode ("It is a depressing world," another member told me in Amsterdam. "We do this because we don't know what else to do"). Nonetheless, the group's forceful tone and emphasis on action cast it in a heroic role. Faced with intolerable conditions it endeavors to respond directly, refusing to stay silent or to sacrifice the present to a longer perspective.

Moral clarity, however, can come at a price, particularly if unaccompanied by reflection or doubt. Functioning as politics, amid political expectations, humanitarianism's moral force threatens to erode into reactive moralism. Divorced from a particular sense of knowledge, it is easily co-opted and its rhetoric redeployed by established interests. As Didier Fassin astutely observes, humanitarian intervention can dispense a soothing balm of self-satisfaction, the intoxicating assurance of being humane.[36] Its most concentrated form can justify military adventure, not simply as part of a longer lineage of moral crusades and just wars but as a political and legal claim to a post-sovereign norm in international relations. Much like the language of humanitarianism itself, a right to intervene can serve as a principle for the expression of power as well as a source of moral opposition to that power's inhuman effects.[37]

THE PROBLEM OF CRITIQUE

Here etymology again proves instructive. The root term for *crisis*, Reinhart Koselleck reminds us, once included the act of rendering judgment, as much a subjective exercise as any recognition of objective reality.[38] An ethical perspective, then, should recognize the claim of crisis around emergency, involving critical reason alongside reaction. Critique too has a history, which Koselleck strongly identifies with the European enlightenment response to an absolutist state and the rise of bourgeois society. In that context the critic could stand apart as a moral sovereign and appeal to utopia. The results were not all salutatory in Koselleck's larger analysis, resulting in a division between moral and political spheres, to the detriment of the latter. An unreflective critic now spoke to the political world by passing judgment, without enduring conceptual risk. Amid the continual crisis of modern conceptions of history, such judgments secured themselves in the future, forever exempt from the imperfections of present action. Turning points and choices might punctuate time, but the critic judged at a safe remove, detached by certainty.

By contrast, conceptual risk requires not only recognizing the burden of decision inherent in claims to crisis but also remaining troubled by it. To illustrate I will add a historical thread to my earlier theoretical allusion. Despite expressing frequent misgivings about the category of the intellectual, Foucault clearly functioned as one in the French terms of his era. A central expectation of that role was to speak at moments of crisis—events of apparent political significance. The turbulent atmosphere of the 1970s offered many opportunities for such public performance: marches, statements, study groups, letters of protest, and expressions of solidarity. It also, however, introduced a greater measure of reflection and doubt. Following the abortive upheaval of 1968, decolonization, and the increasingly obvious impurities of state socialism, it grew harder to maintain inherited categories of ideological struggle. Foucault's later writings on ethics indicate a restless desire for continual interrogation, a politics capable of animated skepticism. Discussing a volume entitled *The Age of Ruptures* in 1979, he called for an "ethic of discomfort" in the face of revolution as well as rising conservatism. Beginning with Immanuel Kant's confrontation of enlightenment, the text closes with a nod to Maurice Merleau-Ponty, suggesting that the essential philosophical task is "never to consent to being completely comfortable with one's own presuppositions."[39]

The son and grandson of surgeons, Foucault's connection to medicine ran biographically as well as conceptually deep. Most tellingly, he wrote about life and politics in the same milieu within which Médecins Sans Frontières emerged. Like a number of prominent French intellectuals of the day, he joined several of Bernard Kouchner's public campaigns during the period, notably traveling with him to Poland to deliver medicines in support of the Solidarity movement. Shortly before his untimely death, Foucault apparently expressed a desire to go on a mission with Kouchner's successor organization, Médecins du Monde.[40] Noting such connections is not to collapse significant differences between the two men (the latter of whom fully and fatefully embraced the life of a politician), let alone between a practice of critical thought and that of humanitarianism. However, it does underscore a certain confluence of desire—the desire to act, to tell truths, to find virtue in opposition—as well as theme. In an era of ruptures and disintegrating certainty, medicine became an influential referent for politics.

MSF too pronounced its own ethic of discomfort of sorts in accepting the Nobel Prize. This discontent may fall within the narrower limits of evaluating the good relative to a humanitarian precept of life. Nonetheless, it seeks a form of moveable action, if not moveable thought.[41] In an effort to provide a minimal definition of humanitarianism at the end of the cold war, the group pointed not only to the preservation of life and human dignity but also the need "to restore people's ability to choose."[42] Framed in the language of liberalism, this statement posits autonomy and choice as natural conditions, if not necessarily individual ones. The assertion also places the legitimate center of politics elsewhere, beyond the reach of a humanitarian organization. If the stakes of crisis are ultimately those of assessment and decision, MSF refuses a full wager. "Humanitarian action comes with limitations," the Nobel address warns repeatedly, adding, "It cannot be a substitute for political action." Just what form this politics might take—beyond preventing genocide—the group cannot say. Medicine offers an array of temporary specific measures, not a lasting, general prescription. Over time it might also have to adjust to its own effects.

As mentioned, MSF prides itself on fostering an internal culture of reflection, debate, and critique. Publications that circulate in-house regularly feature confessions and denunciations as well as jokes and cartoons. One of my favorite drawings addresses the group's reputation for arrogance and knee-jerk opposition. In it a young woman asks a grizzled aid veteran how MSF manages things. "Oh, not like that!" he replies airily. "Not like that either! No, no, not like that!" When she repeats her question he finally responds, "Well, not like that but better! Another question?"[43] The humorous deferral reflects a deeper tension: within a world of crisis and an ethic of refusal, it is hard to say more.

A Secular Value of Life

For what matters today is not the immortality of life, but that life is the highest good.

HANNAH ARENDT, *THE HUMAN CONDITION*, 1958

DECEMBER 1971

The photograph shows its age now, black-and-white details fading into the distance. A group of men sits around an oval conference table in a large office. Drapes frame the window behind them and a bookcase guards one wall. The men wear jackets, most with ties, although a few sport turtlenecks and unruly hair in keeping with fashion of the times. Details of skin, style, and dress suggest urban Europeans on a reasonably cold day. They appear to be in animated discussion as they sit, several gesticulating with their hands. Each has papers spread before him, and several grasp pens or cigarettes, holding them aloft with a practiced air. In one corner a leather briefcase rests on the tabletop, and in another what looks like a flip chart. It could be any meeting during or shortly after the tumultuous end of the 1960s, although the expressions and posture of the group suggest deep engagement.

Dating the image to the end of 1971 helps reconstitute a frame. The official news of the year featured the usual range of events large and small, their significance varying according to perspective. A retrospective selection of headlines runs as follows: In January a general named Idi Amin had deposed the president of Uganda, Milton Obote, and taken his place. In February, Switzerland had finally granted women the right to vote, while Britain shifted to decimal currency. In March a group known as the Weather Underground placed a bomb in the U.S. Capitol, and West Pakistan invaded its eastern cousin, which declared independence as Bangladesh. April saw the death of François Duvalier in Haiti, and the succession of his son, known as "Baby Doc," as president for life. In May polls showed the majority of the American public against the war in Vietnam, and in

June the *New York Times* began to publish the secret Pentagon Papers. That same month the United States dropped its trade embargo against China, and in July it lowered the voting age to 18; rock star Jim Morrison died in Paris at the age of twenty-seven. August saw the Concert for Bangladesh, in which a group of prominent musicians led by George Harrison and Ravi Shankar raised money for those suffering from the previous year's hurricane and the ongoing war. Construction began on a stadium in New Orleans known as the Superdome, even as it ended on the second tower of New York's World Trade Center. Prison riots at Attica shocked the American public in September, while in October Disney World opened in Florida and the Democratic Republic of Congo was renamed Zaire. In November the People's Republic of China took a seat on the United Nations Security Council. In a development that would gain significance retroactively, a small company called Intel released the first microprocessor. By December the Khmer Rouge intensified its attacks on the Cambodian government, and after a short, decisive war India drove the Pakistani army from Bangladesh.[1]

The men in the room would have known much of this, though their focus would likely linger on developments related to health and politics as perceived from France. Several were deeply concerned with events on the Indian subcontinent, while others had experience in Africa, working as Red Cross doctors in the breakaway region of Nigeria known briefly as Biafra. Although that conflict had ended nearly two years earlier, the associated agony—particularly mass starvation among the civilian population caught in the political struggle—continued to mark those who had witnessed it. They had gathered in the Paris office of a French medical journal to form a new organization, one that would offer swift assistance in the face of medical need. They imagined it as an independent association, unburdened by formality or religious ties. With such a group doctors could engage with suffering wherever it might arise, bypassing political obstacles to stand with afflicted populations worldwide. They decided to call it *Médecins Sans Frontières*.

There are many ways to tell the history that leads to that moment. Within the organization capsule summaries usually commence with an origin myth involving Biafra and then proceed rapidly through the ensuing years, pulling each decade out like a file drawer and then quickly closing it and returning to the present. Such a timeline customarily features landmark missions, internal turmoil, and significant crises. Following Biafra, it might mention Cambodia and an organizational schism before turning to a doleful litany of disaster in Afghanistan, Ethiopia, Somalia, Rwanda, and beyond. Here I provide a version of that myth and likewise summarize the decades through a list of landmarks. However, I will also cast the net somewhat deeper and wider. Médecins Sans Frontières emerged from a longer European lineage and against a broad backdrop of concern for human suffering. Upon closer scrutiny, both its core humanitarian value of life and its secular sensibility—the very things that might suggest an ethical framework beyond history—appear more remarkable than we might have assumed. Whatever common human feeling might stir between strangers, it has not always taken the specific form of providing aid, let alone inspired the establishment of an organization to do so on a global scale.

The novel elements behind the photograph have now grown familiar, making them all the harder to recognize. Indeed, the very possibility of undertaking contemporary humanitarian action assumes a great deal. MSF came into being alongside satellite telecommunications, jet travel, and new forms of emergency medicine extending hospital care closer to the scene of accidents. It emerged amid a political context of cold war, decolonization, and generational turmoil. Between superpower tensions and around the edges of ebbing empires, a growing group of intergovernmental and nongovernmental organizations now waved flags with their respective icons and acronyms. By 1971 some of these were already well established, even as a new generation of idealists had come of age after the Second World War. Like any other human activity, the provision of aid occurs amid particular conditions as well as those expectations that render it conceivable in the first place. The first task, then, is to recognize that MSF's moral concern for saving lives has its own history.

"A BEING NOT MEANT TO SUFFER"

MSF's fundraising brochures now regularly feature variations of the catchphrase "You can help save a life." Positioned amid bold graphics of red and white, stark images and impassioned reports, the commanding words suggest even a modest sum might contribute to vital action. Such brochures belong to the genre of humanitarian appeal, seeking to transmute concern for others into charitable revenue. According to a sample solicitation from 2008, contributing $35 provides "all the medical and logistical supplies to supply 40 people a day with clean water," while a more generous $500 translates into a "medical kit containing basic drugs, supplies, equipment and dressings to treat 1500 patients for three months." Beyond specific calculations and accounts of current projects, such brochures assert the primary value of human life. They assume that the lives of people around the world are precious and something to be saved through human intervention. Indeed, they radiate urgency: faced with such knowledge, how could a decent human not act?

The trope of connecting an emotional response to suffering to a moral claim about humanity has a distinguished pedigree. Europe's tumultuous eighteenth century not only laid the groundwork for new forms of political and economic organization, it also established a framework for sentimental reason. Historians deliberate over the precise terms and conditions of this turn toward feeling in public life, connecting it to developments ranging from new forms of narrative and mourning to capitalist exchange.[2] Whatever the precise causes, this legacy complicates simplified portrayals of liberalism that focus solely on an autonomous, selfish individual. For an example let us turn to the pillar of economic rationality himself, philosopher Adam Smith. When evaluating the moral weight of human sentiment in 1759, Smith famously included a propensity for sympathy near the heart of human nature. "That we often derive sorrow from the sorrow of others, is a matter of fact too obvious to require any instances to prove it," he wrote, "for this sentiment, like all the other original passions of human nature, is by no means confined to the virtuous and humane, though they perhaps may feel it with the most exquisite sensibility." After all, even "the greatest ruffian" could be prone to pity and compassion, at least at moments of weakness.[3] At the same time Smith recognized that sympathy varied in accordance with the attachment of a spectator to a scene. Only by knowing about and identifying with suffering could one react with feeling. Moral sentiment thus involves affective imagination. Once one could see through distance, however, suffering strangers, if properly presented, might also evoke sympathy and inspire a philanthropic impulse.[4] Smith's assumption continues to echo through contemporary fundraising documents.

Nonetheless, humans have not always sought to maintain life or alleviate suffering. The long sweep of history offers many examples of our having inflicted intentional death and pain, not all identified as moral failings within a given code of conduct. Indeed, in certain contexts suffering represented a form of virtue. To take a famous example from Europe's claimed Greek heritage, Spartan youth were subjected to extreme discipline and undesirable infants were left to die. Classical scholars debate the exact nature and extent of these infamous traditions. Nonetheless, ancient Sparta left behind both an adjective for austerity as well as a well-worn legend of a boy who avoided dishonor by allowing a stolen fox to gnaw his entrails.[5] The ancient Spartans, it seems safe to say, would have little time for humanitarian appeals. Nor, presumably, would a grubbier group of apprentices torturing a cat in prerevolutionary France or a crowd picnicking at a public hanging in frontier California.[6] From a comfortable contemporary perspective— particularly one shielded from the blunter aspects of death and food production— such habits appear categorically barbaric. Humanitarian mailings reflect a moral order that expects children to survive into adulthood, animals to be well treated, and the force of punishment to be kept out of public settings. But we should not forget that violence and suffering have featured in many moral systems and popular pastimes. Humanitarian sensibilities are neither timeless nor invariably natural, however much they appeal to human universality. The concern for life, in other words, has a history.

Indeed, suffering can define morality through its presence as well as its absence. A loss or ordeal might invite celebration rather than condemnation. Beyond the now disreputable litany of blood sports, violent spectacle, and public executions, we should also recall the greater tradition of sacrifice. By offering up something precious, sacrifice seeks to pay homage, request counsel, offer recompense, or otherwise maintain the order of things. Forms of sacrifice abound in anthropological accounts of religion; peoples the world over have hardly shied away from disemboweling chickens or slitting the throats of goats at moments of ritual need. Some have offered up human bodies as well, on occasion in dramatic fashion. Most readers of this work would likely find the raw physicality of such acts repulsive and their moral implications abhorrent. Suffering belongs in the controlled space of a gym, perhaps, carefully building bodies rather than destroying them. Moreover, to a liberal conscience pain should be a personal choice. Yet if feats of endurance have migrated from spiritual experience to physical improvement, a sense of sacrifice nonetheless remains attached to certain forms of moral action. A person involved in good works should avoid indulgence, and thus an aura of religious sobriety clings to aid work, especially when life and death appear at stake.

Sacrifice, as the term itself suggests, involves an appeal to sacred things. Its violence seeks purification, just as suffering might promise spiritual cleansing. Through an ordeal comes the prospect of vision and reorientation. The general point extends beyond formal religion. From the secular perspective of social science, moments of sacrifice reinforce the essential bonds of social connection, as Henri Hubert and Marcel Mauss suggested at the end of the nineteenth century.[7] The sacred things become social things in which a contractual relation is renewed or redefined. I will return to the theme of sacrifice in a later chapter. For now I wish simply to suggest that some forms of destruction run deep in human traditions of connection, both with the world and each other. Suffering and sacrifice played a particularly pronounced role in Christianity, the religious tradition most immediately framing this European story.[8]

By contrast, MSF's humanitarian perspective not only formalizes Smith's sentiment of compassion into a moral precept, but also reverses its relation to humanity. In the mid-1990s Rony Brauman, the influential former head of the French section, could define the human as "a being who is not made to suffer."[9] Such a statement—clearly intended as a provocation—is historically remarkable. Although few other humanitarian organizations would state their rationale in Brauman's stark terms, their very framework for aid delivery presupposes both that human suffering requires response and that it should take the form of material care. Rather than seeking justification for suffering through an appeal to religious value, social cohesion, or political gain, humanitarians meet human misery with attempts at direct assistance. In a more radical inflection, the sort favored by MSF, such assistance opposes the established order born of such justifications.

This particular form of sympathy, fashioned into principle and extended into an organization, requires a bit more explanation than Smith's appeal to human nature. Sympathy not only indicates a human propensity; its active form defines the humane human. The medical variant of humanitarian action approaches suffering emphatically in the name of life itself. Mercy here does not imply euthanasia or easing of pain through a coup de grâce. Whether or not the being "not made to suffer" might find release in death, moral value here accrues from preserving existence and thereby "saving a life."

To illustrate this last point, I offer a handful of historical sketches. My account is less a genealogy than an outline of trajectory, and its goal is both to suggest precursors for the aid doctor and to distinguish MSF's particular attachment to life from other relevant points of possibility.[10] Two key figures are mythic in their own right: the concerned Christian gentleman turned battlefield nurse and the medical missionary finding virtue in a tropical hospital. Before examining them, however, I will briefly gesture toward other classic conjunctures that frame Europe's Enlightenment. During an age defined as much by feeling as reason, caring for others established itself as a public as well as private good. Between the larger tides of capitalism and liberalism, a surge of empathy coursed through the violent upheaval of revolution and the drawn-out struggle over slavery. Indeed, even as Smith contemplated moral sentiment in Scotland, a dramatic expression of it took shape in response to disaster, framed by the moral austerity of Protestant Geneva.

THE SECULAR SENSE OF DISÁSTER

On the morning of All Saints' Day in 1755, while the churches stood crowded, a massive earthquake shattered the city of Lisbon. The event quickly became the talk of European polite society and inspired theological speculation as well as concern for the victims. Did the catastrophe signal divine wrath? Was it a response to Portuguese sin or Catholic failing? The French author known as Voltaire, then in exile in Geneva, composed a poem upon hearing the news. In it he dramatized the senselessness of suffering involved, using the unhappy moment to discredit the view that events in the world can be justified by virtue of their existence. This poem figured in several philosophical disputes of the day, while serving as a literary stepping-stone toward his later master fable, *Candide*. Alternatively sardonic and portentous in style, the work displays an embryonic humanitarian sensibility. Voltaire emphasized the moral significance of arbitrary pain while rejecting any easy theological justification for it. It is a classic moment—perhaps the canonical moment—of secular enlightenment.[11]

Other luminous figures of the era likewise found inspiration in the event. The young Immanuel Kant wrote a pioneering text on seismology and contemplated the sublime. The even younger Johann Wolfgang von Goethe reportedly encountered doubt at the tender age of six. Jean-Jacques Rousseau read Voltaire's poem and wrote a long response. He had recently returned to his native city of Geneva and re-converted to Calvinism. Earlier that year he had sent his older and more famous neighbor a copy of *Discourse on Inequality*, receiving a characteristically caustic reply. In rejoinder to Voltaire's poem, Rousseau pointed out that faith could serve purposes other than rational explanation. "This optimism that you find so cruel," he wrote, "consoles me while I suffer the very pains that you describe to me as being insupportable." Moreover, the destruction stemmed from the human habit of urban living, as "it was not nature that piled up there twenty thousand houses of six or seven floors each." Rousseau pointed out that had the inhabitants of Lisbon dispersed across the countryside, "The destruction would have been less, and perhaps insignificant." Rather than properly valuing their natural life, however, the unfortunates had been blinded by the allure of goods and civilization and rushed back to their doom in hope of rescuing clothes, papers, or money. "Can't you see that the physical existence of a human being has become the least important part of themselves, and that it seems to be scarcely worth saving when one has lost all the rest?"[12] Life, Rousseau in effect suggested, was the real good, and humans should rediscover its simple virtue.

If a minor document in the history of philosophy, Rousseau's letter presages both the social science of disaster and the humanitarian response to it.[13] Events such as earthquakes, hurricanes, and tsunamis are primarily disasters inasmuch as they destroy a built environment, and hence those caught within it. They afflict urban dwellers far more than nomads, and those in poorly constructed buildings most of all. Even more crucially, perhaps, Rousseau identifies physical existence as an overlooked value within the panoply of civilized life. Beneath the encumbrance of clothing, knowledge, and wealth one could find a lost natural being: the human who suffered and yet might be saved.

Recounting this well-known episode recalls one critical stake of claiming a secular perspective. Rather than ascribing suffering to moral failure or appealing to the greater wisdom of an omnipotent deity, human anguish could appear senseless. Redemptive value, then, would come only from efforts to prevent or alleviate it. In his pioneering work on the anthropology of secularism, Talal Asad notes that pain "enables the secular idea that 'history making' and 'self-empowerment' can progressively replace pain by pleasure—or at any rate by the search for what pleases one."[14] The term *secular* here refers not to a condition of disbelief, but rather a conceptual reconfiguration that distinguishes between religion and politics, differentiating between the ethics of public and private life. Pain anchors this distinction quite precisely when it takes the form of collective catastrophe. The idea that legitimate public action concentrates on relief of suffering—whatever personal views or beliefs might dictate—establishes a secular framework for the actions of both atheists and faithful adherents alike. In this respect MSF stands firmly in the enlightened tradition of the Lisbon disaster. Brauman's portrayal of the human as a "being not meant to suffer" echoes Rousseau's understanding that misery enters the world through history rather than nature, thereby justifying efforts at worldly redress.

Secular concern for misfortune extended well beyond disaster. Most crucially it established new political terms for everyday as well as exceptional anguish. The French Revolution, as Hannah Arendt decreed disapprovingly, birthed a "politics of pity."[15] Rather than classic ideals of liberty or justice, the condition of being a victim came into political focus, dividing those who suffered from those who did not. Political energy thus diverted into what Arendt termed the "social question" as Rousseau gave way to Robespierre and the eventual fury of Jacobin terror. In this roundabout manner, suffering produced another kind of sacrifice, cleansing a new order with the blood of the old. Out of it emerged new political vocabularies and assumptions for liberalism, a language of left and right, of rights and revolution. Just as disaster might require earthly explanation, misery might claim political redress. The revolutionary way forward, however, appeared to lead through the guillotine. To what extent would its inheritors follow a similar path?

The question of violence suggests a significant tension between a politics of pity and human concern for misery. To the extent that it categorically seeks to mitigate suffering, a humanitarian perspective stands in sharp contrast to the violence of popular upheaval. Humanitarianism—even French humanitarianism—is thus hardly a simple extension of revolutionary politics. Indeed, strands of the larger tradition exhibit a distinctly conservative cast and paternalistic sensibility. Nonetheless, aspects of MSF's oppositional vision, as well as its style and rhetoric, echo the French revolutionary tradition.[16] At times the group has approached something like a politics of pity on a global scale, even while reacting vigorously against suffering produced by would-be revolutionaries. It has done so, however, as an element of what political theorists like to call "civil society"—the coordinated efforts of ordinary citizens rather than a state. In this sense it recalls another eighteenth-century landmark of humane sensibility, the abolition movement, in which some at the center of the European empire came to recognize the suffering of distant slaves as a moral injustice. The long struggle against slavery provides an enduring point of reference for later forms of activism. At the same time, it is important to note that the overriding European sentiment toward the Haitian revolution remained one of horrified refusal. Freedom might be granted but not seized through violence.[17]

Although colonial war might disrupt empathy, a direct antecedent to MSF's humanitarianism did emerge amid the carnage of a European battlefield. Unlike most individual gestures of compassion this would inspire an influential movement, one that established an enduring complex of institutions known colloquially as the Red Cross.[18] If well worn through repetition in canonical accounts, the story still merits close attention. As Susan Sontag noted, the combination of mechanized weaponry, conscript citizen armies, and war reporting presented a dramatic new stage for "the pain of others."[19] Moreover, since war stood at the edge of law it positioned this drama as an exceptional experience. Alongside natural catastrophes, humanitarians found a ready object for sympathy in human conflict, in which they could likewise identify needless suffering. Even if this vision only slowly extended beyond European theaters, it provided a critical precedent for more expansive forms.

BATTLEFIELD PASSION, MEDICAL MISSION

On the evening of June 24, 1859, a Swiss civilian named Henry Dunant stumbled onto the battlefield of Solferino. The pious son of a Genevan family of means, he had pursued the French emperor to Italy in order to lobby for his business interests in Algeria and had little experience to prepare him for what he saw. Following a heavy day of fighting, the wreckage of both French and Austrian armies littered the field. Wounded men groaned miserably, a combination of hot weather and poor provisioning adding thirst to their shared torment. A nearby church received some of the wounded, and Dunant spontaneously made his way there to offer what assistance he could. Although a stranger to military combat, he was no newcomer to charitable endeavors; active in a movement to unite Christians and Jews, he had also played a prominent role in organizing the first world conference of the YMCA in Paris in 1855. The plight of these stricken soldiers touched a new chord within Dunant. He threw himself fervently into the work and for several days labored alongside women from the town and assorted travelers he pressed into service.[20]

The experience inspired Dunant to publish a short memoir describing what he had seen. Entitled *Un souvenir de Solferino* (*A Memory of Solferino*), the book proved widely influential. Its author launched a crusade to improve care for wounded soldiers and quickly received invitations to capitals all over Europe. He imagined a relief effort of committees led by well-born volunteers, who, since they were motivated by noble sentiments alone, would prove more reliable than paid help. Military professionals remained alternately intrigued and skeptical of Dunant's proposals. Even his counterpart Florence Nightingale doubted their suitability, arguing that this was the proper responsibility of governments and that substituting for them might make war too easy. Nonetheless, Dunant's plan found fertile ground in his own city. Along with a retired Swiss war hero and two doctors, a wealthy lawyer named Gustave Moynier joined the cause and began the practical steps needed to realize the organization. In 1863 the first of a series of international conventions met in Geneva. It established a set of resolutions to authorize committees that would assist with the care of wounded in the time of war, and a uniform sign—a red cross against a white background—that would render its members distinctive.[21]

Although Dunant was but one of a wave of reformers horrified by the effects of modern warfare, it was his legacy that defined the kernel of an international system. The Red Cross eventually expanded into an array of organizations undertaking a variety of missions. In addition to separate national societies, a league emerged to coordinate their greater union. At the same time the International Committee of the Red Cross (ICRC) continued its own path in Geneva, becoming a fixture of international law by virtue of overseeing the Geneva Conventions. The collective purview of these entities grew to include far more than the care of wounded soldiers, gradually encompassing sailors, prisoners, and civilians, as well as responses to natural disasters.

Told as a triumph of human spirit over barbarity, Dunant's story features prominently in progressive accounts of the aid world. Given that the Red Cross is a defining component of the aid apparatus and the Geneva Conventions a landmark in international humanitarian law, such attention seems only due. When considered relative to MSF's concerns for life, however, Dunant's moment on the battlefield exhibits crucial differences. In the first place, Dunant's inspiration derived more from heartfelt faith than from secular reason or medical sensibility. A deeply religious man, he appealed openly to Christian sentiment in his effort to "civilize" warfare. The men who joined him in Geneva were not only prominent citizens of the city, but also notably devout; emerging from a Protestant milieu, they framed their endeavor as an ecumenical concern. The very symbol used by the organization carried religious connotations, a fact which would prove a source of lasting controversy when the Red Cross expanded beyond Europe.[22] Dunant's group also imagined war in terms of formal engagements between national armies, at a moment when the destructive force of weaponry and the flesh of conscripted citizens combined into mass martyrdom. Thus, although the initial vision of the Red Cross came from ordinary citizens offering battlefield care, it focused on easing death alongside saving life.

This last point merits particular amplification. Dunant's short book includes a good deal of impassioned description, combining romantic visions of battlefield heroism by dashing, aristocratic officers with heart-rending accounts of the agonies of wounded common soldiers.[23] Some have faces "black with flies" and others are "no more than a worm-ridden, inextricable compound of coat and shirt and flesh and blood." Here a swollen tongue hangs from a broken jaw, there a skull gaps open, there a back quivers red, furrowed by buckshot.[24] Faced with this suffering, Dunant and his companions offer cool bandages, sponges, warm compresses, a drink of water or—once his driver forages supplies—lemonade. At times their primary gift is companionship, offering a hand to grip, a prayer or reassurance. "I spoke to him," Dunant wrote of a stricken soldier who raged against his fate, "and he listened. He allowed himself to be soothed, comforted and consoled, to die at last with the straightforward simplicity of a child."[25] In Dunant's rendering the suffering of the dying at Solferino was not only a physical matter. Many soldiers, realizing they might expire, begged for a letter that would inform their families of their fate and ease their mothers' distress. Death here was not simply an individual concern but also a social fact, an event that demanded appropriate recognition. In response, Dunant's small band of volunteers offered the comfort of communication, whether in the form of a farewell letter or a promise to convey the tragic news.

Dunant famously made no distinctions on the basis of nationality, and the women with him proclaimed a brotherhood among the wounded. A "moral sense of the importance of human life" drove him, but it found expression in simple gestures. It also inspired a frenzied mix of relentless activity, cold calculation, and sudden heartbreak at an unexpected detail that "strikes closer to the soul."[26] Although much of his turmoil echoes through contemporary humanitarianism, Dunant's mission remained one of mercy. Washing wounds and whispering comfort, he prefigured Mother Theresa as much as MSF. To Dunant, life meant the life of a larger person, the end of which extended beyond a particular body. Compassion included ensuring dignity in death.

The movement constructed by others around Dunant's vision certainly addressed itself to physical suffering, helping equate its symbol with medical care in many parts of the world.[27] Nonetheless the core organization in Geneva retained an attachment to the wider, narrative sense of life, involving itself in such activities as registering prisoners and tracing missing persons. It played a significant role in nascent international law and strove to achieve a variety of internationalism constructed around political neutrality and the possibility of appeals for decency across religious and cultural difference. On the basis of these accomplishments, Dunant shared the first Nobel Peace Prize in 1901.

Neither the Red Cross nor the Geneva Conventions initially encompassed the colonized world.[28] When the organization did gingerly extend beyond Europe later in the twentieth century, it encountered another form of humanitarianism. Medicine had played an increasing part in the colonial drama during the nineteenth century, both as a "tool of empire" and as an arm of colonial service and authority.[29] The specifics varied by region, empire, and period. Nonetheless, with the emergence of germ theory and the advent of modern research-oriented medical practice—what anthropologists term *biomedicine*—combatting diseases endemic in the tropics offered one potential path to scientific glory. Such work was also a matter of practical concern for European military forces and colonial administrators. Charged with governing mobile forces and increasingly interconnected populations, they faced a constant threat of epidemic. After a long era of astonishing death rates, the health of European troops in tropical postings improved dramatically by the early twentieth century. The well-being of colonial populations, however, remained a continuing and vexing problem. Diseases like sleeping sickness inspired determined health campaigns involving medical officers in the most remote regions and connecting the project of empire to a microscope. Such efforts were clearly political in the larger sense of the term. They derived from grand schemes and affected myriad local interests. They incorporated the lives and welfare of remote peoples into the calculations of government and the apparatus of rule, albeit more as objects than as subjects. The motivations behind them, however, were often complex, mingling altruistic sentiment with desires for profit and control.

In Africa missionaries played a significant role in offering medical care, particularly in the British case. From David Livingstone on, the image of a heroic white doctor toiling in darkest Africa struck a romantic chord for Europeans.[30] Although the increasing focus on physical health alongside spiritual states generated some tension, the larger narrative of salvation remained intact. Missionary work appeared a particularly noble and self-sacrificing form of altruism. Hospitals, moreover, in which the labors of a worldly healer might suggest the value of a more glorious physician at work in a "Great Dispensary in the Sky," provided a ready venue for proselytization.[31] Missionary medicine walked a line between sacred and secular care, removing tumors and cataracts in a public flourish, mixing treatment with prayer, and constructing and staffing clinics and hospitals, many of which remain in use today. Even as Africans encountered Christianity through health care, the European reading public encountered Africa through reports of suffering on the "sick continent." In materials from the early twentieth century we find tropes common to contemporary aid brochures, such as calls to "adopt" a patient or appeals to send funds for doctors because "Congo boys and girls are dying."[32] Yet the focus on life remains within an explicitly Christian frame.

Illustrative of this point is an exceptional figure from the middle part of the century, one who came to exemplify the medical mission as a moral calling. Born in Alsace, Albert Schweitzer was first a theologian and subsequently a doctor. An appeal from the French Protestant Missionary Society in Paris inspired him to study medicine at the age of twenty-nine. Leaving his university post, he completed the new degree and then devoted himself to running a hospital in what was then French West Africa. Rather than simply talking about the gospel of love, he would "put it into practice." In return, Africa would give Schweitzer his signature understanding of purpose. As the official presentation of his Nobel Peace Prize recounted, "One day in 1915—he was forty years old at the time—while traveling on a river in Africa, he saw the rays of the sun shimmering on the water, the tropical forest all around, and a herd of hippopotamuses basking on the banks of the river. At that moment there came to him, as if by revelation, the phrase which precisely expressed his thought: Reverence for life."[33]

This sense of "reverence for life," together with its expression through efforts on behalf of suffering Africans, provided a moral exemplar for the waning days of European rule. Aspects of Schweitzer's mission, particularly his pragmatic focus and emphasis on protecting life, continue to resonate in secular humanitarian projects. However, the "reverence" in his case was literal and the impulse fully sacred. Even after becoming a doctor, Schweitzer remained a theologian.

The new doctor's turn to missionary medicine, however, occurred prior to his moment of vision. Unlike Henri Dunant, unexpectedly hurrying about a battlefield, Schweitzer prepared himself professionally before embarking to treat the afflicted. Health care, he felt, would provide him with a broad passport to utility, deeply purposeful and mobile.[34] His conception of this "path of service" was deeply humanist, if not quite secular. For Schweitzer, medical care was not simply a tool for conversion in the narrow sense. Rather, it was the means to realize the humanistic promise of Christianity, and in so doing to offer a measure of redemption for what he perceived to be the failures and sins of civilized rule.[35] Moreover, his thought derived from meditation on experience, not rational exposition alone. He cast his reverence for life quite broadly, feeling concern for the well-being of nonhuman animals and even plants. It was an attitude, not a specific creed, focused primarily on awareness. Schweitzer had few illusions about a natural basis for mercy. The duty of humanity was not a given; rather it derived from the challenge of dedicated spiritual work and difficult practice. In a modest way, the theological doctor sought to change the world by emphasizing matters of the heart.

At the same time, Schweitzer's relations with African collaborators proved complex. He asked his staff to move heavy palm trees to spare them from cutting—a philosophy that struck them as "perverted"—while maintaining rigid divisions between Europeans and Africans. It appeared to many that he only fully accepted the latter as patients, sick and needy.[36] In later years his work would be criticized not only for its paternalism and social remove, but also for its resistance to change. When it came to questions of both political and medical progress, the hospital Schweitzer founded struck a distinctly cautious note. While emphasizing the survival of his patients and his forest hospital, the good doctor still kept one ear cocked for "the sound of bells in a Christian country."[37]

Schweitzer's vision, like Dunant's, positioned moral sentiment about humanity beyond politics. A Protestant from Alsace with a Prussian wife, he had to tread carefully in a French colony, promising to remain "mute as a carp" on religious matters and paying his expenses through private fundraising.[38] Unlike the Red Cross, which operated through states, the missionary doctor did not expect governments to take up the "duty of humanity" as an official policy; instead he relied on religious congregations and individual charity. Moreover, Schweitzer's work differed in the slower pace of its peacetime setting and in its broader emphasis on life. As on Dunant's battlefield, a better death might arrive through care, the soul's passage accompanied by the relief of prayers as well as physical comfort in the mission hospital. However the force of *reverence* lay with the living and the recognition that life came "each day as a gift." To take up this path required more than a willingness to engage in acts of mercy, or even medical training: ultimately one needed a properly contemplative worldview. "There are no heroes of action," Schweitzer maintained, "only heroes of renunciation and suffering."[39] Life, from this perspective, was the essential ground for sacred understanding and not simply a good in itself.

DISCOVERING A THIRD WORLD

When searching for antecedents to MSF in the Red Cross or among medical missionaries, we must also recognize conceptual shifts between eras and activities. The term *humanitarianism* itself came into being only in early-nineteenth-century England and has meant different things over time.[40] First applied to describe a theological position stressing the humanity of Christ, it subsequently covered efforts to alleviate suffering or advance the greater human collectivity. As such it reflected broad concern about ruptures associated with modern industrial life, as well as the ambition to improve conditions across a wide range of institutions such as hospitals, prisons, and schools. Humanitarian ideals included philanthropy, suggesting the uplift of poor and benighted peoples would come through the moral leadership and financial generosity of the wealthy and enlightened. Distinctions between relief and development did not always apply, and activities now described as "humanitarian" did not always receive that label. Critical elements of contemporary understanding—human rights, genocide, a world of nation-states—only appeared in the aftermath of the Second World War and came into alignment a generation later. To imagine action "without borders" requires not just a secular sensibility about life, but also a particular form of division and interconnection between humans.

By the time Schweitzer won his Peace Prize in 1952, the bells of Christian empire rang less certainly. In 1944 the Nobel committee had chosen the ICRC for that same award, just as in 1917. Yet the second bout of world war found the Red Cross struggling with fresh problems and responsibilities related to the advent of a more total form of conflict. The group had forwarded millions of parcels, letters, and messages and distributed many tons of relief goods. Still, the conflict had produced a new scale of destruction and civilian suffering that exceeded all these efforts. The Red Cross, moreover, faced its own uncomfortable ethical legacy. In October 1942, after due deliberation and discussion, the International Committee had decided against issuing a public appeal over the Nazi concentration camps. Concerned about jeopardizing its delicate web of relief efforts on behalf of prisoners of war, and doubtful about the practical efficacy of speaking out, it stayed quiet, leaving diplomacy and denunciation to others. However difficult to evaluate in historical terms, the decision would haunt the organization in ensuing decades.[41] Whether or not a Red Cross statement would have affected the course of events, the absence of one appeared a moral failure to later generations for whom the Holocaust represented a new epitome of evil. The Red Cross also found itself on one side of a widening cold war chasm, dismissed as a "bourgeois organization" by the socialist alliance.[42]

Beyond redrawing political maps, the war reworked the conceptual and organizational terrain of international affairs. A wave of institutions came into being in its wake, headed by the United Nations. These established new mechanisms for international governance and provided critical elements of a moral language centered on the figure of the human. The 1948 Universal Declaration of Human Rights not only enumerated a lengthy list of ideals, but it also affirmed the "the inherent dignity" of all members of the human family.[43] Under a term coined and championed by a Polish Jewish lawyer named Raphaël Lemkin, the newly named crime of genocide expanded the category of "crimes against humanity" featured in the Nuremberg trials so that it applied to times of peace as well as war.[44] While the reach of these developments may have remained limited even in rhetorical terms, the universal human became available for later reference.

During the postwar years this nascent moral discourse about rights and needs remained overshadowed by two other geopolitical phenomena: the cold war standoff between American and Soviet spheres of influence and the decolonization of European empires. France struggled to maintain a degree of autonomy between the new superpowers. Unlike Britain, it parted reluctantly with its colonial possessions, fighting bitter wars in Indochina and Algeria and endeavoring to maintain a sphere of influence in Africa. For their part, the new states emerging from anticolonial struggles also maneuvered between Eastern and Western alliances, as well as the receding colonial powers. In 1952 a French economist named Alfred Sauvy introduced the term *Third World* to describe this new, largely postcolonial terrain. An allusion to the three estates of the French Revolution, this new tripartite substituted the West for the church, the East (ironically enough) for the aristocracy, and ex-colonials for the commoners. As Odd Arne Westad notes, both American and Soviet ideology focused on the betterment of humanity, and each sought control primarily through forms of aid and improvement rather than direct domination and administration.[45] Discourses of development moved directly into the political spotlight, and new institutions, bureaucracies, and armies of experts maneuvered to spread rival gospels of modernization.

The cold war ran considerably hotter across the landscape of this new Third

World than it did in Moscow or Washington. Stumbling from crisis to crisis, the United Nations gradually added agencies to provide for suffering civilians.[46] The Red Cross too strove to address the new landscape, sending missions to Palestine, Indochina, Algeria, Korea, and other sites of conflict. In 1967 it added Nigeria to the list. There, following a series of coups and rising ethnic tensions, the southeastern region of the country proclaimed independence as the Republic of Biafra, and a bitter civil war ensued.

From the perspective of humanitarian organizations, the Biafran conflict would later appear a watershed. Although many of the elements involved—including the infamous manipulation of suffering and aid—were not entirely new, they came together in a newly evocative and disturbing way. As the Nigerian army slowly strangled the rebellion over the next three years, images of starving children spread worldwide through the new wonders of satellite transmission as well as older media. Improvements in air transport and emergency medicine fostered a new sense of the possible when it came to intervention. The political alignments surrounding the conflict were complex (France, Portugal, South Africa, and Israel supported the rebels, whereas Britain, the United States, and even the Soviet Union backed the government), yet the separatist government mounted a highly effective campaign to influence public opinion, highlighting civilian suffering and warning of genocide. A number of aid agencies became deeply involved in attempting some form of relief. The majority of the afflicted civilians came from the largely Christian Igbo people, and Catholic missionaries played a significant role in advocating for attention and shaping media coverage.[47] But the primary rationale of media engagement that emerged from the conflict was a secular appeal: *lives* were at risk and had to be saved.

Biafra proved deeply traumatic for several of the groups involved in the conflict. The ICRC, which sponsored airlifts, vaccinations, and food programs on a massive scale, had never raised and invested so much money. In addition to Swiss delegates, it fielded a team of doctors recruited from national Red Cross societies, including a significant French contingent. The group abided by its traditions of neutrality, even if the sympathies of its field staff were plain enough that several were killed by Nigerian troops. When the government clamped down on relief flights and terminated its cooperation, the group protested privately but reluctantly withdrew, with new doubts and expectations. Entering the conflict as a relatively stodgy collective overseeing the Geneva Conventions, it emerged as a full-fledged relief organization. Other groups like Oxfam were similarly shaken. Even if the predicted genocide did not materialize, the scale of suffering remained immense as both the federal government and the rebels sought to use starvation for strategic ends. Caught up in the drama, aid workers agonized over their limitations and raged at restrictions imposed on them by the prevailing order. Later some would wonder whether their actions had helped prolong the suffering. But at the time many embraced the ethos of spectacle and found moral energy in its immediacy. A generation came of age in Biafra, and several new nongovernmental organizations emerged in its bitter wake. The most ambitious of these would be Médecins Sans Frontières.[48]

THE CALL OF BIAFRA, THE ALLURE OF A NAME

Of the men assembled in Paris for the 1971 photograph, five had been Red Cross volunteers in Biafra. One of these, Bernard Kouchner, was destined to become a charismatic force in international humanitarianism and French political life. Passionate and telegenic, he was already emerging as a public figure at the time, and his later fame would help wrap MSF's origins in an additional layer of legend. In the mythic version of the group's birth, it came into being through Kouchner's rejection of Red Cross silence. The large arc of the story rings true, as MSF came to embody an alternative Red Cross, shaped by youthful rebellion and the media age. The historical record, however, offers more qualifications and details. The break with traditional discretion actually occurred over a period of years, and the initial impetus for the group's founding came from several directions, including the vision of a pair of restless journalists and the hunger of suburban French doctors for charitable adventures. Even among the Biafran veterans Kouchner was hardly alone. Several of his colleagues were by then old hands at aid work and played a more prominent official role in MSF at the outset. And several of his younger successors were actually closer to the generational moment and would do more to realize the organization's institutional potential. But it was Kouchner who articulated the group's vision most grandly and left the largest mark. Years after parting ways with the organization his name remained attached to it; even when his successors took issue with his public positions they could never quite break free from his legacy. It is only fitting to follow his story first.

The child of a Jewish doctor and a Catholic nurse, Bernard Kouchner entered the world during the uncertain lull at the onset of the Second World War.[49] He grew up in a France shadowed by that conflict and infused with the cult of the Resistance. Haunted by the Holocaust, particularly after learning of the death of his own grandparents, Kouchner easily gravitated to Leftist politics, and he joined the Communist student union in 1959. He opposed the Algerian war and defined himself through antifascism. Although studying medicine, he nursed journalistic aspirations and published several pieces of commentary.[50] He visited Yugoslavia and Cuba and even met with Castro. In the middle of the decade, however, the party tightened its control over the student group, excluding Kouchner and his associates. Some went on to form small Maoist and Trotskyite collectives. For his part Kouchner helped edit another Leftist publication and finally finished his studies in gastroenterology in May 1968. That very month the Latin Quarter in

Paris erupted in a student revolt. Although later identified with this historical moment, Kouchner was actually nearing thirty at the time and had already passed through one political baptism and disillusionment. Amid the tumult in the streets he heard a different call and joined the Red Cross in Biafra.

Between September 1968 and January 1970, some fifty French volunteers made their way to a hospital in Biafra for varying stints of medical duty. Kouchner would go three times, growing increasingly passionate about the cause. As he would later recall, the general idea for what would become Médecins Sans Frontières first emerged in conversations there. When back in Paris he agitated for the Biafran cause and signed an open letter to diplomats attesting to the suffering involved. On October 23, 1968, together with his senior colleague Max Récamier, Kouchner published a testimonial in the French newspaper *Le monde,* the first of a series of such efforts by members of the team. Although a departure from silence, this publication remained a modest one. As Anne Vallaeys notes, it focused on medical issues, and far from denouncing the Red Cross, exhorted would-be humanitarians to join the mission.[51] Nonetheless, it marked a break with humanitarian discretion. It also demonstrated a point of continuity in Kouchner's own personal trajectory: the medical student had become a journalist, and the journalist found new voice as a doctor.

Récamier and Pascal Grellety-Bosviel, the doctors who oversaw the Biafran team, were older than Kouchner. Both had prior experience in aid work—including a Red Cross mission to Yemen, where they struggled with an early version of a prefabricated clinic—and had come of age in a milieu of Third World solidarity that largely featured religious organizations.[52] Récamier's humanitarian convictions derived primarily from Christian charity, not the revolutionary tradition that had shaped Kouchner. Nonetheless, the two found common ground in the face of what they thought to be genocide, foreshadowing later humanitarian alliances.

Following the collapse of Biafra, the former volunteers started a group with the ungainly acronym of GIMCU (*Groupe d'intervention médicale et chirurgicale d'urgence*). Their idea was to have it serve as a sort of expeditionary brigade for the Red Cross. The new group's associates included Jacques Bérès, a surgeon who had volunteered for Biafra but not made it there in time, and Xavier Emmanuelli, another former Communist and future politician, who had worked as a doctor in the merchant marine and after an accident began to nurse a vision of rapid intervention.[53] Members of GIMCU participated in some abortive missions in 1970, arriving late after an earthquake in Peru and attempting to provide assistance during the Jordanian crackdown on Palestinians. When a hurricane struck East Pakistan, they waited in vain for a call. The situation spiraled into secession and civil war and neither Pakistan nor India showed much willingness to cooperate; still, the Red Cross did not send them. Récamier, however, saw an appeal in the medical journal *Tonus* for volunteers to form an emergency group. Fatefully, the Biafran veterans decided to respond.

Tonus was hardly a radical publication, being directed primarily toward suburban general practitioners. Its editor, Raymond Borel, however, was something of a restless soul. The author of several novels, he had lived in Brazil and spent time in Hollywood as an aspiring scriptwriter, becoming friends with John Wayne. Back in Paris after the Korean War, he worked for the magazine *Détective*. In 1963 he received an offer from an American-backed venture to help create a new medical publication. Its niche would be social issues, addressing the place of doctors in a rapidly changing world. Borel signed on and recruited Philippe Bernier, a freelance journalist caught up in the abduction of a Moroccan opposition leader and consequently jailed. Protesting his innocence with a hunger strike, he wrote a series of articles for *Tonus* that detailed his physical and mental state. After his release, Bernier joined Borel's journal. It occurred to the two that some young doctors might seek a more inspirational way to spend their vacation than lying on the beach and so would be ready to volunteer for humanitarian missions if asked. In November 1970, just as East Pakistan became a disaster zone, Bernier authored the first of what would be several calls to arms, enjoining doctors to volunteer and aid victims of disaster. Bearing the provocative title "Are We Mercenaries?" it featured a doctor who had witnessed scenes of chaos and bureaucratic impasse following a recent earthquake in Yugoslavia. In response, the doctor imagined a medical strike force that could mobilize quickly and freely, thereby saving lives. French doctors, he was sure, were not mercenaries.[54] The end of the article—next to an advertisement featuring a product for diaper rash—included a form to sign and send to *Tonus* as an indication of interest. Similar appeals followed, and a year later Bernier could report that 182 readers had enlisted in a volunteer group now titled *Secours Medical Français* (SMF, or French Medical Aid).[55]

One of these appeals caught Récamier's eye and emissaries of GIMCU visited the *Tonus* office. Although different in style as well as trajectory (Kouchner apparently did present himself as a "mercenary," albeit of emergency medicine), the two ventures quickly found common ground.[56] The members of GIMCU had grown frustrated with Red Cross caution and were eager for a more independent association. They would join SMF. Borel and Bernier, for their part, were impressed with the worldly air and energy of their new partners. A meeting was set and in anticipation the *Tonus* team reviewed its nascent organization over whiskey. *Secours Medical Français,* they belatedly realized, might have an unfortunate ring in former colonies. Turning the initials over and over, they at last came up with another permutation: Médecins Sans Frontières. On a gray December night in 1971, the new collective assembled. Borel and Bernier brought their lawyer as well as several doctors and surgeons who had responded to their appeal. Kouchner and his compatriots joined them around the table, and together they agreed to establish a new association and settled on a charter. The Biafran precedent and Kouchner's preferences notwithstanding, this initial charter—largely the work of Bernier—included the Red Cross principle of neutrality and adhered to the tradition of medical confidentiality and public silence. Still, a new alliance between journalism and medicine was now official. "The answer to all who doubted you," *Tonus* proclaimed proudly to its readers on January 3, 1972, beneath a photo of the eleven men around a table. "'Médecins Sans Frontières' has become a reality."[57]

In the triumphant article announcing the new association's birth, Bernier suggested that the movement's existence rendered its genesis "superfluous." This rhetorical flourish anticipated the group's later impatient style and nonchalance about history, even its own. MSF embraced action, counting on speed, improvisation, and daring to overcome obstacles. As the organization grew, quarreled, and split, however, the founding moment became subject to considerable reworking and dispute. Read with an eye to their outcome, past events could provide an aura of justification as well as precedent. As Kouchner's star rose, other names receded. And as MSF established a reputation for outspokenness, the line from Biafra to testimony grew straighter and straighter.[58]

Despite erasing historical detail, the mythic version of MSF's emergence does capture the extraordinary, mobile allure of its name. The shift in acronym from SFM to MSF may or may not have eased the burden of colonial history. It did clearly open a new rhetorical horizon for global claims. The phrase *sans frontières* was to resonate widely, first through France, where it described a whole movement of new organizations—*sans frontièrisme*—and subsequently worldwide. In English translation, "without borders" eventually became a gloss for globalization. The expression may have appeared in the late 1960s as the name of a youth travel agency in France or a rebranded European game show.[59] But MSF popularized it. Moreover, it established a new form, serving as a prototype organization that adopted a borderless sense of space together with an ethos of direct intervention and media involvement. Alongside Doctors, the world has gained Reporters, Pharmacists, Engineers, Animals, Magicians, Knitters, Sociologists, and even Clowns Without Borders. The translation of *frontières* into "borders" would remain a point of slight contention. To adherents of MSF the name denoted a general willingness to expand and overcome barriers in general, not a simplistic dismissal of national borders. Even when yielding to the international dominance of English as the language of world governance, as well as expanding far beyond France, the organization retained its original acronym. Nonetheless, "without borders" conveys its epochal ambition. Henceforth, doctors would go anywhere.

The choice of an emblem proved less straightforward but revealing in its own way. In MSF's early bulletins several symbols received consideration, including a flying bird.[60] MSF eventually adopted a variant of the cross in red and white, tilted against a red swatch. It would retain this insignia until the mid-1990s, when—facing legal action by the ICRC—it switched to a stylized "running man" in red and white. Like its name, the evolution of the group's symbol is to some degree instructive of its larger trajectory. Where the roots of Dunant's organization were clearly Christian, those of MSF filtered through a figure of humanity. Founded as a "free association" under the relevant French law of 1901, part of the secular legacy of French Republicanism, MSF presented itself without reference to religious tradition. At the same time, it absorbed the influence of religious as well as political opposition movements, offering a point of convergence around a common concern for life.[61]

JACOBINS WITHOUT THE GUILLOTINE

The initial profile of MSF was hardly revolutionary. As it did with the charter, the *Tonus* group took the initial lead when it came to filling offices. Max Récamier became vice president but most other positions went to those who had responded to the SMF appeal, and the presidency to a man named Marcel Delcourt, Borel's neighbor, who was also a Gaullist. From a distance the selection might appear incongruous, but at the time it seemed strategic. First and foremost the new group sought legitimacy, and thus it cast the most respectable members in public roles and emphasized professional restraint. A few days after MSF's birth, one of its new officers, Gérard Pigeon, emphatically affirmed the group's commitment to silence: "The doctor does not leave as a witness."[62] The Biafran veterans might disagree, but at the outset they went along quietly.

The early years of MSF's existence were filled with enthusiastic dreams and heated discussions but relatively few effective missions. The vision of the time remained that of a voluntary association of medical professionals, a band of adventurers ready to rush to assistance. At first the collective functioned like a placement agency, gathering would-be volunteers and sending them to work with other groups in Third World settings. Many organizations seeking medical volunteers directed their efforts toward longer-term development, however, leading to ongoing debate over the extent to which the group should respond to "chronic emergencies."[63] It became apparent that to take action in the wake of disaster, MSF would need to become directly operational. In December 1972, the group finally launched its first mission, responding to an earthquake in Nicaragua. Thanks to Kouchner's daring and connections, the team managed to hitch a ride with the French military, but again arrived too late to provide much in the way of actual medical care. The theatrical episode did garner press attention, if not all of it favorable.[64] In the short run MSF's relations with the Red Cross suffered, and its members acquired the image of being medical hippies. In the longer run it had at least taken a step, however modest, toward running its own missions.

Members of MSF continued to volunteer for other organizations. Another early venture to Honduras was similarly inconclusive, and fundraising remained on a modest scale, targeted at medical professionals rather than the general public. Tension increased between the Biafran and *Tonus* factions. Members of the former came from a hospital milieu and favored emergency missions; the latter were largely engaged in private practice and held a wider view of medicine. They also tended to be more politically and socially conservative. A trip by Kouchner, Récamier, and Bérès to aid Kurdish rebels in Iraq in 1974 precipitated a struggle over proper conduct for the organization. Eventually the Biafran contingent emerged victorious. Bernier quit and MSF moved more decisively in the direction of publicity and engagement, if remaining ragtag in its organization. In 1975 a team left for Vietnam, and as Saigon fell they drove about in a white VW van marked with crosses.[65] The following year in Lebanon MSF launched a more substantial operation, supporting a Beirut hospital. By this point MSF counted 780 adherents and a budget of around 300,000 francs.[66] It also now testified more openly, describing the mission's work under fire and beginning a tradition of more active witnessing.[67] Moreover, the close of 1976 saw MSF embrace wider publicity in the form of a pro bono ad campaign on its behalf (appeals to medical professionals alone having yielded limited results). Posters featuring a dark-skinned child with wide eyes and the memorable slogan "Two billion people in their waiting room" raised the association's profile considerably, setting the stage for success in public fundraising.[68] The posters also captured its increasingly militant spirit. In keeping with the French Revolutionary tradition, MSF clearly intended to make waves.

As the group solidified and grew, it gained a new generation of adherents. Having come of age politically during May 1968, they combined leftist orientation with skepticism and confrontational style. Several had gone to medical school together at Cochin in Paris. They also shared the common experience of encountering MSF as an existing entity and approaching it from the perspective of field missions. One prominent presence was Claude Malhuret, who like Kouchner would later transform into a politician, becoming a French minister and eventually mayor of Vichy. As a student he matched his medical education with socialist politics and *tiers-mondiste* ("third-worldist") sympathies. He first heard of MSF in 1974; its name reminded him of the May rebellion.[69] Malhuret then met Emmanuelli and eventually worked for nearly a year in refugee camps in Thailand. There he grew disillusioned with leftist justifications of the regime in Cambodia and frustrated with MSF's inability to provide much support.

A second key figure was Rony Brauman, who eventually emerged as the group's most defining leader. Born to Polish Jews in Jerusalem, his childhood carried a deep imprint from the Holocaust, and it would remain a central referent in much of his writing. As a student he gravitated toward anarchism and then Maoism, spending a period as an activist. Tending further left than Malhuret, he responded more skeptically when first hearing of MSF, suspecting it of bourgeois tendencies.[70] Moreover, on his initial approach Emmanuelli famously turned him away. He went instead to a rural hospital in Benin with a Catholic organization, and later to an urban hospital in Djibouti. These experiences deepened his growing humanitarian convictions, though, as he recalled years later in Paris, he still sought a group "that wouldn't have religious discourse, even if activist."[71] Joining MSF at last, he also went to a camp in Thailand. The Khmer Rouge episode in Cambodia brought Brauman, like Malhuret, to break with political ideology and refocus on human suffering.

Viewed at a distance, all these figures—Kouchner, Emmanuelli, Malhuret, Brauman—exhibit considerable similarities.[72] While elements of biography, approach, and style varied, all found their deepest engagement with the world through the secular faith of medical care. Their interest in politics shifted form and tense: rather than focusing on a utopian future, they increasingly concentrated on suffering in the present. Unlike Schweitzer they were restless, mobile, and combative. Life became their key value, but their spirit proved more radical than reverent. Their horizon also stretched beyond a single hospital: as Kouchner infamously put it on a television show, after May 1968 they "discovered" the Third World and its misery.[73] Responding in 1978 to an interviewer's question as to whether he was tempted stay put like Schweitzer, Kouchner replied with characteristic cheek: "It's a respectable image, but one that belongs to the domain of charity rather than medicine. However, if a *médecin sans frontières* looks into the essence of himself, he will certainly encounter the secret desire to be the Good Samaritan. Jesus Christ, perhaps."[74] Malhuret, along with Emmanuelli and Brauman, shared Kouchner's ambivalent view of charity but desired a more comprehensive and instrumentally effective organization: a lighter and more activist Red Cross. In keeping with Kouchner's distinction, their common model of humanitarian engagement would remain medical rather than charitable. The refugee camp, however, rather than the battlefield or the hospital, proved the defining terrain.

SCHISMS AND EXPANSIONS

The subsequent trajectory of MSF only deepened its focus on the moral significance of saving lives, even as its protagonists struggled over how best to achieve this end. A second mythical moment came in the form of a schism, when in 1979 Bernard Kouchner lost power and departed to found the rival Médecins du Monde (MDM, or Doctors of the World). As with MSF's founding, there are multiple interpretations of this episode, and feelings remained raw for decades. The drama unfolded not only within the group's modest meetings, but also in the public eye. Malhuret had rapidly risen to a position of leadership, partly with Kouchner's blessing. It soon became apparent, however, that their views diverged. Where Malhuret took inspiration from the functionality of the Red Cross, Kouchner strongly rejected the prospect of becoming "bureaucrats of misery."[75] The precipitating event came in late 1978, when Malaysia denied entry to a boatload of Vietnamese refugees in full view of the media. The image of thousands suffering aboard the *Hai Hong* resonated in France and inspired a project to send a "Boat for Vietnam" to demonstrate solidarity with the refugees. This appeal became the occasion for a remarkable display of solidarity across France's own political divides: most notably, long-time opponents Jean-Paul Sartre and Raymond Aron both signed on, joined by a host of other intellectual luminaries such as Roland Barthes, Simone de Beauvoir, and Michel Foucault. Humanitarian concern provided new common ground.

Kouchner naturally championed the venture and expected MSF to provide medical services for it. Malhuret and others who had spent time working in camps in Thailand were skeptical, seeing the mission as more of a publicity stunt than an effective aid project. Tension between the factions grew. Then Emmanuelli aligned himself with Malhuret, publishing a scathing, sarcastic article attacking the project, calling it a "Boat for Saint-Germain-des-Prés" and implying that it had more to do with Parisian self-image than meaningful assistance.[76] Kouchner was furious, feeling betrayed. In the event, the boat—christened *L'Île de Lumière* (The Isle of Light) no less—sailed without MSF's sanction, but with Kouchner and associates on board. Rather than rescuing refugees it became a hospital ship, anchoring off an island and offering medical services. It also received considerable media attention. At a stormy board meeting in 1979, Malhuret called for a more professional and less spectacular organization, one that included compensation for volunteers, as "the time of Doctor Schweitzer is over." Kouchner countered that MSF was effectively dead, killed by "bureaucrats of misery and the technocrats of charity."[77] He then walked out, followed by his allies. They left MSF for good, founding MDM the next year. However, the majority of MSF's members stayed and the group continued to expand rapidly. From the perspective of the original organization, Kouchner's departure marked the end of a chapter, not a conclusion.

In retrospect, it is easy to read this split, as most MSF versions of the story do, as the ascendance of pragmatism and professionalism. The elements are certainly there, since the schism allowed a largely younger generation to seize control and reshape the organization over the ensuing decade. By contrast, Kouchner's new group would narrate the same event as an origin story, emphasizing purity of principle. However, it would be a mistake to overstate the differences between MSF and its new rival. MDM would align itself more emphatically with human rights, media advocacy, and the beau geste. It would also retain a more amateur

feel and trail its older sibling in fundraising, logistical expertise, and medical innovation. Nonetheless, despite personal animosities and periodic clashes over
particular issues, the two organizations underwent a largely parallel evolution.
Indeed, one of MSF's first actions under the new regime was its own controversial
beau geste: a celebrity march to the Thai border to protest the aid policies of the
Cambodian government. Both groups intervened in Afghanistan's civil war, riding mountain trails with the mujahedin, and together entered the consciousness
of the American press of the day as the "French Doctors." Amid the romance of
running clandestine missions, any pretense of adherence to neutrality and discretion vanished. "Like our forerunners in Biafra," Brauman would later write, "we
had implicitly picked our side."[78] Legitimacy came not from international law, but
from the moral worth of providing services where there were none, in a war where
"a million died." If the rival strands of French humanitarianism had each "chosen
a truth," in Borel's words, those truths were less different than some may have
imagined at the time.[79] MSF was only seven years old when the schism occurred—
the "age of reason," as Emmanuelli noted in an issue of the organization's bulletin
just before the fateful board meeting.[80] Its real growth had only just begun.

In 1982 Brauman became president of MSF, a post he was to hold for the next
dozen years. During that time the budget increased exponentially, as did the
number of volunteers and missions. MSF adopted increasingly sophisticated
fundraising techniques, some self-consciously borrowed from the United States.[81]
It established administrative and logistic structures to manage both people and
supplies. Although still an informal and sometimes haphazard affair, it began to
exhibit greater professional expectations and to resemble more of a machine. In
the space of just two decades, the group grew to match its global claim, its flag
fluttering in all manner of remote outposts.

Not all of this growth emanated from Paris. As early as the 1970s MSF had
begun to explore the possibility of internationalization implicit in its name.[82] In
1980 a young Belgian named Philippe Laurent, who had volunteered for MSF in
camps in Thailand, proposed establishing a branch of the group with some associates in his home country. Despite concern over legal issues, the Paris leadership
generally supported the initiative, and a similar one in Switzerland shortly thereafter. From a Parisian perspective both were Francophone countries and seemed
natural extensions, analogous to MSF's regional "antennas" in French provinces.[83]
To the surprise of the French, however, the group in Brussels not only grew rapidly but also began to assert independence. The Belgians mounted a major operation in Chad, taking over much of the health service in that country. To the
French, their approach appeared overly close to development and shared its illusions about the future. The Belgians saw their work as part of a different humanitarian strategy, one focused on growth and the use of institutional funds. They
also increasingly resented what they perceived as French arrogance and meddling,

such as when the French spoke out on behalf of two Belgian hostages without first consulting the Brussels group. In 1984 a branch of the movement opened in Holland. Jacques de Milliano, a Dutch doctor who had volunteered with the Belgians in Chad, met with colleagues in Amsterdam and decided to open an office. The Brussels office was supportive, Paris far less enthusiastic. French qualms notwithstanding, MSF was becoming international and for the first time exceeding the bounds of the French language.[84] With the founding of a Spanish section in 1986, as well as a smaller offshoot in Luxembourg (also sponsored by Brussels), it became undeniably European.

MSF struggled to define a political frame for its evolving sense of humanitarianism. Although many of the key figures had roots in Leftist politics, their experience in refugee camps led them to break with their former assumptions about international solidarity. As Brauman himself later noted, the period between 1975 and 1980 was an era of expanding Soviet influence in the Third World. With the eruption of one refugee crisis after another MSF took an increasingly anti-communist turn.[85] In 1984 the French membership agreed to launch a foundation to reflect on humanitarian issues, and in January 1985 Brauman and Malhuret announced the birth of a think tank known as Liberté Sans Frontières. LSF quickly established itself as a center of controversy, taking a public stand against the leftist tradition of *tiers-mondisme* and accusing it of romantic misrepresentation. As well as upsetting much of France's intelligentsia, LSF also provoked consternation among MSF's field staff and loud opposition from the Belgian office, which saw this as an autocratic veer into politics, and right-wing politics at that. Relations between Paris and Brussels grew increasingly cold. The Belgians suspended relations and attacked LSF in print. For its part the French leadership filed a lawsuit to block the Belgians from using the MSF name. To complete the soap opera, Kouchner and fellow founding fathers Récamier and Bérès hastened to loudly support Brussels. The suit failed, and slowly and gingerly the movement reassembled itself as an international coalition. LSF quietly disbanded in 1989, though not before involving several significant figures in the French humanitarian world.[86]

Even as this internecine struggle played out in Europe, other clashes erupted on the ground. In Ethiopia a devastating famine captured considerable international attention and inspired massive humanitarian response, including the famous concert known as Live Aid. MSF-France and MSF-Belgium both sent teams to Ethiopia. The French grew suspicious of Ethiopian government policies, particularly forcible resettlement, perceiving in them the political manipulation of the famine and international relief. They began to express their opposition publicly, a stance that created significant uproar in the aid world. The Ethiopian regime was likewise displeased and at the end of 1985 evicted the French team. The Belgians stayed on, preferring to remain quiet and offer care. The French continued to agitate, questioning the larger humanitarian operation. This position met with considerable denunciation at the time—Bob Geldorf suggested in *Le Monde* that MSF had become a "political organization," and both the French ambassador to Ethiopia and Bernard Kouchner disapproved of its stance—but the incident enhanced its public profile and later became central to the group's mythic self-conception. A new tradition of speaking out was now enshrined.[87]

During the Ethiopian conflict critics still dismissed MSF as an amateurish operation. Over the second half of the 1980s, the group continued to improve its operations and cultivate a more professional profile. It developed a new logistics system and established an epidemiological wing known as Epicentre. At the same time it became increasingly sophisticated about its media presence and fundraising, even setting up an in-house production unit for short films. The organization also began working in Western Europe itself, focusing on outcast populations such as the homeless and drug addicts. By its twentieth anniversary in 1991, MSF-France boasted 700,000 donors and 850 volunteers in the field, while deriving two-thirds of its funds from private sources. MSF-Belgium nearly rivaled it in size, though it drew more of its operating funds from institutional donors. Next came MSF-Holland, followed by the smaller Swiss and Spanish sections, Luxembourg, and a tiny, newly formed Greek section to fill out the ensemble.[88] The French had also sponsored a New York office the year before, focused on fundraising and recruitment.

Gradually a true international structure began to emerge. There would be five largely autonomous "operational" sections that sponsored missions: France, Belgium, Holland, Switzerland, and Spain. The big three established "partner" sections around them to provide assistance with finances and human resources. These developed somewhat haphazardly and initially functioned like colonies or subsidiaries of a crime family. France and Holland assembled the most profitable empires. The French claimed Japan (1992) and Australia (1994) in addition to the United States (1990). The Dutch planted their flag in Canada (1991), the United Kingdom (1993), and Germany (1993). Belgium assembled the less lucrative array of Italy (1993), Demark (1993), Sweden (1993), Norway (1996), and Hong Kong (1994).[89] In between a small and relatively weak international office appeared. Established in 1991 in Brussels, it eventually shifted to the aid capital Geneva the following decade. Despite periodic attempts to improve coordination between the operational sections, they would find reason to quarrel as often as to collaborate.

With the dissolution of the Soviet Union and the unraveling of cold war geopolitics, the larger international system of humanitarian agencies also came into its own during the 1990s. UN peacekeeping and relief missions increased and NGOs propagated exponentially. For its part the MSF collective continued to grow while stumbling from one catastrophe to another. The series of conflicts in the

Balkans and the Rwandan genocide proved particularly traumatic. In Rwanda MSF found itself reduced to working under the ICRC, and in frustration the French section eventually called for military intervention. In the ensuing refugee crisis in Zaire (present-day Democratic Republic of the Congo) it infuriated its Belgian and Dutch cousins by loudly and unilaterally withdrawing from the camps. Following an international gathering held in 1995 at Chantilly, relations between the sections gradually improved. When it won its Nobel Prize, the MSF collective had united enough to plunge into an advocacy campaign for pharmaceutical equity and to begin committing itself to AIDS care.

By the time of my encounters in the 2000s, then, MSF was a large, complex, transnational federation. It boasted a combined budget of hundreds of millions of dollars that was rising steadily toward the billion-dollar mark, and it mounted seventy to eighty field missions a year. In addition to sponsoring some two thousand international volunteers, the group engaged around ten times as many local staff at project sites. It had begun to recognize, uneasily, that the status of local staff might mirror older colonial divides, even as it worried yet again about devolving into a business. It likewise fretted over the expansion of its office personnel and planned to devolve management of some field missions to partner sections. Although the Paris office might still assume primacy, its hegemony rarely went unchallenged and English increasingly served as a lingua franca. To fuel these many operations, the group relied largely on small donors. Rather than relying on institutional grants, it depended profoundly on the moral force of "saving lives."

SECULAR HUMANITARIANISM AND SACRED LIFE

Viewed from within, the MSF movement can appear as an evolutionary transformation of generational experience. In the spirit of self-mockery, a 2001 article in *Dazibao,* the internal broadside of MSF-France, suggested that the group's real charter dramatically shifted over time. In 1970, an original "community of friends" offered "love to Third World populations" along with residual Maoist principles and hallucinogenic substances. By 1980, "mercenaries" of a private organization offered food aid to "Ethiopians, Afghans and other victims of the Moscow Olympics boycott." In 1990, a "profitable multinational company quoted on the unlisted securities market" offered assistance to populations victimized by disasters and was so overwhelmed as to "no longer know where help is needed most." By 2000, the e-charter of MSF.com championed both the 35-hour work week and the right to "full and free on-line access for anti-retroviral drugs."[90] Beneath this satirical representation ran the recognition, troubling to more than a few within the organization, that MSF had moved from being an oppositional and marginal presence to an established institution now entering middle age.

Although the French section of the group flirted with liberal ideals during the mid-1980s, what emerged from this period was less any certain ideological stand than a focus on life itself. The various strands of the organization and its offshoots struggled fiercely over terms of engagement but agreed on the value of human life. Rather than considering crisis from the long-term perspective of utopian history, they perceived it in relation to the immediate needs of those affected. Moreover, they reinforced this fundamental consensus powerfully in their operations. During the 1970s and 1980s refugee camps presented these humanitarians with clarity at the level of practice. Instead of political abstractions, their action could focus on particular bodies suffering in particular times and places; they could both speak out and actively intervene at the level of health. Thus MSF focused its energies on providing a direct response to suffering, wherever it might be found and whatever its origin. By the early 1990s the group, now part of a growing trend of nonprofit professionalization, had a global network in place and had become more technically proficient. Even if underlying conditions remained unresolved, emergencies proved conducive to both technical response and moral denunciation.

What, then, distinguishes this secular humanitarian concern for life? In comparison with Dunant's ministrations to wounded soldiers, MSF expends relatively little attention on the needs of the dead and dying or the larger social world they represent. Rather, its focus rests firmly on clinical bodies and the populations they compose. Unlike Schweitzer, MSF has spent little time elaborating a philosophy of life as such. This is hardly due to an absence of reflection in general; as we shall see, the group has devoted an impressive measure of reflective attention to other abstract concepts, such as its version of ethical witnessing. Life, however, is simply to be saved. In this sense Brauman's radical definition of the human as "a being who is not made to suffer" provides an accurate categorical touchstone. The humanitarian response to suffering presents itself as action, not contemplation. At the same time MSF remains a deeply realist organization, fully committed to responding to the shortcomings of an actually existing world. The point in "saving" life thus lies not in denying death per se, but rather in opposing *preventable* deaths, the view that "people shouldn't die of stupid things." This list of stupid things has grown varied and long, ranging from conflict and disaster to a range of diseases that might be averted with sufficient political will. Common to all of these is the prospect that with modest medical action, they need not prove so lethal.

MSF's sensibility gelled over time. The record of its early years shows comparatively little talk of humanitarianism per se and much of heroic medicine. In the initial announcement Bernier portrayed its creation as an act against "all the borders that still rise up between those whose vocation is to save, to care, and the victims of human barbarity or natural disturbances."[91] Salvation here involved professionals returning to the moral roots of their occupation and offering their services to any in need. They would do so freely, as unpaid volunteers, without thought of personal reward. If need be they would accept suffering to relieve suffering. Whether in response to sudden catastrophe or the "chronic emergency" of the Third World, the work of each *médecin* "sans frontières" defined a fundamentally medical mission.

By the end of the 1970s the term increasingly described a collectivity rather than a collection of individuals and the group became known by its acronym, MSF. This collectivity shifted to public exhortation, both in the sense of testimony and fundraising. After bitter struggles it professionalized, supporting its volunteers monetarily and improving its technical reach. It internationalized and became a plural institution, developing routines and traditions along with a legacy of dissent. It also developed a distinctive conceptual vocabulary around its version of humanitarianism. In contrast to the ideological divide of the cold war, the group emphasized moral protest. Since this protest took the form of medical action, it had a ready measure of relative achievement: lives saved. If some would donate and others act or stand aside, then more would live. All could participate. When confronted by preventable fatality, MSF increasingly framed its action in terms of witnessing and advocacy. Humanitarian medicine, after all, offered little redemption for loss of life, the inevitable long-term outcome of any clinical case. Once life was extinguished, meaning could only come from memory or appeals to prevention. Absent a soul or utopia, it is hard to transmute a stupid death into a good one.

In its secular medical version, then, humanitarianism has increasingly concentrated on a distinctly material project of salvation. In addition to being a biological matter of existence and a political object of concern, life emerges as a key moral value. The life at the center of humanitarian concern appears as a common quality, shared by all humans. However, it is also non-fungible and so eludes exchange; one life cannot substitute for another, anymore than could an immortal soul. In this sense it is sacred, not as a substitution for the soul in Christian theology, but perhaps as a secular "reoccupation" of its significance.[92] In lieu of an alternative higher good, focus rests on actions to maintain existence and enhance prospects for survival. As a matter of practical morality, then, the worth of this form of life derives precisely from saving it.

PART TWO

Global Ambitions

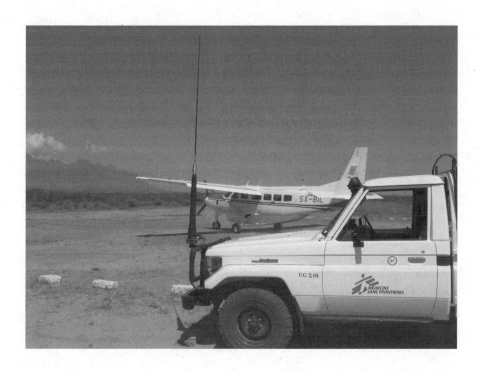

3

Vital Mobility

Speed saves lives.
MSF FUNDRAISING BROCHURE, 2005

THE "PUNCH"

On my initial trip to an MSF field site, I experienced the minor drama of a flat tire. The Land Cruiser was carrying a full complement of patients as well as staff members, though I was the only non-Ugandan aboard. When the tire blew we lurched and began to bump. Mohammed, the driver, quickly slowed down and pulled to a stop. I leaned out the window and confirmed that the left rear tire looked flat. A staff member clambered out, peered glumly at the wheel, and assured Mohammed it was indeed to blame. One by one the rest of us, except for one patient on crutches, joined him on the road. At the end of a day no one seemed particularly eager to leave the modest comfort of a seat or accept that our journey might be delayed. Mohammed, however, was in his element. A middle-aged but athletic man, he swung himself with practiced ease atop the vehicle to loosen the spare and slide it to the edge of the roof. Directing his male colleagues and passengers to hold the heavy object in place, he jumped down and helped us navigate it to the ground. Mohammed swiftly set the jack, scratching the dirt several times to level it properly before raising the car. Off came the old tire and on went the new, with just the slightest hint of effort. After lowering the vehicle Mohammed heaved the old tire on top for later repair. As we began to climb back inside he dusted his hands and gave a broad smile, clearly pleased with his performance. It had indeed been a thing of beauty as far as repairs go—quick, assured, and accomplished, displaying a minimum of extraneous effort. Later Mohammed would tell me that he had raced in a 1970s cross-country rally, where he had, as he put it laconically, "really learned to change a tire."

While our driver displayed his skill with a jack a small crowd of bystanders gathered around the vehicle. First children arrived running, quickly attracted by any sign of excitement. Their elders followed more slowly, drawn from the steady trickle of people trudging under heavy bundles. One by one they paused to inspect the unusual sight. This remote stretch of road carried mostly rickety bicycles, and the battered trucks that occasionally passed invariably sagged under their cargo, no match for our comparatively gleaming machine. A live foreigner such as myself was likewise an oddity, especially outside a vehicle. As I helped struggle with the wheel, a girl of about ten in a striking green and black print dress maneuvered cautiously to get a closer look. Others concentrated on our transport itself, some standing on their toes to peek inside from a safe distance. The patients meanwhile kept close; if their conveyance suddenly vanished, it would leave them with a long walk home. Those staff not occupied with the tire lounged proprietarily by the doors. Their supervisor, a well-dressed Ugandan nurse, impatiently inspected her nails. The air was still and no one spoke. Where before the engine had roared and wind whipped through the open windows, now all was quiet. For a brief moment we were all on the same ground, passenger and pedestrian alike.

Then Mohammed's show was over. We reloaded and were off, the bystanders dispersing behind us in our rear window. Conversation picked up immediately, and for the first time staff and patients chatted and laughed together, all clearly relieved the interruption had been so brief. We dropped the patients at their homes, one by one, and then drove back to the office. Along the way we passed through the modest, dusty hometown of Idi Amin. Amid the long evening light its inhabitants plodded through the shadowy streets, some wobbling along on laden bicycles. They paid us little heed. Two small boys by the roadside played with toy pull trucks fashioned ingeniously out of old cans and scrap metal. Absorbed in their game they only briefly glanced up and did not run or wave. Our vehicle was far less interesting when in motion.

Back at the office we dispersed for the evening. I dined with Mohammed at a local eatery that featured a television, sharing a meal of sweet potatoes and beans as a James Bond movie played on the video player, periodically interrupted by the machine's request for head-cleaning. The young boy in charge finally substituted another, cruder action film with an inexhaustible supply of bodies. Mohammed seemed to enjoy the distraction, even as we both laughed about the absurd rate of gunfire. Being tired, we talked little until I mentioned the flat. He then grew animated, recalling different moments in his life behind the wheel. The puncture (or "punch," as he memorably referred to it) led to a series of stories, most featuring far greater adversity. Mohammed had worked for many years as a truck driver, including a stint across the border in the Congo. There, he assured me, the roads would melt in the rains, trapping everything in thick, impassable mud. Even in good weather, some stretches were in such poor shape that it took him two or three days to travel a mere ten kilometers. By comparison, he found rural Uganda smooth sailing.

As Mohammed retold his exploits, I contemplated punches and punctures. The more I considered the terms, the more they seemed to summarize the event of the day. Our impatient passage over the landscape, usually so careless, had come to an abrupt halt. The hole deflated not just a tire, but also the larger medical mission invested in the vehicle; when brought to a standstill we were simply another group of people on a rural road with a lot to carry. For a brief moment this minor incident revealed the extent to which the team's travels—and its work in general—depended on a delicate web of support systems. Normally seamless and reliable, this fabric of infrastructure became visible when ruptured. Standing on the warm red earth of the roadway, far from our destination, the Land Cruiser came into new focus. Mundane and ordinary in motion, it grew extraordinary when immobilized, its vital importance on full display.

GLOBALIZATION ON THE GROUND

Imagine all the little things you have to do to go on holiday, then scale them up a few thousand times, and you will soon realize why it is that about half the people MSF sends on missions are non-medical.

PETER MORRIS, "LOWDOWN ON LOGISTICS," *SANS FRONTIÈRES* (MSF-AUSTRALIA, 1996)

By the time of its Nobel award, MSF enjoyed a reputation within the aid world for excellent logistics. One of the organization's great boasts was its ability to mobilize emergency aid to almost any part of the planet within forty-eight hours. While this claim might founder against the reality of certain political boundaries, or lapse in embarrassing mistakes, it contained a significant measure of demonstrable truth. MSF had developed the material capacity to be remarkably mobile. Such mobility depended on preparing and perfecting an assemblage of equipment—like the Land Cruiser—that could travel rather literally to the ends of the earth. The resulting web remained not only thin and fragile, but also expensive. Designed to be a temporary structure, forever impermanent and easily relocated to fit shifting demands, it required a ready flow of revenue to operate. At the same time it embodied the medical form of global connection implicit in MSF's name.

Mobility by itself, of course, hardly represents a general panacea for all human afflictions. Nonetheless, it has long stood as a vital principle in the domain of emergency care. From Larrey's "flying ambulance" during the Napoleonic wars in Europe, on through the equipment in any emergency wing of a contemporary hospital, mobility stands for a rapid link between patient and treatment. To realize this medical equation, one of these two elements has to move. Moreover, that movement must be rapid, as battlefields and accidents dictate haste. A fundraising slogan often used by MSF in recent years—"Speed saves lives"—carries a literal edge: when dealing with a severe physical trauma or an outbreak of disease, chances of survival compete against the clock. The slogan likewise reflects something of the organization's longer lineage in emergency medicine and its general ethos of perpetual crisis. When life is on the line, medical response appears a natural and unquestionably powerful response. Yet many procedures in modern medicine rely extensively on equipment, often in large arrays and rarely transportable. For humanitarian doctors to operate in remote locales, they first had to learn to make their tools travel.

Over the decades following the Second World War, a global infrastructure emerged to respond to human suffering amid conflicts between superpower proxies. Even as weapons like the AK-47 proliferated, enlarging the terms of destruction for local and regional disputes, new technologies of care altered the terms of survival.[1] Sharing a common lineage with military and industrial logistics, this humanitarian apparatus derived from reconfiguration as much as innovation. Nonetheless, by the final years of the cold war it had coalesced enough to offer stable objects and routines designed for emergency settings. If hardly a remedy for the upheaval accompanying geopolitical contestation, the new humanitarian equipment did offer a means to temporary, piecemeal relief. It thus promised literal, as well as symbolic, sanitization.

The general arc of this history emerges through the story of MSF's own logistical epiphany: the group's discovery of preparedness in the form of the humanitarian "kit." A kit, of course, is a mobile repository of potentially useful implements. Varieties of it feature in the long history of military equipment as well as the toolboxes of craft production. Humble medical versions populate many corners of ordinary existence, the most familiar being small boxes labeled "first aid" and stored in anticipation of minor emergencies.[2] The humanitarian form expands on this theme, casting the problem of first aid on a global level. By prepackaging equipment and guidelines, MSF and its kin performed the miracle of standardization, reducing the time and expertise required to reproduce a generic response. The organization could thus translate its actions between settings more fluently while also accommodating turnover in personnel. Like emergency medicine in general, the kit has proven a remarkably powerful antidote for many urgent health problems. Other conditions, however, have remained beyond its reach and continue to suggest its limitations. When diseases prove chronic, when installations settle in place, when questions become more singular—in short, whenever problems slow down—the kit system loses its transcendent magic.

PRECURSORS AND PROTOTYPES

To understand the nature of the equipment MSF eventually set in place, it is help-
ful to return to two orienting moments: the recognition of a need for baseline
equipment and the normalization of emergency care in civilian life. Humanitarian logistics has many obvious lines of descent, from military supply lines to industrial food distribution, or, amid colonial encounters, the naval surgeon's chest.
Aerial warfare too has a long lineage, particularly in the colonies.[3] But the two
historical strands crossed emphatically during the Second World War. As large-
scale bombing entered military strategy, it produced a shattered landscape and
civilian casualties. Amid the rubble of European cities during the 1940s, the importance of portable medical infrastructure became critically visible. A key antecedent for MSF's later global kit thus appeared in the fading centers of empire
newly pulverized by bombers.

The degree of devastation in the Second World War presented the Red Cross
with a significant technical problem. Composed of a mosaic of national societies
as well as the Swiss-based ICRC, it had formed a Joint Relief Commission to better
coordinate its disparate efforts. This commission, however, soon found itself at a
loss in the face of massive aerial bombardments that left civilian populations in
urban centers medically bereft:

> "There is a total lack of medical supplies here." It was by a summary appeal of this
> kind that the Joint Relief Commission of the International Red Cross was asked in
> the beginning of its activities to send medical relief to a capital which had just un-
> dergone an air raid. Such a request, put so tersely, left us somewhat nonplussed.
> What should be sent? What medicaments would be required by a large city which
> had been devastated by an air attack? What quantity of each medicament would be
> required? No statistics were there to enlighten us, no document on the problem was
> available. We had to improvise.[4]

How best to provision a devastated landscape? Most urgently, what medications to provide after the destruction of health infrastructure? The commission
first surveyed the national Red Cross societies about the medical requirements of
their respective countries. The response was, however, "surprisingly diverse, one
might almost say, disconcerting." No simple uniform agreement could be found.
The commission quickly marshaled medical experience and science in an effort
to determine what was "absolutely indispensable to ensure medical care and to
meet the emergency needs of a population which has been deprived of food and
medical supplies."[5] Newly sensitized to local culture, the commission highlighted
the fact that both national preferences and therapeutics varied across the European continent. The Red Cross, then, needed a catalogue that would be simultaneously encompassing and precise, allowing for regional differences and yet conducive to medical and pharmacological accuracy.

The Joint Relief Commission took it upon itself to compose a model inventory of sorts, entitling the condensed Latin result the *Materia Medica Minimalis* (*MMM*). Suitably anchored in a classical language, the work subsequently appeared in French, German, and English editions. For a Europe embroiled in war, the legacy of Rome served as neutral ground as well as a convenient means of scientific expression.[6] Balancing this scholarly touch with quartermaster's eye for practical detail, the authors estimated quantities necessary to treat a "population unit" of 100,000 persons for six months. They based their figures on the consumption of medicaments in Switzerland, recognizing that these numbers might prove a controversial standard and require later alteration. The urgency of the situation, however, demanded calculation, however rough or temporary. Since "circumstances and difficulties" can affect delivery, they further divided the *MMM* into two categories of drugs, the first of which should receive priority. The list itself included only pharmaceuticals; bandages, cotton, and surgical instruments were to be handled in separate consignments. Nonetheless, its content lived up to its name, defining a minimalist baseline for medical infrastructure.

The *Materia Medica Minimalis* marks a catalytic moment in humanitarian thinking. Although the Red Cross had featured training activities and addressed medical techniques at some of its past international meetings, with the *MMM* it had produced something more: a mobile, self-supporting template. Crisis response could now involve a principle of flexible standardization and operate in a medical vacuum. The final report of the Joint Relief Commission, reflecting on its wartime invention, mused that this work, though "called into existence by the needs of the moment, possessed a usefulness which it seemed would outlast the war period."[7] The assessment would ultimately prove prophetic. Although the *MMM* itself never became an icon of relief work, its conceptual descendants proliferated in the following decades.[8] When later European humanitarians began to recognize crises beyond their own continent, they encountered what they would come to describe as "resource-poor settings." The provision of medical infrastructure emerged as a central problem in international health. In emergencies its absence grew acute. Effective assistance for all manner of disasters required basic medical materials and guidelines, preferably planned in advance. The global mobility of biomedicine depended on it.

The close of the Second World War ushered in a new geopolitical configuration, along with categories and institutions for its governance and through them new cadres of experts. Medicine likewise changed. In addition to new materials such as antibiotics, the mass mobilization of military experience offered training and templates for the reorganization of medical care. Like science, biomedicine grew increasingly "big" and technologically focused: the era of house calls gave way to that of hospitals.[9] Not all of these developments were novel or unanticipated. The longer development of emergency medicine depends on late-nineteenth-century

medical concepts of shock and trauma, the reorientation of care following accidents, and the catalytic effects of the First World War.[10] In terms of transport,
civilian ambulances owe an obvious debt to military medicine writ large. Other
figures, such as the traveling ship's surgeon and the missionary doctor, would also
surely feature in a more comprehensive story of medical mobility. But for the
generation that shaped MSF, the Second World War can serve to mark the critical threshold of a shifting medical approach as well as expectations. Once across
it, the field of emergency expanded in both material and conceptual terms.

One story about MSF's background merits particular mention. Between the
1950s and the 1970s, emergency medicine grew into a professional specialty, and
emergency care became a norm across developed medical settings.[11] In the French
context it took institutional shape through the establishment of a national service
known as the *service d'aide médicale urgente,* or SAMU, deploying teams of the
service mobile d'urgence et de réanimation, or SMUR. The SAMU system emphasized mobile intensive care units that could offer rapid treatment by doctors following an accident. As such it actually stayed true to the nominal ancestor of
the ambulance, the *hôpital ambulant* of the Napoleonic Wars (which functioned
something like a MASH unit), to a greater degree than did the American model
of paramedic transport to the emergency room. Here a doctor traveled—at speed—
to the patient, offering care directly in the field. Both at the conceptual level of
defining emergency and the technical level of providing delivery, the SAMU
system provided a model for MSF, as several of its key protagonists have duly
pointed out.[12] Through the deployment of mobile SAMU teams and equipment—
wailing down an improving road network—every citizen of France might increasingly expect expert care at a scene of distress. For French doctors training and
practicing in or after the late 1960s, this would become a normal part of their
professional vision. With the evolution of air travel into a routine form of rapid
transport, this vision realistically extended worldwide. Suffering, whether near or
far, could now elicit response.

THE NEED FOR AN APPARATUS

At the outset MSF existed largely on paper, hastily reaching the field by piggy-
backing on the interventions of others. By the end of its first decade, however, it
had begun to mount short interventions into areas afflicted by natural disasters
and war. From a humanitarian perspective its services were very much in demand. Even as the group found its collective calling, the geopolitics of the cold
war struggle shifted increasingly in the direction of proxy wars following the end
of U.S. involvement in Vietnam. Alongside the paralyzing shadow of nuclear
apocalypse during the 1970s and 1980s, irregular armies fought savagely in settings like Angola, Mozambique, and Afghanistan. These confrontations only

enhanced the international flow of conventional weaponry, fueling ancillary conflicts and alliances while prompting the displacement of civilian populations. The number of refugees worldwide grew exponentially during these decades, providing a surplus of humanitarian need well beyond the capacity of UN agencies. A nongovernmental group with a global vision thus had plenty of opportunity to offer medical assistance.

Three early episodes proved particularly formative for MSF's technical operations. First, and most fundamentally, the exodus of people from Vietnam and Cambodia under the Khmer Rouge set the ground for an ethics of action in refugee camps. Working on the border of Thailand, young MSF volunteers became radicalized through encounters with suffering rather than dreams of revolution. The refugee crisis soon emerged as a natural habitat for medical humanitarianism: massed populations in need of urgent, basic clinical care provided a ready stage for moral dramas of suffering. After the boat people episode prompted the schism within MSF, this younger generation took control and sought to expand the organization's technical focus and capacity. Rather than simply dispatching volunteers to a site of need, the new goal was to ensure that they could offer useful services once there. The camps of Southeast Asia provided a critical laboratory of sorts in this endeavor, as we will see shortly.

Next, the Soviet invasion of Afghanistan only further confirmed the French humanitarian rupture with state socialism. MSF undertook clandestine missions in the Afghan mountains, experiencing its own romance of Third World solidarity. The Afghan adventure marked an extreme in MSF's break with Red Cross discretion, as well as in its participation in cold war politics. The militant adventure also involved a striking degree of local adjustment; in contrast to later practice, mission volunteers immersed themselves in the populations with which they worked, living and traveling in the same manner. Transport involved the torturous navigation of mountain passes with pack animals, medicines carefully packed in small parcels. Teams were isolated and resupply difficult. In this case solidarity did not ultimately translate into political influence; the organization watched with dismay as its erstwhile partners pursued their respective power games, and the country disintegrated into civil war following the Soviet withdrawal.[13] Over time, MSF would throttle back on the romantic version of *sans frontiérisme*, emphasizing independence and operational efficacy instead.

Finally, during the mid-1980s famine in Ethiopia, the original French branch of MSF found itself evicted after denouncing the Derg regime's policy of forced resettlement. The episode, occurring amid the televised glamour of Live Aid, helped establish the group's outspoken reputation. At the same time, MSF faced attacks of its own as critics suggested that it was long on hot air but short on actual capacity.[14] The charges stung enough that MSF redoubled its efforts to improve its technical abilities and professionalism. By the end of the decade it had a new logistics system and an epidemiological subsidiary in place. Once the French section grudgingly accepted its newer European relatives as equal partners, the collective emerged as a truly multinational operation. Increasingly it would be known not only for flamboyance, but also for speed and efficiency.

The group's initial venture in Uganda, which occurred between the three episodes outlined above, illustrates the technical problems that prompted MSF's logistics revolution. The eventual setting of my flat tire was never a central front in the cold war; its postindependence turmoil and the rise and fall of Idi Amin had deep colonial and regional roots. Nonetheless, the Ugandan crisis occurred at a transitional moment in the evolution of humanitarian aid. It also holds the comparative advantage of falling outside of MSF's mythic self-narrative, combined with a detailed record of inefficiencies at the time.[15]

At the beginning of the 1980s, the Karamoja and West Nile regions of the country experienced extreme famine. The crisis in Karamoja, an arid area bordering Kenya and peopled largely by photogenic cattle herders with a fierce reputation, received a good deal of media attention. A number of aid agencies responded to images of starvation by rushing teams and materials into the field. Amid the volatile aftermath of the fall of Idi Amin, the general situation in Uganda was, in the words of a UNICEF official of the time, "at best chaotic," and the relief operation quickly encountered a host of problems. Subsequent analysis by a group of scholars and humanitarian workers identified a long list of specific setbacks as well as some general issues. Prominent among these were lack of coordination and turf struggles between different organizations (and even branches of the same organization), a landscape of need extending beyond the targeted recipients of aid, and a "disaster within the disaster" regarding food supply and distribution.[16]

A former representative of another UN agency observed that many of the people who were alongside her in Uganda had participated in major relief operations elsewhere over the previous decade. Their discussions revealed a repeated pattern of failure and identified a root cause: "One of the recurring themes was that time and time again the same problem arose in every disaster situation: logistics."[17] She imagined creating a "strike force" of reservists within the UN system, a cadre of experienced professionals with access to stockpiles of equipment, who could be ready to leave at a moment's notice. The UNICEF official similarly concluded that responses like this must be "quick, rational, and experienced" rather than "prolonged" or "irrational" but doubted that his own agency, created for long-term activities, would be suitable for the task: "To use a metaphor, such a rapid shift in activities and allocation would amount to demanding a shipping company to turn into an airline overnight."[18]

MSF joined the many organizations briefly present in both the Karamoja and West Nile. At the time it was not yet ten years old and still a relatively minor, if flamboyant, entity in the world of humanitarian affairs. The missions to Uganda were its first in a famine zone and did not prove a particular success. As a lead participant noted dryly in an interview with me, "In that era we improvised; later we'd become more efficient." A report written for the group's bulletin at the time summarized the situation with one graphic image: a bullet-ridden loader sitting useless, its brand new tires stolen by raiders to make sandals.[19] Only a decade, however, MSF had grown into a large and complex organization, fully capable of both technical innovation and logistical efficiency in crisis settings. The system it developed went a long way toward fulfilling the UN administrator's vision of a global humanitarian strike force.

THE GLOBAL KIT

The concept of the kit has a long military and medical lineage. The *Oxford English Dictionary* suggests that by the late eighteenth century the English term had expanded from meaning a wooden vessel or container to indicating the collection of articles in a soldier's bag. An equipment case or chest had long been the steady companion of ship surgeons and other mobile healers, and by the early twentieth century groups like the Red Cross assembled first aid kits. These were all-purpose collections that encompassed essential materials in a more modest version of the *MMM* list described above.

The humanitarian variant would be more comprehensive, recombinant, and ambitious: collections of supplies designed for a particular need and preassembled into a matrix of packages. The organization could then stockpile these packages and ship a relevant set rapidly to any emergency destination in the world. As the mature MSF logistics catalogue later summarized the conceptual approach it embodied: "A kit contains the whole of the needed equipment for filling a given function. Intended for emergency contexts, it is ready to be delivered within a very short time frame."[20] Thus the diffuse problem of acquisition was effectively translated into a concentrated one of transportation, which could be more easily solved from a central office. Essential materials no longer had to be hastily assembled anew in response to every crisis or uncertainly negotiated on the ground amid fluctuating availability, quality, and price. Moreover, by preassembling materials with a checklist, the kit could function as a form of materialized memory whereby previous experience extended directly into every new setting without having to be actively recalled. For an organization facing crisis settings with a constantly shifting workforce of volunteers and temporary employees, not all of them equipped with the same professional training, such continuity would prove especially valuable.

From the perspective of MSF, the kit system derived from a few early masterminds, now receding into organizational legend. Its immediate origin lay in the experience of a French pharmacist named Jacques Pinel, who was responsible for Cambodian refugee camps on the border of Thailand in 1980. Prior to that time MSF team members—usually part of a larger, often chaotic operation—had rotated responsibility for logistics; now that they were running their own independent mission they created a new category of supervisor positions.[21] Guerilla raids over the border led to periodic Vietnamese bombing runs, whereupon the Thai army would seal the camps, preventing access for several days at a time. In due course the MSF teams learned to assemble essential equipment until they had the process down to a system. As the main protagonist recalled in 2004, this evolved less from any grand design than the "banal" practice of packing a bag for a series of weekend trips and translating experience into anticipatory habit:

> The kit, it's nothing more than someone who's leaving for the weekend . . . who needs his backpack with something to drink, something to eat, something to put on his feet if they get sore. He needs all that. So, how does he do it? The first time he imagines what will happen, and assembles his bag with that imagination. And then after that first experience, he sees that there are things that didn't amount to much and others he was missing. And then after the second, third time, he'll finally have a perfect bundle and he prepares it before the weekend, checks it, and then leaves and it works.[22]

In its initial form the proto-kit was a relatively heavy box made by local carpenters, carried in the back of a pickup truck and hence nicknamed "semi-mobile equipment."[23] Built along the lines of the French SAMU emergency system, its originality stemmed less from its form or content than its adaptation to the setting in which it was deployed. Reworking a guide from the UN High Commission for Refugees and a nutritional package from Oxfam, MSF volunteers eventually assembled standard lists of medicine and supplies for a kit that could meet the needs of 10,000 people for three months, as well as instruction manuals for its use. The project of procedural simplification on site grew into one of standardization between locales. As Pinel would later recognize, the kit responded to the specific "ecology" of humanitarian emergency exemplified by the refugee camp, where a large number of people lived in temporary and often precarious conditions, receiving care from a shifting group of personnel, not all of whom were familiar with the setting or its diseases.[24]

Following this experience in Thailand, Pinel went on to coordinate MSF-France's new central logistics operation in 1982. Together with associates he began to apply the kit model to analogous situations elsewhere. The key principle lay in dismantling a problem (be it disease or disaster) in technical terms, identifying its critical potential components, and developing specific responses to each. For example, cholera is a common health concern for displaced people living in crowded conditions. Anticipating this problem, the MSF logistics team developed a general kit for the disease:

> We know that we are going to have a cholera epidemic there. OK, we get together people who have already worked on cholera, when we get there there's nothing of what we need to put in place for a cholera epidemic. So, we need a cholera camp, that is to say an isolation tent. . . . If there are thousands of people that's too many, so we'll create a unit to treat 500 patients. . . . What will be necessary? Some tents, OK, how many tents? OK, we'll need 100 50-square-meter tents. We'll have perfusions because we're going to give infusions and on average there are those [patients] who get 2–3 liters and then there are those who get up to 20 liters. So we'll say 10 liters on average, OK. Out of 500 patients there are how many who will receive 10 liters . . . OK, there will be 100. . . . When we finish planning, *voilà*, we have the kit. We try to really make this kit, in order to see how it is, how it fits into boxes, how much it weighs. We physically create this kit, and then we use it in the next cholera epidemic . . . and then [we do] an evaluation. And then we revise it. . . . That's how the kits advanced, succeeded, not so much because of the notion of the kit, which is really something supremely banal, but following many years where we imagined the kits and evaluated them in numerous situations. And then we divided the operations up like sausages, we cut, we sliced. That is to say, there's a cholera epidemic, a measles epidemic, put in place in a dispensary of a refugee camp. In doing all that, all the units like that, then when it's necessary to mount an operation we have all our equipment.[25]

Through this combination of organic practice and assembly line routine, MSF created a more global component variation of the Red Cross medical index. By the latter part of the 1980s the concept of the kit became central to the group's emergency work.

To gain a sense of the level of detail involved, let us briefly examine MSF's mature cholera kit, Kit 001. Although designed for refugee camps, with modifications it can adapt to either rural or urban displaced populations. Built on a unit of 625 treatments, it weighs in at just over 6,000 kilograms. Its contents include an array of medicines (e.g., 6,500 sachets of oral rehydration salts and 10,000 tablets of the broad spectrum antibiotic doxycycline) as well as materials for taking patient samples (e.g., dissecting forceps and a permanent black marker) and performing basic medical procedures (e.g., surgical gloves, tunics, trousers, and boots of several sizes; ten 500-gram rolls of cotton wool; twenty-five arm splints; and catheters and bandages galore). But the kit does not stop there; it also features support items, such as well over 100 buckets and 100 disposable razors, not to mention logistical articles like notebooks, pens, wire ties, and even two staplers. Simply put, the degree of anticipation contained within this collection of trunks and boxes would put most Boy Scouts to shame.[26]

MSF has matched its kit system with guidelines: short, informative instruction books and pamphlets detailing responses to practical problems. The group makes these available in English, French, and Spanish; some are also available in Russian and Arabic. The subject matter centers on clinical and engineering dilemmas volunteers might encounter in the field, such as how best to conduct minor surgery in a war zone or how to set up a simple water sanitation system. The guideline system acknowledges that even volunteers with established general expertise may possess inadequate technical background for unfamiliar conditions. Neither a nurse from Lille nor a logistician from Toronto, for example, is likely to have much training in combating cholera or building a pit latrine. The guides further seek to address audiences with different levels of knowledge, and in a concentrated way that obviates the need for larger libraries. Simple to copy or replace, in the pre-digital era their minimal form guarded against the potential hazard of disintegration that threatens expensive books in humid climates.[27]

Around the kits, MSF also developed its own mobile infrastructure. Once Pinel took over logistics for the group's operations in 1982, he realized that Thailand had been a relatively easy environment in which to operate. There the team had been able to acquire vehicles and drugs locally, and the phone system worked. Much of Africa, however, proved a different story, as its crisis zones generally lacked phone service, transport, and even basic drugs. Pinel and his associates created a radio communications network, standardized drug lists, and a vehicle pool. They restricted vehicle purchases to Toyota Land Cruisers, already deployed in many Red Cross and UN missions, both to simplify their parts list and to be able to use the workshops of these other organizations.[28] Simplification and standardization remained their watchwords. In 1986 MSF-France also established a main logistics center and depot in order to provide a standing reserve of equipment for emergency operations. One of several "satellite" organizations created around that time , the depot moved between locations in France before settling near the Bordeaux airport. From this base the logistics team could—political conditions permitting—quickly launch mission material toward any corner of the world via a chartered plane. The kits in the plane's cargo bay would then provide the vital organs of emergency response in adverse conditions: tools for setting up a camp, ensuring transport, and providing basic health care.[29]

Over time MSF's different operational sections have pursued slightly different logistics strategies. MSF-France, MSF-Switzerland, and MSF-Spain all use the central depot in Bordeaux, known as MSF-Logistique. MSF-Belgium maintains its own center in Brussels called MSF- Supply (formerly Transfer), founded in 1989. Both of these units also offer products to other organizations in the humanitarian market. Conversely, MSF-Holland has gone a more decentralized route; instead of sponsoring a proprietary logistics center, its procurement department relies on agreements with established outside suppliers. Nonetheless, the core logic of approach remains the same. All seek to ensure the availability of standardized materials on a flexible, rapid-response basis.

A similar logic extends beyond logistics to medical action. MSF not only established its own training programs and guideline series, but also produced publications for a broader professional audience, such as a guide to refugee health.[30] In concert with its epidemiological affiliate, Epicentre, the organization sponsored an in-house periodical entitled *Medical News* and encouraged staff to submit material to peer-reviewed publications. The goal was both to generate applicable knowledge and to foster a culture of exchange, transmitting technical innovations and standards across far-flung missions. The need was real. Describing a 1983 mission in Sudan, an MSF veteran recalled the challenge of adapting surgery to field settings. Trained for optimum operating conditions, they had to let go of "a certain disciplinary rigor that—though established for good reason in the operating room—was fairly incompatible with mission life."[31] Moreover, he recalled, it proved unexpectedly difficult to harmonize practices around a common standard. Coming from different training backgrounds, the surgeons had different habits, even at the level of suture thread. Although their overall practice might share a common approach with military surgery, the humanitarian form labored without the same disciplinary norms or resources. MSF also faced problems when it came to patient populations. Unlike wounded soldiers, civilians arrived in a wider range of shapes, conditions, and ages, from very young to very old.[32]

The kit system expanded throughout the organization to produce a set of relatively stable forms. Kits are now available for all manner of eventualities. The Toyota Land Cruiser, the workhorse vehicle for MSF and many other NGOs, comes as a kit. Standard modifications outfit it for either cold or warm climates, although, unlike other many other organizations, MSF proudly shuns air conditioning. Yet another box contains a collection of stickers and flags to mark the vehicles' affiliation. Members of a mission can order an Emergency Library Kit and request items from a field library list that includes such assorted titles as "How to Look After a Refrigerator," "Human Rights in a Nutshell," and "Blood Transfusion in Remote Areas."[33] Governing the overall design are principles of quality, efficiency, and simplicity of maintenance. In some domains a spirit of standardization dictates a particular brand of product (Toyota vehicles, for example); in others a desire for flexibility of procurement allows substitution of any generic equivalent (most articles are "open" rather than brand specific). Indeed, the sheer proliferation of kits and the flood of guides poses its own challenge for anyone new to the work. "The real problem now is where to find information," a logistician told me in Brussels. "It can be overwhelming for a person on the ground."

The group's kit assemblage reflects the increasingly technical orientation of the aid world. Partly derived from military and health planning, as well as the artifacts of other organizations, MSF's logistics system has in turn influenced the operation of the larger humanitarian enterprise. In 1988 the World Health Organization endorsed MSF's classic kit by adopting it as the "new emergency health kit."[34] During the Rwandan genocide, members of an ICRC surgical team were impressed by the speed with which a kit could be unpacked. Several former MSF logistics personnel eventually migrated to the Red Cross, which also adopted some of MSF's guidelines.[35] Unlike the WHO's slower efforts to glean knowledge from formal research, MSF's approach was emphatically operational in outlook and appealed directly to teams in the field. The cholera kit, for example, diverged from WHO's model in part because it incorporated the group's experiences in Malawi instead of relying on the findings of a research institute in Bangladesh, as WHO did. Since MSF was running emergency programs and had encountered higher rates of cholera than expected in its own epidemiological studies, the group emphasized treatment of acute cases and included more intravenous treatments relative to oral ones.[36] Early editions of MSF's guidelines invited users to copy them; consequently, borrowed elements circulated widely. MSF tacitly approved "borrowing" in general, favoring wider circulation over copyright protection. Some MSF guidelines even eventually appeared as part of WHO's growing repertoire. However unorthodox its initial approach may have been, MSF's journey to professional respectability now appeared complete.

VARIATION, ADJUSTMENT, AND LIMITS

The kit system has never operated in a vacuum. MSF also boasts a long tradition of improvisation and modification of designs to fit its needs. For logistics staff in one of MSF's central offices this primarily implies working to simplify systems and reduce their cost. Innovations include such items as insect netting on vehicle grilles to simplify maintenance and experiments to improve a portable system for mixing food used in nutritional therapy. As the logistics director of MSF-Belgium told me in 2003, "One of MSF's luxuries is that we have the means to do R & D. Many others don't, but we have both the will and the resources. . . . The market usually favors things that are expensive and use a lot of energy. We want to try and find things that are less so, for example [things that use] solar panels or a bike as an energy source." The drive for innovation inhabits field settings as well. At one project in Uganda a member of the team showed me a clever container for contaminated sharp instruments. Made out of simple PVC tubing, it could easily mate with the tube to a larger disposal dump, providing a quick, inexpensive solution to one problem of sanitation under adverse conditions. The device, I was told, owed its existence to an inspired logistician working in Thailand. Once its value was recognized, the idea circulated back through the network.

At local mission sites logistics personnel commonly tinker and improvise. Indeed, the classic image of the MSF "log" is emphatically that of the handyman *bricoleur,* deploying the means at hand to achieve a desired result.[37] Placed in charge of a wide range of equipment and often dealing with unreliable local conditions, the logistician must constantly negotiate to solve problems. In early years MSF's supply chain was intermittent and advice far away, meaning that one had to make do with imagination and the materials in inventory. If less pronounced in an era of improved communications, professional training, and ubiquitous guidelines, a capacity for improvisation remains essential to the position. As a logistics coordinator in Uganda told me emphatically in 2004: "Either you do the job or you don't do the job." He was referring to a temporary structure he once had to construct with logs and mud in the complete absence of recommended materials. The result did not conform to guidelines and was hardly pretty, but it functioned. What more, in the end, could one really ask of something temporary? Moreover, he had found the challenge personally rewarding. "Part of MSF is that people want to reinvent the wheel," he admitted. A completely standardized environment would "spoil the fun."[38]

A French logistics overseer—known as a "superlog"—suggested to me in 2001 that the real key to logistical success was being "someone who knows the difference between the possible and the impossible." He pointed out that the work really required less personal mastery than an ability to supervise. In many settings labor and even technical skill were readily available. "Throughout Africa," he observed, "there are people who can fix a fridge." The important thing was to be able to recognize who did good work and then to oversee it in a way that would achieve timely and reasonable results. One of his colleagues went even further, emphasizing the value of curiosity, since circumstances continually changed. "Situations are always different," he told me. "Even the same place a year later is different." Thus for all the merits of standardization, one should never adhere to it too strictly. Curiosity mattered even more for the most fundamental part of the work: understanding people. "Tools," he noted, "are not *always* useful." Indeed, in practice they could create problems as well as solve them. For example, a radio could prove a vital connection or an alienating distraction. Being glued to a handset might save your life, but it also distanced you from local surroundings and the information they contained. Warming to the theme, he described the overemphasis on technology and technical fixes as a spreading plague in the humanitarian world. He felt MSF increasingly relied too much on computers. "Do you really need one [when] dealing with the Dinka?" he wondered. Computers might be valuable for calculating budgets and writing reports for donors. Humanitarianism, however, confronted issues that exceeded software algorithms: "Ultimately the question is that some people decided some other people were not important. And that is not a technical problem."[39]

For all the value of the kit system, then, it also displayed limits and came with potential side effects. Not every development could be anticipated or every response preplanned. Once in the field, kits would be pulled apart, partially used, and reordered at a local level. The vast improvement in humanitarian equipment had produced greater efficiency and raised the measurable quality of care. That very success, however, might threaten to overshadow human relations and consequently the basic moral motivation itself.

A deeper challenge to the mobile constellation of kits came from locality itself. Once an MSF mission remained in situ for an extended period, it became increasingly subject to the greater gravity of place. Uganda again provides illustration of this point. Two decades after the initial fumbling forays there, several sections of MSF ran a variety of programs in the country. One of these was a workshop to maintain and repair vehicles.[40] Located in Kampala, the workshop owed its existence to Bernard, a taciturn and dedicated French logistician. Amid MSF's many short-lived interventions and ever-shifting personnel, Bernard nursed his garage as a longer-term venture. Knowing that each new head administrator would review existing projects, requiring justifications for their continued existence, he tried to keep one step ahead in assuring its value. Beyond servicing the vehicles of MSF–France and MSF–Switzerland in the country, the workshop also cared for some in less stable neighbors like Sudan and the Congo, where parts were unavailable, and undertook contract work for other NGOs.

Well equipped with standards, catalogues, and a computerized ordering system connecting it to MSF's logistics center, the workshop exemplified stabilized humanitarian infrastructure. At the same time, however, it remained under continual threat. This threat stemmed not only from turnover in MSF's fluid administration and the varying visions of its representatives, but also from the pressures of competing interests. Once trained, the local mechanics who labored at the workshop would often depart for better-paying positions. Even when on the job they did not always work with the humanitarian fervor the director expected. He did not blame them for this but found it complicated his role as a manager, leaving him poised somewhere between maintaining a moral cause and justifying a bottom line. The workshop regularly faced competition from commercial garages that threatened to undercut it. Bernard also struggled against the impatience of field personnel in project sites, who often wanted to circumvent central control and make purchases directly. "It's a constant battle," he acknowledged, especially since some parts could be found in local markets more cheaply, and the quality there was improving. Although a firm believer in the value of the kit system and the advantages of using standard, well-selected materials, Bernard emphasized that MSF's logistics network was really designed for emergency settings. A stable entity like the garage regularly interacted with the local economy, each small transaction pulling it away from the institutional orbit.

Efforts to address specific diseases and broader health inequities similarly altered MSF's technical circulatory system, exposing its limits in the process. As the organization took on a wider range of diseases, it also altered the logistical work of procurement. Pharmaceutical orders, once largely routine, grew more complex and harder to fill. An article published in 2005 in MSF-France's house journal *Messages* provides a summary of the shift:

> For many years medicines were considered "consumable operational tools" simply requiring a regular supply, like . . . spare parts for a Toyota. Medicines arrived from MSF Logistics, who bought the generics from producers based in the North. Very few questioned the quality issue, and national authorities allowed these importations, especially for refugee programs which made up the majority of our programs at the time. Drug management in these programs was facilitated by the fact that we treated a limited number of pathologies using standard protocols that called for essential medicines that were often old, well-known, and inexpensive. In just a few years all this changed: the arrival of new diseases such as AIDS, resistance to usual medicines, markets opening, deregulation, patents, counterfeit medicines, artificially elevated prices of recent products, the stop of production of less profitable drugs and of applied research into tropical diseases. The Campaign for Access to Essential Medicines was born, and an international coordination of pharmacists was created.[41]

The head of MSF Holland's logistics team took a more apocalyptic view of this turn of affairs. "The old system is crumbling," he told me grimly in 2002. "Bulk orders are growing versus kits. If more than 40 percent of the content isn't useful then why not order more tailor-made assemblies of goods?" Pharmaceutical products, he said, were his biggest headache. Drug companies, even generic producers like Cipla, cared about market penetration, not humanitarian issues. "That's a big factor. The PR desks of companies want to be on the good side of public prices. We find out that the guys in sales, in production, don't know what's going on, however. . . . The basic logic is simple, but the application complicated."

In the event his dire assessment proved premature, MSF continued to send kits and found ways to move drugs. Nonetheless, the problem of drug procurement involved legal issues as well, and heightened customs regimes slowed border crossings. Two years later, at the logistics center in Bordeaux, an employee in charge of drug orders reflected on the changing nature of his job: "Traditionally—that is, five to seven years ago—it was quite easy to send things, just a matter of connecting MSF and the local government. Now there are more and more additional entities, agencies, protocols, etc. This is especially true with the medical end of supplies; there are more links now between different actors. It's not an issue of transport, but the administration of supply. All a question of having the right documents and timing them so it works."

He noted that during an emergency, bureaucratic oversight was usually "very light," both on the part of local governments and within the organization itself. Since the focus was on speed they would just send a kit. For regular program orders, however, they would go item by item. For materials like psychotropic drugs, they now needed to complete an order form for the French health ministry. It thus was not possible to "just make a kit."

The specificity of a disease also holds implications for logistics. The recent rise of state concern over "biosecurity" has amplified interest in outbreak diseases.[42] Although frequently caustic about the inflated fears surrounding emerging diseases, MSF actively participates in responding to them. When Ebola surfaced in Uganda in 2000, MSF specialists joined with counterparts from international and local agencies to combat it. If a relatively small part of the group's activity, these efforts and the wide publicity surrounding them contribute to the organization's medical reputation.[43] Moreover, such threats of a sudden outbreak fit readily into the kit system. MSF's logistics catalogue now includes a kit for Ebola (also deployed for the Marburg virus in Angola in 2005), and it developed a SARS kit based on its experiences in Vietnam in 2003.

Diseases that operate on a slower timeline, however, rupture the bubble of emergency response. In so doing they bring the kit system back to the ground, exposing the limits of its capacity to remain disconnected. Consider two brief, complicating snapshots from Uganda. In December of 2004, I visited a cholera treatment center MSF-Switzerland had opened near a displacement camp in the north of the country. The enclosure, with its wooden palisade, resembled a small fortress, and a large flag with the organization's logo flew just outside. Access to the area was strictly controlled, and upon entry and exit each and every person had to pass through a disinfection station. Inside the enclosure, several large tents sheltered patients lying on beds, as well as their attendants, plenty of clean water, chlorine, and simple medications. The cholera outbreak was subsiding, and few actual cases now appeared amid new arrivals with diarrhea. Soon MSF would move its equipment and redeploy it to other ends. The camp itself remained overcrowded with both residents and aid workers. Although the organization had sponsored a few short-term improvements to hygiene and the water supply, it would not attempt to address the deeper problems, particularly in a setting with many other aid actors. At a nearby health center a Ugandan doctor presented the results of a modest statistical study he had just conducted on the outbreak. Out of several hundred cases only eight had resulted in death, he reported happily, ascribing this success to the rapidity of MSF's response. The organization's cholera coordinator agreed readily, noting that here a rapid, preventative response had worked. He also added drily, however, that MSF had not worried about cost. Since this was an emergency, the organization hadn't asked him to calculate or justify expenses beyond ordering the requisite kits. Poverty might remain beyond his reach, but cholera, so to speak, could come and go in a box.

Earlier that year I had made a return visit to the French AIDS project further to the northwest. Part of MSF's ambitious wave of antiretroviral projects at the turn of the millennium, it sought to demonstrate the feasibility of treating poor people in poor places. In this sense the AIDS program represented something of a meta-kit: by combining experience from multiple locations, MSF could create a mobile set of treatment protocols, less dependent on full-scale laboratory support and adapted to shifting personnel. No one project would be open to the charge of representing an anomaly, since the larger chain was clearly replicable. In another sense, however, the AIDS program rapidly revealed the limits of the kit approach. MSF initially committed to five years of treatment. The therapy provided, however, would need to last a lifetime, since the drugs produced temporary remission rather than a cure. MSF's approach depended heavily on imported materials, personnel, and funding, none easily substitutable in a provincial town. As I detail in a later chapter, team members at the Ugandan end of the project worried about these issues even as they worked frenetically to expand patient rolls in the face of tremendous demand. The translation of treatment from rich to poor countries could not alter the economic imbalance between the two contexts. That particular crisis simply exceeded the boundaries of a shipping container.

MSF's logistics system, then, achieves only a partial and temporary state of universal mobility. Nonetheless, the guides serve as "mini Bibles of practical spirit," in the apt phrase of an epidemiologist in Uganda. "When faced with cholera," he summarized cheerfully, "just wash everything in chlorine and it works fantastically well." If not a universal solution, this procedure provided an expansive point of reference. The kits have proven similarly resilient. Even when emptied and enjoying an unplanned afterlife—such as the bench I once sat on in northern Uganda—their battered modules testify to the enduring scope of this network.

MOBILE MEDICINE

What then to say about MSF's logistical creation relative to its ethic of valuing life? First and foremost, the kit system represents a self-consciously *global* system, in the sense of being mobile and adaptable worldwide. While flexible in application, the result is not at all fluid in terms of community involvement.[44] Indeed, the kit system is the exact opposite of local knowledge in the traditional sense of geographic and cultural specificity in place. Rather, it represents a mobile, transitional variety of limited intervention, modifying and partially reconstructing a local environment around specific artifacts and a set script. In practice it may require considerable negotiation to implement, necessitating the cajoling of both patients and instruments to perform their proper roles. But its very concept strives to streamline that potential negotiation through provisions that reconstitute a minimal operating environment. The cold chain system used in vaccine distribution serves as a useful general analog in this regard. Just as refrigeration extends the essential environment of a vaccine alongside the vaccine itself, the kit system extends the operating environment of biomedicine into a landscape of need. To insure reliability and quality, MSF is willing to ship almost anything anywhere during an emergency.

Deeply invested in a practical logic of standards, the kit system reflects something of Bruno Latour's analysis of circulating inscriptions as "immutable mobiles."[45] MSF's constellation of guidelines and toolkits collects and distills specific clinical knowledge into a portable map of frontline medicine. Developed and refined through practice, its many elements connect one outbreak or crisis to another. In this sense the cholera epidemic in Thailand travels to stabilize the cholera epidemic in the Congo. Together, in a vast chain, the assembled kits standardize disaster by responding to it. Such a characterization reveals the degree to which biomedical knowledge and practice depend on infrastructure and the background work necessary to translate treatment into a new setting. MSF's classic emergency formation generated a "culture of standardization" (as one logistician proudly put it to me) in which speed and control were paramount. Beyond obvious incompatibilities, local concerns could emerge later. During the emergency they would be held at arm's length or bypassed to the degree possible.

The kit system did not stem from corporate or state need but rather from moral imperative coupled with medical judgment. To be sure, standardization has a long history in military and business settings. Here the critical rationale, however, derives from valuing human life over profit or political strategy. The kits respond to emergency settings: conditions of apparent rupture in which the instrumental goal is temporary stabilization. Standardization is thus never an end unto itself, nor part of a conscious effort to reshape or capture economic terrain. Humanitarian planning of this sort remains attenuated by its very mobility. Beyond emergency settings, MSF missions reenter a larger world of exchange and circulation. Once there, the regime of standardization melts away.

At times the kit can appear as a constraint, the organization's self-created barrier to creativity. A humanitarian affairs officer with MSF-Holland described the general dilemma this way to me in 2006: "The kit made us good specialists in a closed camp setting. . . . We just don't seem to know what to do with open settings. Whether urban Rio or Chad, when we have low density and widely dispersed populations we have more problems. What I see is an institutionalization of closed settings. . . . We're used to thinking we have to have a kit to act."[46]

A pointed blog posting for MSF-France's research arm in 2009 related a caustic anecdote from field experience in which a triumphant headline about the donation of "60 metric tons of essential drugs" from a UN agency translated into just one meager and hastily delivered box on the ground. The Congolese aid workers who unpacked it found themselves mystified by the language of its instructions and determined that its contents conformed to outdated protocols. The post's author queried the bureaucratizing force of what he termed "kit culture," noting that "in Congo as well as many other places, the kit has become more than a tool, it is increasingly the embodiment of *the* humanitarian gesture itself, as if dropping a kit constitutes the raison d'être of humanitarian interventions." UN agencies, he added meaningfully in conclusion, were hardly alone in this regard.[47]

Discussing MSF's kit system with me in 2003, Rony Brauman described it as "an apparatus in Foucault's sense" as well as "a logic for action."[48] Widely read and resolutely critical, the former president of MSF-France attributed a degree of strategic coherence to the organization's material engagement, however contingent its origins and practice. Its goal, as he reiterated at the end of the 2006 documentary film *L'aventure MSF,* was not to transform the world but simply to assist people in moments of distress so that they might be alive for any future reconstruction. For this end the kit system has proved an admirable asset, at least for certain conditions. Yet how does this small action, not to mention the broader "kit culture" of humanitarianism, fit into a larger ethical and political calculus?

Over the final decades of the twentieth century, humanitarian operations became a normative part of international affairs. At the same time, personnel involved in aid projects professionalized, following career trajectories spanning multiple agencies as well as formal degree programs at universities and specialized institutes.[49] With the circulation of personnel and ideas, practices and technologies standardized. The result was a limited and temporary infrastructure, highly mobile and concentrated on immediate needs. Amid the debris of decolonization and superpower struggles, humanitarians devised a means for crisis response, one that proved simultaneously effective and ephemeral. The essence of modular mobility, the kit is ultimately an open container for a closed world. Like humanitarianism itself, it remains available for appropriation into a wide range of projects related to health and issues well beyond.[50]

The establishment of a fast and efficient logistics system for humanitarian action changed everything and nothing at all. Particular lives can now be spared, at least in the short run, from certain forms of distress. The situations that imperil them, however, too often find return rather than resolution. Given the degree to which the demographics of suffering usually outweigh any response, it would be a gross misnomer to call the greater humanitarian apparatus anything like a "solution" to global states of disaster. Like the simple bracelet used in nutritional assessment, MSF's assemblage of tools register human agony by trying to alleviate it. In this sense humanitarian kit culture represents nothing more—or less—than a "Bracelet of Life" for a suffering planet.

FOLLOWING THE MONEY

MSF's mobility is not simply a matter of technical capacity, but also the result of business acumen. At a practical level the question of funding remains unavoidable for any operational endeavor. Given that moving people and things around the globe costs money—particularly if done quickly—medical humanitarianism requires a substantial source of revenue. Longer-term projects might offer the relative benefits of local sourcing, but at the price of continuing commitment and obligation. Even a "corporation not structured around capitalism" (as one veteran put it in Brussels in 2001) has to have something of a business plan, must maintain accounting books and keep a close eye on them. Moreover, as an aid fundraiser observed to me early in my research, the humanitarian enterprise remains ever precarious. Since its dominant financial idiom is the gift, not commerce, it depends on generosity rather than self-interest. Donors can easily lose patience or change their minds.

By the standards of nonprofits, MSF has proved remarkably successful; in just four decades it has established a high profile and grown comparatively rich. Furthermore, it managed to achieve this status largely through swaying individual members of the public rather than depending on states or foundations. Unlike many "nongovernmental organizations" it receives relatively little government funding, focusing instead on amassing personal donations large and small. Consequently it stands relatively free from the dictates of institutions. The focus on public support constitutes a point of pride for the organization, which sees it as permitting a degree of independence from powerful interests. However, the considerable funds that flow through its financial statements are never completely "free." Once coaxed from donor pockets, resources require shepherding. Is the money "well spent"? What about waste or corruption? Receiving and giving entail obligations along a greater chain. MSF must guard its public profile, attending to the sensibilities and expectations of those who contribute to its cause. In this sense money constitutes an intensely moral matter, not simply a profane necessity. The movement of funds across borders fuels the aid world but also generates deep anxieties. When tied to mobility, even independence carries burdens as well as opportunities.

MSF's international expansion was only partly haphazard. The development of partner sections also reflected strategic planning tied to fundraising as well as the recruitment of skilled volunteers. Whereas the tumultuous period of the 1980s produced a handful of loosely associated rival sections, the following decade saw a period of more pragmatic consolidation and expansion. This produced a dependency between the older "operational" cores and their newer, peripheral "partner" subsidiaries. The economic relation between the two resembled the classic dyad of empire, in the sense that resources flowed from colonies to metropolitan centers. Partner sections in the United States and Japan fed Paris, for example, whereas those in Canada and Germany sent their tribute to Amsterdam. As these outposts expanded they grew restive, however, and expected a larger say in how MSF conducted its work. By the time of my research, an initiative to devolve more authority, including some mission oversight, to these junior partners was well under way.

At the same time the organization fretted about its own phenomenal growth, fearing that it was becoming less medical and field-oriented.[51] Mindful of the significance of Islam and concerned about relations between global north and south, it also hoped to direct future growth toward parts of the world where it was less well known or had only maintained a field presence.

The fundamental logic of MSF's network, however, reflected the humanitarian financial circulatory system: money flowed from rich arteries toward poorer veins, powered by a sensitive and sometimes fickle heart. From this point of view, a middle-income country like Brazil or South Africa offered donor possibilities that a poor state like Chad or even Uganda simply did not. The United States proved a particularly lucrative claim. Securing an office there helped the farsighted French section wean itself from state support and UN contracts relatively early, and then advocate that its European neighbors do the same. Although not all American funds went to Paris, enough did to provide a good 40 percent of the French budget in 2003.[52] As its income increased, the organization naturally underwrote more expenditures, which in turn raised fundraising expectations for the following year. Given the vast expanse of human need, all pressures were inflationary.

The French section also displayed a flair for domestic publicity and fundraising, beginning with the ad campaign that defined its profile in the 1970s. It continued to experiment and tinker. After realizing that the average donation hovered near 300 francs, it launched a campaign encouraging donors to contribute "a franc per day," adjusted after currency conversion to "a euro per week." This campaign had proved a veritable gold mine, the French director of fundraising assured me in 2003, both increasing the donors' sense of involvement and costing less money to run. By the time of our conversation the organization analyzed giving carefully, noting patterns and seeking to tailor particular appeals (for example, sending fewer solicitations to someone who regularly gave only once a year). Even as its donor base expanded, MSF annually lost around 3 percent of its previous supporters, either due to financial constraints or disenchantment. As the director noted cheerfully, an organization that embraced controversy had "lots of opportunities to piss people off." The same group that once delighted conservatives by denouncing the cold war excesses of socialist regimes, for example, now criticized pharmaceutical companies and the American war on terror. MSF's calls for a Rwanda inquiry had angered some contributors, and every time the Palestinian question came up it regularly infuriated others. The vast majority of donors, however, stayed remarkably loyal, year in and year out. Whereas humanitarianism in general might suffer from a growing atmosphere of competition, overkill, and scandal, MSF still appeared professional and trustworthy. One could give to them with a clear conscience.[53]

For all this consistent popular support, the funds the group receives still carry a heightened expectation of virtue. Unlike some forms of religious donation, giving here involves a direct sense of contractual return.[54] Watchwords like *transparency* and *accountability* reflect the general assumption within contemporary philanthropy that donors have a continuing interest in their contribution—like investors—along with a right to know how it is used. Donation involves not merely an act but a relationship, one that the organization hopes will continue in an aura of trust and good feeling. Although the donation might not produce profit in an economic sense, it does presume a continuing sense of propriety and ownership. A recipient should avoid actions that might reflect badly on a donor.

The donation page of MSF-USA's website makes this amply clear by outlining the organization's "commitment to our supporters."[55] After thanking contributors for their gift, it offers extensive assurances of "how MSF uses your donations to reach people in need in the most effective and cost-efficient manner, while adhering to stringent fundraising ethics." The group spends judiciously and transparently, making every effort to comply with donor wishes. Contributors can expect to receive news from the field and are welcome to make inquiries. Should a program close or funds exceed need, the organization consults with donors of restricted contributions. MSF seeks to ensure that funds serve real needs and reach their targeted recipients by making its own operational assessments and managing its programs directly. Furthermore, staff demonstrate restraint by receiving modest salaries (the largest not to exceed three times the lowest) and making careful expenditures. The vast bulk of donor contributions can thus travel to the field as a pure gift, unsullied by personal, state, or corporate interests.[56]

Moving money, however, exposes these virtuous ideals to the pressures of circulation. This is particularly true across borders as the easy clicks of a donation web page translate into the sluggish terrain of the field. In settings where most transactions now occur electronically, one forgets that physical currency carries its own material weight. This realization becomes less avoidable, however, when dispersing funds for missions that operate in a financial void. During the initial years of Musevini's government, for example, the absence of banks in Uganda forced aid groups to manage their own chains of distribution. One veteran of the period recalled how MSF volunteers used to arrive with bills stuffed into their pockets; between the small denominations in circulation and the high rates of inflation, he found himself responsible for 70 kilograms of paper money to pay staff salaries. Even in less extreme circumstances, money casts shadows of mistrust and temptation. Where material resources are scarce, their presence becomes sharply visible, like an oasis in a desert.

For most aid organizations, national governments appear as prime suspects for theft and corruption.[57] This anxiety stems partly from the crystalized residue of anecdote and historical experience, as well as ideological faith in market rather than state forms. But it also derives from stories and expectations circulating within mission sites themselves. In settings where promised salaries and materials arrive only sporadically, people readily speculate about where they may have gone. The fact that someone—say, a government minister—builds a remarkably large house makes for lively gossip. In settings where both unemployment and kin obligations run high, it is not surprising that people make demands on anyone with a job. Given the stark inequalities of daily life and periodic examples of larger injustice, the moral certainty that MSF and its contributors attach to donations can falter in translation. How to identify a partner in virtue? How much should one person benefit while another does not?

To follow a donation from solicitation to use, then, reveals an ethical maze rather than a straight line. When one of MSF's fundraising brochures suggests that a modest $35 contribution will provide "all the medical and logistical supplies to supply forty people a day with clean water," it collapses the considerable gap between monetary equivalence and actual drinking.[58] Ensuring that forty people do enjoy a day of water requires movement, work, and continual negotiation. The point is not to discredit fundraising rhetoric or even a commitment to fiscal transparency. Rather, it is to highlight the moral anxieties attending humanitarian funds as they flow through the world. One memorable story I heard involved an unnamed Dutch aid worker who loudly proclaimed to national staff in Sudan, "This money is from my grandmother!" Simultaneously self-righteous and plaintive, the line reflects the moral investment carried by personal donations. Although the story presents an example of egregious behavior, it also exposes a core tension within nonprofit work. The shock expressed by some volunteers that government staff at the hospital where they worked might be selling medicines or running another business during working hours reflects more than an individual loss of innocence. It also reveals the greater amnesia that permitted such innocence to exist in the first place. As an MSF veteran once commented to me dryly in Amsterdam in 2002, "The luxury of the Western world is not having to consider moral dilemmas with even the smallest actions." Circulating money unsettles things, including the purity of humanitarianism.

THE PRICE OF INDEPENDENCE

Private donations represent a significant source of independence for MSF, freeing it from the potentially compromising control and funding cycles of institutional donors. Like the kit system, fundraising undergirds the group's capacity to act and mount operations worldwide. As the American donor website notes, by controlling its funds the group can define its own mission, choosing where to intervene "on medical needs alone." It can operate worldwide, quickly and with minimal constraints. It can even decline funding it finds inappropriate. And it can innovate, taking up a new challenge like AIDS without waiting for others. A buffer of six months' reserve provides some insurance against downturns or unexpected costs. Beyond that the organization promises to pour any excess into its field programs, "expanding the reach of its programs in the years to come." For MSF, independence is a vital ethical principle, one that allows it to claim humanitarian integrity.

Nonetheless, this revenue stream exerts its own tidal forces, fluctuating dramatically according to publicity and the emotive power of crises. In general, major natural disasters produce the greatest waves of charitable donations, as their graphic visuals obviate the need for advocacy or advertising. By contrast, longer-term campaigns targeting specific diseases or health inequities at a structural level—the very sort of thing that private funding has permitted MSF to address—require substantial investments of time, money, and image-making. They also yield relatively less in the way of income, not to mention the possibility of tidy closure. Individual donors prefer to give "spontaneously" rather than in response to solicitation and respond better to tangible stories than statistics.[59] They have expectations, not only regarding how their money might be spent, but also about what the organization should be doing. Whenever a crisis fills the news, they assume humanitarian organizations will be there. "It's great to be financially independent," a member of MSF-Holland told me in 2002, "but it's still public money. They expect us to be in Afghanistan, Kosovo, and so on." She went on to outline the problems of trying to work in high-profile settings while also calling attention to less publicized disasters.

The most dramatic example of sudden largesse came with the Indian Ocean earthquake and tsunami at the end of 2004. In response to appeals for help, money simply poured into charitable coffers—over $3 billion in the United States alone.[60] Commentary on tsunami giving has noted several factors propelling this astonishing swell of humanitarian contributions. Not only was the event a dramatic natural disaster whose victims appeared innocent of any wrongdoing, but it affected scenic areas involved in international tourism. Furthermore, the tsunami occurred at a high point on the religious calendars of wealthy Christian nations, amid a holiday identified with gift exchange. Thanks to both professional and amateur fundraising, giving opportunities rapidly proliferated through commercial contexts. In a surprisingly short space of time, tsunami relief defined the very impulse of philanthropy and consequently the currency of humanitarianism.

On New Year's Eve, MSF announced that it would no longer accept donations earmarked for the tsunami. Coming a mere week after the event itself and at a moment of heightened public concern and record fundraising, the group's statement took both the professional aid community and members of the contributing public by surprise. The moral moment seemed to demand the generosity of contribution and self-sacrifice. However, MSF had already far exceeded its fundraising goals and foresaw only a limited role for its medical expertise in this catastrophe, which produced considerable death, destruction, and suffering but relatively little disease. The organization asked contributors to redirect donations else-where, otherwise offering to return the money.

MSF's decision to halt its fundraising provoked considerable criticism from many quarters and confused some of its own contributors. How could a humanitarian organization refuse donations for a worthy cause? Others, however, were impressed by what they took to be the organization's renewed commitment to its moral authenticity. After all, MSF had long embraced controversy in the name of a greater good, and part of its stature derived from appearing rigorously virtuous.[61] Indeed, a marketing analyst might point out that MSF's public refusal to fundraise in this case furthered the group's iconoclastic reputation—its brand profile—and in that sense could ultimately appear strategic. The director of MSF-USA at the time assured me that the decision actually was easy for the organization, and the budget hardly suffered. Nonetheless the episode illustrates the two-edged nature of media exposure: what was vital for fundraising could constrain independence as well as permit it. To determine its own course, MSF had to swim against the tide.

Its commitment to supporters notwithstanding, MSF has generally resisted efforts to create standard codes of humanitarian practice. It remains wary about such trends, fearing that they might suffocate operations and curtail independence. Still, increased expectations about oversight and auditing have seeped in along with rising donations. Balancing the expectations of fiscal oversight against the imperative to spend funds can prove a challenge. As a member of MSF-Belgium told me in 2003:

> Last year we had little margin for initiative; the focus was all on reviewing programs at headquarters. . . . The problem was that at end of the year we spent less money! This is a problem because we're supposed to spend the money we're given, not put it in the bank. So for the last three months we have been told, please, if any you have any idea, then go for it. This whole situation is clearly a consequence of increased management. Before we had less than model management. But if you don't leave a certain space for freedom, you're always under expectations. Now we're back to a Maoist "let a hundred flowers bloom."

Certain figures have grown crucial, however, amid the flowers. In each budget MSF must demonstrate its commitment to field projects, aiming to exceed the 80 percent allocation level that has become a nonprofit gold standard.[62] If it is launching new advocacy programs or publishing materials about an issue, it needs to frame these endeavors as part of its greater "social mission." It also cannot build up a large reserve without raising questions. Every program needs to demonstrate its value and report something that might count as an outcome, however difficult "success" might prove in humanitarian settings. Like bureaucratic order, management has become a norm, even without institutional mandates.

The group also faces constraints in its public appeals. Although a number of staff told me they cringed at fundraising imagery—dewy-eyed, nameless children in particular—such faces continue to loom on publicity posters and travel through the mail. Whatever ethical qualms they might raise, these images seem to work.[63] To afford its treasured independence, then, MSF must conform to aesthetic expectations. It also faces the limit of its own self-image: a group known as Doctors Without Borders can hardly stop traveling or reacting to crises worldwide. Its system rests on a steady stream of volunteers circulating from project to project, participating directly in medical work and reporting on their experiences. To depend on partner organizations—let alone states—would disrupt this vision and its ethical claims. Morality here derives from immediacy, and hence continued mobility.

All aid groups face financial pressures and limitations, and MSF is no exception. The scale of the problems it confronts far surpasses its reach and would do so even if it were stretched less thinly around the globe. Humanitarianism lacks an internal principle of limitation and thus poses inflationary demands. Just as people can never be too healthy or too secure, from a humanitarian perspective they can never survive too long or suffer too little.[64] Nonetheless, by virtue of its relative success in building and funding an infrastructure for intervention, MSF has the wherewithal to do something when facing crisis. In contrast to most other aid organizations it does not have to contact partners, submit proposals, or wait for donors. This comparative capacity to act presents its own ethical challenge: the decision of where and how to deploy. Yet this choice is never quite free and the organization soon confronts its limits and inability to achieve resolution. In effect, MSF determines the course of its own continuing frustration. It should thus come as no surprise that the group embraces discontent and periodically expresses outrage.

4

Moral Witness

My duty is to speak out; I do not wish to be complicit.
EMILE ZOLA, "J'ACCUSE . . . !" 1898

WITNESSING DISASTER

A Spanish doctor once told me a different story about MSF's Nobel Peace Prize. Some members of the group, he said, had fantasized about using the prize money to sue the UN Security Council for failing to intervene in the Rwandan genocide. He had been working in the region at the time, and the prospect of such an action clearly resonated deeply. Nearly a decade after the events, passion still flickered in his eyes recalling the moment, and his voice constricted when referencing the country. Aid organizations had inadvertently turned civilians into bait there, a horror that would live with him forever. "In Spain people didn't die because of me," he remarked bitterly. Later, over a dinner, he confessed that he sometimes thought of entering forensics, a specialty where death marked a beginning rather than an end.

No doubt such a lawsuit would have proved a satisfying, cathartic moment for others as well. However unlikely or unreasonable in legal terms, what a defiant gesture for justice! It recalled a defining moment in the European history of public intellectuals: Emile Zola's famous "J'accuse" letter regarding the Dreyfus affair, wherein the author publicly indicted the French establishment for its anti-Semitism. In an otherwise unjust world, surely the only moral position would be to speak truth to power. Even if Zola had to flee to England, he appeared on the right side of history when Dreyfus was at last exonerated. The fantasy lawsuit would have fully embodied MSF's conceit of practicing "rebellious humanitarianism." After all, the group had come to define itself partly through its willingness to speak out, its defiance of Red Cross discretion. During the genocide MSF had frantically issued public statement upon statement, even while its remaining

98

members in Rwanda worked desperately under the Red Cross flag. Given the hapless impotence of medical action, a legal protest on behalf of those slaughtered could appear relatively effective, if only as commemoration.

The organization's actual choice for the allocation of those funds, however, illustrates the degree to which it increasingly valued expert knowledge alongside humanitarian sentiment. By designating its fledgling drug-access campaign as the recipient, MSF pushed its public presence in novel if less dramatic directions. The focus on medical materials brought new actors into view: corporations as well as states, international trade treaties, and pharmaceutical laboratories. It likewise stretched the group's timeline beyond the mercurial humanitarian present, introducing the slower rhythms of scientific research and policy negotiations. Although widely supported by most people I met in the organization, the initiative also created unease. Addressing structural inequities in health care shifted the focus away from the clinic and toward public health. To embark on such an advocacy venture required developing new forms of expertise, which some worried might gradually undermine MSF's attachment to the field. It also entailed a heightened degree of collaboration, which might threaten the group's fierce tradition of independence.

This moment of contrast between the fantasy lawsuit and the actual campaign— one suffused with raw human emotion, the other with professional distance— captures an essential tension in MSF's endeavors. What to do beyond clinical work, particularly when facing an impasse or obvious failure? The group's general answer had been to practice *témoignage,* or witnessing. By the 1990s this French term appeared across MSF's polyglot sections to designate a loose and shifting array of advocacy efforts, including public speech. It had become a maxim for the organization that while words might not always save lives, "silence can certainly kill."[1] The degree to which witnessing involved expertise above and beyond a good heart, however, was less clear. MSF tended to stick close to its areas of medical specialization and to derive its knowledge from its field operations. But did one need to marshal more specific, technical knowledge to make an effective case? Or was witnessing fundamentally a matter of human solidarity, the simple expression of the most basic sense of humanity?

Following such questions helps to place MSF's particular trajectory in a longer arc of claiming public speech. It also reveals the ambivalent position of medicine between ethics and politics, as well as the growing weight of expertise. Collective actors like NGOs now commonly play a significant role in fashioning moral discourse, seeking headlines in the manner of public intellectuals. They do so, however, armed not only with a passionate appeal for justice—a "cry of the soul," as Zola put it—but also an array of reports, often remarkably dry and marshaling the results of studies they themselves conducted. MSF's defense of life and dignity takes shape in specific facts as well as general truths. It alternately produces heart-rending narratives of suffering and dispassionate arrays of statistical analysis. Recognizing such claims to knowledge requires a heterogeneous category in which passion and dispassion intermingle. Here I refer to MSF's wider testimonial tradition as a genre of "motivated truth."[2] With regard to humanitarian concerns the figure of the doctor occupies a privileged place, positioned not simply as humane but also expert in matters of suffering.

DISCOVERING *TÉMOIGNAGE*

When asserting itself as a moral witness, MSF could draw on a French Enlightenment tradition stretching back to Voltaire. Moreover, the "duty to speak out"—as Zola had put it—hardly ended with the Dreyfus affair but reverberated on through the twentieth century. The French experience of the Second World War in particular shadowed later events. Like the question of Dreyfus's innocence, resistance to Nazi rule served as a litmus test of character, revealed in speech and actions. Truth had a moral and political edge. The cold-war period amplified the Revolutionary legacy of political left and right and complicated it when French colonialism entered a bloody endgame in Vietnam and Algeria. In such a context, intellectual heroism could be personified by more than one literary figure. Two iconic authors, sharing a common root in the Leftist tradition and opposition to Fascism, provide a useful contrast. Jean-Paul Sartre enthusiastically sparred with conservative counterparts, trumpeting truth in the form of direct political resistance and opposition to colonial rule. Albert Camus, a lonelier thinker compromised by his connection to Algeria, emphasized truth in the form of moral integrity amid political disaster.

MSF would, in a sense, follow in the tradition of both these examples, combining Sartre's public volume with Camus's moral focus. A text by the latter author, however, best prefigures the orientation of the organization, one quite in keeping with its professional profile. Frequently read as an allegory about fascism, Camus's *The Plague* details the efforts of a doctor to combat and chronicle an epidemic afflicting his city. He does so simply by practicing medicine and keeping a record. Throughout, his manner combines skepticism with consistent devotion, a series of small acts rather than dramatic heroism. The key to this attitude is maintaining a fundamental sense of "honesty" or "decency." As the work's central character, Dr. Rieux, explains to a journalist who has decided to join him, "However, there's one thing I must tell you: there's no question of heroism in all of this. It's a matter of common decency. That's an idea which may make some people smile, but the only means of fighting a plague is—common decency."[3] He continues to define this decency as a matter of simply "doing my job." In his case the métier of a physician dictates providing care, a sign of devotion not only to bodies but also to human dignity. Amid extraordinary conditions, the most ordinary of behavior can translate into a supremely moral act.

This passage from *The Plague* resonates with MSF's "ethic of refusal"—a position that advances no universal or utopian solution beyond consistently rejecting "the apparent futility of the way the world is."[4] Facing crisis, the moral thing is simply to carry on. Camus's appeal to decency further echoes in a comment by James Orbinski, then the president of MSF's international council. In a video made in the run-up to the group's official receipt of the Nobel Prize, he states emphatically, "There is nothing heroic about being a decent human being." The central humanitarian conceit finds precise location in formal humility and its moral avatar: the responsible ordinary person, doing what should be done. However flamboyantly performed, MSF's appeal focuses on this fundamentally common conception of moral value.

The union of efforts between a doctor and a journalist featured in *The Plague* likewise anticipates MSF's own hybrid birth and development. Rather than the literary author donning the mantle of civic virtue or drafted into wartime reporting, here medical practice provides the most legitimate avenue to public speech. Confronting an eruption of illness, Dr. Rieux could document its devastating effects in clinical detail. But whereas Camus's fictional affliction arrived to his protagonist's doorstep, the historical actors who created MSF looked outward. From the outset the organization saw its stage as one of worldwide disaster. In an era of decolonization, the suffering that appeared most egregiously visible and compelling to it lay in the Third World. The agony of ordinary people caught in political circumstances beyond their control—the hot edges of the cold war—provided a new kind of romance. Amid civilian suffering the virtuous doctor would learn to testify.

The practice of testimony, however, adhered uneasily to the professional role. As attendants to the suffering, doctors would appear well positioned to voice the "misfortune of others."[5] However, the medical profession carried its own legacy of official discretion. The Hippocratic Oath famously admonished restraint, given that physicians might easily learn too much in the course of practicing their art. "And about whatever I may see or hear in treatment, or even without treatment," it read, "in the life of human beings—things that should not ever be blurted out outside—I will remain silent, holding such things to be unutterable."[6] MSF's initial charter of 1971 defined it as an assembly of doctors and health professionals who agreed on their honor to uphold a list of shared principles, including this tradition of confidentiality. The new *médecins sans frontières* would likewise refrain from expressing public opinions "with respect to events, military forces, and leaders who have accepted their assistance."[7]

In the mythic version of MSF's origins, the group emerges in open revolt against humanitarian silence. As noted earlier, the historical record suggests a more gradual and muted departure from the Red Cross fold. Like its ancestor, MSF too opposed "the horrors of war" and largely preserved Red Cross principles. But the myth does capture a shifting sense of moral duty when facing atrocities. For a generation aware of the burden of genocide, the Red Cross failure to speak out about the Nazi concentration camps—whatever it may have meant at the historical moment—proved increasingly haunting. Although Bernard Kouchner hardly founded MSF singlehandedly, he indeed gave it voice. The breakaway Nigerian enclave of Biafra provided a compelling tableau. As Kouchner memorably summarized the experience, "We did not consent to being medical alibis for the massacre of Biafrans."[8] Upon returning to France, he and his companions spoke out against this perceived instance of genocide in the run-up to MSF's founding. That their first publication in Le Monde did so modestly detracts little from its symbolic afterlife. That the new group explicitly forbade such practices likewise matters little when viewed at a historical remove. Over time témoignage could appear as organizational destiny.

REFINEMENTS AND CONTESTATIONS

As MSF expanded, the question of bearing witness grew central to its activities and internal debates. At the same time the form and object of this endeavor shifted subtly across eras and a growing range of engagements. While témoignage became a recognizable tradition, it remained open to reinterpretation and reinvention. Was it a matter of individual conscience or collective policy? Was its purpose to identify human rights abuses or to agitate for particular state action? Should it take the form of narrative testimony or medical data? Did it address itself to a general public, to an audience of targeted specialists, or even to some abstract moral domain of history? Would the group serve as a literal witness in a legal sense, providing testimony for court proceedings? Some of these questions appeared in reflective discussion, while others simply emerged in practice.

MSF's initial, avowedly amateur decade featured short, chaotic missions and frequent disputes. By 1975 the Biafran veterans had claimed ascendancy, and the question of témoignage was back on the table. In an editorial for the group's second bulletin, Kouchner's ally Max Récamier raised the question of whether to abandon medical neutrality and embrace media testimony as an effort to "treat the disease and not only the symptoms."[9] Operations soon exceeded the formal charter. As a retrospective article later noted dryly, "The principle of adhering to strict neutrality was soon overtaken by practice."[10] Indeed, a small mission had departed to assist the Kurds in northern Iraq in 1974. The following year the group conducted a minor sortie into the war zone of Vietnam, and in 1976 it undertook a more significant stint in a Beirut hospital. On the occasion of MSF's fifth anniversary Kouchner celebrated with his own presidential column in the bulletin. MSF, he proclaimed, practiced "active neutrality" on the side of victims: "For us, suffering children in the Third World are neither of the right nor left."[11] The cover of the same issue featured the organization's first advertising billboard, a sign of the coming significance of public exposure and fundraising. Not long afterward, the question of public speech played a central role in the schism of 1979. The faction that deposed Kouchner and his allies emphasized action over publicity. Nonetheless, that faction subsequently embarked on a public march for Cambodia, citing familiar concerns about genocide. Witnessing had arrived to stay.[12]

The action in Cambodia marked part of an antitotalitarian turn for the 1980s, during which MSF increasingly identified suffering amid the ruins of socialist dreams. Opposing the Soviet invasion of Afghanistan, the group undertook a particularly impassioned intervention. Actively partisan and clandestine, the "French doctors" cast Red Cross neutrality aside and joined the CIA and Osama bin Ladden alongside the mujahedin. MSF—particularly its original French branch—embraced controversy on an ever-increasing scale. This was highlighted by its eviction from Ethiopia after it denounced the regime's actions during the famine. The Ethiopian experience traumatized MSF-France, becoming a point of continual return and reference. For once its sortie into public speech had produced significant drama, resulting in expulsion and leaving it exposed to counteraccusations. At the same time, the fact that the group had only gradually grown aware of links between aid and Ethiopian government policy suggested that it had flirted with complicity itself. The role of the witness had been put to a dramatic test, with a resulting loss of innocence.

Other unsettling experiences would follow. The newer Belgian and Dutch sections of the organization, which had generally favored "silent diplomacy" over speaking out, publicized chemical weapons attacks on Kurds in the Iraqi town of Halabja in 1988. (These accusations took on unexpected political significance when repeated by the U.S. government many years later.)[13] Meanwhile, in Honduras that same year, MSF–France came into conflict with camp committees over the definition of its role in Salvadoran and Nicaraguan refugee camps and again withdrew. Claiming ethics was proving politically fraught. Nonetheless, the practice of *témoignage* had begun to emerge as something more systematic within MSF's ideology. Rather than simply issuing episodic denunciations, members of the group would strive to become "troublesome witnesses," as Rony Brauman put it in his presidential report of 1983.[14]

While MSF grappled with the political complexity of its ethical appeals, it also adopted a more professional profile in making them. To this end it created satellite offshoots devoted to media production and epidemiology. Given that the group had found its operational habitat in refugee camps, it needed to know more about the populations within them; statistical analysis would strengthen MSF's claims to medical truth about specific forms of suffering. The organization also extended its international scope by establishing partner sections as well as a central coordinating office and began to wean itself away from institutional funding in order to increase its independence. At a collective meeting in Toulouse in 1989, the national sections affirmed the centrality of *témoignage* to their work. They amended the official charter again, underscoring the importance of issuing public statements while retaining a commitment to neutrality. The group then began a more systematic approach to documenting humanitarian crises, sponsoring first a meeting and then a book series on the theme of populations in danger.

The early 1990s brought a series of international debacles in Somalia, the Balkans, and Rwanda. It was likewise an era of acrimonious disagreement between MSF's different sections over how best to respond. The genocide in Rwanda particularly shook the organization. As the carnage unfolded, MSF finally publicly proclaimed its helplessness in a bitter refrain: "You can't stop genocide with doctors." The French section denounced the political and military complicity of its own national government but also issued its first call for military intervention to halt the slaughter. Upset at the flagrant manipulation of aid by the perpetrators of genocide in the aftermath, the French then pulled out of the Rwandan refugee camps in Zaire and Tanzania at the end of 1994. The group subsequently denounced the new Rwandan regime for the forcible repatriation of Hutu refugees and an accompanying massacre. Although other MSF sections followed different strategic lines of action amid heated debate and an exchange of accusations, all eventually withdrew from the camps, publicly protesting the continuing political situation within them.[15] By all accounts, the events in Rwanda left considerable scars. These were only deepened by the exceptional publicity garnered by the group, coupled with the revelation of just how little immediate impact its most passionate protests actually had in the face of genocide. This unease lingered in the supposition within MSF that the organization's Nobel Prize derived in part from a belated and superficial sense of international guilt following the Rwandan crisis.

In 1995, the different component parts of MSF gathered at Chantilly, France, to broker a new understanding of their common enterprise. The document they created went into greater detail and defined the principle of witnessing in the following way:

> Witnessing (*témoignage*) consists of: the presence of volunteers among populations in danger, motivated by concern for the fate of fellow human beings and a willingness to be at their side and listen to them, as well as to carry out medical work among them; and the duty to report on the situation and on the fate of these people. Where MSF is present as a witness to massive and repeated violations of human rights and/or humanitarian law (such as forced population displacements, *refoulement* [forced return], genocide, crimes against humanity and war crimes), then MSF may ultimately be forced to make public denunciations.[16]

The moment also produced linguistic reflection. As English increasingly crept into the group's work, the term *advocacy* became the preferred alternative translation for *témoignage* due to its perceived lack of religious connotations and more militant overtones.

Following Chantilly, the trend toward a greater prominence of public statements continued, coupled with a growing recognition of their limits. By the late 1990s MSF had experienced a full range of humanitarian violations, from murder and manipulation to militarized forms of intervention.[17] The distinctiveness of its action further eroded with the advent of wars conducted in the name of humanitarian ends. Despite its call to arms amid the Rwandan disaster, MSF never signed on to any general "right of intervention" (*droit d'ingérence*) of the sort championed by its founding member Kouchner and implicit in its own name. Rather, it struggled to reclaim the banner of humanitarian virtue from what it saw as co-optation by military forces. The advent of coalitions led by NATO and the United States in Kosovo, followed by Afghanistan and Iraq, proved particularly worrying. As a consequence the group stepped back from making political claims and calls for intervention that might legitimize military action. By 2003 it consciously avoided this "temptation" in Liberia and the Democratic Republic of the Congo and subsequently suggested that such restraint should be a humanitarian principle.[18] When the Rwandan episode eventually appeared to have been an anomaly, not an expansive precedent, the watchword instead became a tighter focus on the provision of aid, along with greater realism about what its actions might achieve.

Even as MSF pulled back from endorsing force as a means of protection, it faced new questions about how to respond to the pursuit of justice. The establishment of special tribunals for Rwanda and the former Yugoslavia, followed by the inauguration of the International Criminal Court in 2002, raised issues about the group's formal legal role and responsibility. MSF had supported the creation of a system to address international war crimes. Nonetheless, as a humanitarian organization it held increasing reservations about participating too closely in any juridical system. Beyond concern over the impact on its field operations, the group was wary of creating legal precedents that might erode its independence. It wanted to see how the court's proceedings played out in practice. During French government hearings about Rwanda and Srebrenica MSF had discovered the degree to which such proceedings could simply fold into state policy, with inconvenient statements either ignored or subject to reinterpretation and manipulation. In any event, MSF decided to distinguish formally between collective testimony and that of individual members. The organization would provide public materials and statements as it saw fit but would only cooperate with legal proceedings when it alone held crucial evidence. Since MSF—unlike the ICRC and the UN—did not require its members to sign a confidentiality clause, however, individuals could follow their conscience in providing eyewitness testimony.[19] *Témoignage* of the legal sort would ultimately be a private matter.

MSF's expanding field of activities gave rise to new concerns. Three initiatives held particularly significant implications for public advocacy, namely the provision of psychological therapy; efforts to expand pharmaceutical access, including access to AIDS drugs; and the identification of violence as a medical problem. All these developments, it should be noted, marked a departure from the organization's tradition of practicing emergency medicine.[20] The recognition of mental and emotional suffering opened new terrain for action, not only in the aftermath of natural disasters but also in settings like Palestine, which had relatively few other medical needs but held strong political appeal. As Didier Fassin has shown, the shift to treating psychological trauma also created new terms for defining actors as victims and new tensions for humanitarian testimony over whose plight to emphasize across a conflict.[21]

Meanwhile, the launch of the Access Campaign in 1999, together with the rollout of MSF's AIDS projects, refocused attention on the structural inequities of health care. An entirely new advocacy arm came into being, publishing a regular stream of reports, press releases, and brochures. The advocacy actions involved included such classic political gestures as letter writing, signature gathering, and coordinated lobbying with other actors. The motivation for the Access Campaign had been MSF fieldworkers' frustration at repeatedly encountering outdated protocols and shortages of crucial but unprofitable drugs. As a member of the public health department at MSF–Holland put it to me, "The more I go to the field the more I realize the work needs to be done in Washington and Brussels." Nonetheless, moving into the domain of pharmaceutical equity departed not only from the group's historic focus on emergencies but also its focus on specific events. The campaign increasingly involved itself in topics like trade agreements and patent disputes, leading some to question whether it strayed too far afield. The campaign also had the effect of repositioning its parent organization within human rights endeavors. Even as MSF stepped back from testifying in court proceedings, it rearticulated something like a right to health at the level of policy claims.

Finally, the group followed a broader aid world trend of redefining war as violence and violence in turn as a medical condition. One effect of this shift was to introduce gender into MSF's criteria for project selection. After first running a pilot project in Congo-Brazzaville, in 2003 the organization recognized sexual violence as a legitimate focus. Given that this form of abuse was often invisible and stigmatizing, confidentiality became a heightened concern. To document and represent sexual violence, MSF increasingly employed statistical studies to bolster personal testimonies, transforming individual experience into an epidemiological state.[22] Thus, the most intimate of violations dictated a less personal response. In this respect MSF's incorporation of sexual violence, along with mental trauma and pharmaceutical supply, reworked its conception of *témoignage*. Upholding humanitarian truth now clearly involved more than the direct display of broken bodies. In these emerging domains it increasingly required expertise.

Meanwhile the familiar litany of disasters rolled on—earthquakes, famines, floods. So too did less publicized suffering at the horizon of world news: long-running civil wars in places like the Congo and the unglamorous misery of impoverished people dying from curable disease. In many bleak settings, aid workers increasingly served as prominent sources for international journalists on the rare occasions that they descended, becoming central nodes in the larger information network.[23] Far from representing an aberration to humanitarian practice, media engagement had become a routine part of it, as routine as humanitarian presence itself.

PLURAL PRACTICE

Like many aspects of MSF's activity, witnessing has remained internally as well as externally contentious. As a consequence even general statements about it reveal a complex and sometimes contradictory logic born of lengthy negotiation. The different national sections of the organization developed somewhat different habits as well as interpretations of their common doctrine. Here I examine efforts by the three largest, Belgium, Holland, and France, to explain *témoignage* to their own members in the wake of the Nobel moment. Although broadly related, their definitions take disparate forms.

In 2001 the research arm of the Belgian section produced a small "reference tool" handbook on the topic. Entitled "MSF and *Témoignage*," it mixes general observations with brief descriptions of historical examples drawn from MSF's greater experience. The current charter, it notes, calls for volunteers to respect "their professional code of ethics" rather than discretion, but it does not mention *témoignage*. The handbook acknowledges this absence to be "somewhat hypocritical," given that witnessing constitutes a fundamental aspect of MSF's mission, but ascribes the absence to the practical realities of negotiating access on the ground. "Omitting *témoignage* from the [MSF] Charter was intended to avoid unnecessary suspicion and conflict with local authorities, as it can easily be interpreted as declaring political intent, even espionage." On the same page, the booklet stresses that bearing witness constitutes a moral and political choice for members, rather than a moral duty imposed on them. "MSF chooses to respond to people's plight by communicating it to others; none of us is legally obligated to do so. In other words, as individuals we can choose to speak out or not, but as an organization we feel morally bound to do so."[24] This particular duty of testimony, then, remains essentially collective.

At the same time the handbook also underscores the importance of the group's autonomy to this collectivity: "When we speak to the international press or lobby local authorities, we do so only in the interest of the victims, and never to further a particular cause of MSF. It is important to note, however, that MSF never asks the permission of a given population to speak out on its behalf. Our reactions to a crisis are our own; this is part of our independence."[25]

Thus, although MSF personnel may be reporting the words of others, their representation is never ethnographic or even juridical in motivation. Through their collective expertise, they verify problems affecting a population and—like any physician—reserve the right to offer an opinion, whether or not it is fully accepted by the potential patient. At the same time the primary objective of MSF's efforts should be to "improve the situation," not to satisfy the group's own sense of outrage.[26] On a practical level the handbook provides what it terms a *"témoignage* toolbox" of strategic options: silent diplomacy, letter writing, media events, overt diplomacy, press communiqués, and public statements or position papers. It also mentions longer-term endeavors to keep an issue alive, such as books and conferences, and the prospect of cooperation with war crimes tribunals.[27] But the work closes on a cautionary note, warning that *témoignage* is "no magic formula for justice."[28] Although fundamental to this humanitarian vision, witnessing may not yield much in the way of satisfaction.

A year before the Belgian effort, MSF-Holland produced an Advocacy Information Kit to orient its volunteers. This short, spiral-bound volume opens with copies of the MSF charter and the final agreement of the Chantilly meeting. These are followed by a review article composed for the Nobel occasion and brief pieces summarizing the place of witnessing and humanitarian affairs at MSF–Holland. The kit also contains a primer on international human rights and humanitarian law, as well as elaborations of core principles (independence, impartiality, neutrality, voluntarism, and governance as an association) and operational values (proximity, transparency, and accountability). Other elements include a guide to data collection (both for routine medical monitoring and for investigation of particular matters of concern), a position paper on female genital cutting (which MSF opposes on health grounds, noting that immunization, oral rehydration, and the use of condoms also represent deviations from "tradition"), background papers on "the right to health" and humanitarian assistance, an outline of the organization's policy on protection and, finally, a reference guide to relevant international legal documents.

The most striking element of the Dutch kit appears as an appendix: sample "witness statement forms" for gathering information about potential humanitarian violations. The first, intended to document specific incidents, guides the user through the process of interviewing someone who has experienced or observed a reprehensible event. Beyond recording basic facts about the witness and the context of the interview, the form prompts its user to request details about perpetra-

tors (distinguishing whether they are members of a military or not), their potential motivation (personal, ethnic, influenced by intoxication), and the incident
itself (weapons used and whether an official complaint was filed). The second
template addresses conditions in a refugee camp. In addition to basic demo-
graphic data, it seeks evaluative statements about general living and security
conditions (improving or not?), as well as circumstances related to refugee movement. The form also includes a section in which to record specific violations and
the response undertaken by camp authorities. In contrast to the Belgian list of
general suggestions, the Dutch forms are specific, directive, and eminently practical. They imply a relatively routine process undertaken under fairly predictable
circumstances. One could be trained to practice *témoignage*.

The French section, by contrast, refused to produce any such set of guidelines.
With characteristic panache it proclaimed witnessing too contextually specific an
activity to ever conform to a standardized algorithm. Instead, the French championed an ambitious series of case studies that would cover key controversial
moments when the group actually engaged in public speech. More chronicle than
guide, the endeavor would contain as much primary material as possible and remain open ended. As the project's editor explained to me in 2003, it was initially
conceived in 1998–1999 as a common resource for all the sections. Actual imple-
mentation proved complex, however. Both the potential scale of the endeavor and
the sensitive nature of some of the events turned out to be daunting. Although the
approach emphasized primary sources and sought to present people "in their own
words," as the editor put it, the result nonetheless became the focus of some controversy within the organization. By focusing on cases that had involved heated
disputes between sections and individuals, the series revived disagreements, even
at the level of fact. Moreover, not all participants were equally prepared to share
their comments publicly. Thus when the casebook series began to appear in late
2003 under the title "Prises de parole publiques MSF / MSF Speaking Out," it remained in somewhat restricted circulation. Early versions included a warning that
their use required authorization by MSF's International Council. Even if anxieties
have since eased, only the introductions and timelines appear on a public website.[29] For that reason I will not quote directly from their contents but simply
describe them as collections that would be immediately recognizable to any professional historian as a valuable resource. Each compiles primary documents and
fragmentary oral histories related to the event in question, ordered only by a map
and a detailed timeline. Not all sources agree or represent the same perspectives.
Rather than presenting post hoc consensus or bullet points of "lessons learned,"
the collections emphasize the complexity of each agonizing dispute.

Taken as an evolving whole, the casebook series suggests a reflective and combative tradition short on certainty and long on argument. The casebooks also
indicate the degree to which the Rwandan moment marked the organization, as

four of the first six editions chronicle the genocide and its extended aftermath in Zaire (now the Congo). In contrast to the Dutch kit or even the Belgian handbook, they are not prescriptive or practical; each demands an investment of time to absorb and yields little in the way of clear direction. The controversy surrounding their contents and its dissemination is equally revealing. *Témoignage* appears less a matter of moral clarity than one of intense dispute. Although members of MSF might share a common vision of the dangers confronting humanitarianism and its intended beneficiaries, they did not necessarily agree on how to respond or choose between the unpalatable options that often confronted them. Even years after the fact they were not quite ready to speak to history.

Within and across the organization, other tensions weighed on the practice of witnessing. Who can speak for medical humanitarianism? Public image notwithstanding, MSF had come to incorporate far more than an association of physicians. A large number of nonmedical personnel worked and volunteered with the organization, including a veritable army of national staff resident in mission countries. All were equally human and presumably equipped with decency. But would they enjoy equal credibility as the face of a medical organization? Similarly, for a long time MSF's partner sections primarily concerned themselves with fundraising, advocacy, and recruitment of volunteers. Would their relative distance from field operations handicap them when it came to determining what, and how much, to say? The concern was hardly abstract, given that the organization regularly produced testimony in contexts where identity mattered. As a humanitarian affairs officer for MSF-Holland observed with a hint of annoyance in 2002, "With the U.S. State Department, they always want an American volunteers from the field to testify."

Even those nonmedical staff most concerned with issues of public presentation—members of the communications departments of the various headquarters—regularly emphasize that MSF is first and foremost involved in field operations. The production of reports should not be taken as its raison d'être. "We are not Amnesty or Human Rights Watch," I was told repeatedly. Witnessing, in this view, emerges as a secondary effect of medical humanitarian action—an essential byproduct, but a byproduct nonetheless. A French operations director, himself trained in law and actively involved in testimonials about human rights abuses in the Balkans, made this point quite strongly: "Thus, for me *témoignage* is linked to action but should never be seen as an action itself. It's not the work of one specialized body. Rather it's the responsibility of everybody. You, me, a doctor, a nurse, a log [logistician]—whoever is on the spot. *Témoignage* is also not just denunciation, it can simply be information. Some people distinguish it from communication, but for me it's something more political to address violence against a population. However, MSF should not become a sort of press agency. That's not our job at all."[30]

Despite such disavowals, a significant part of MSF's actual practice has quite clearly involved public relations. The organization's identity—its moral legitimacy and corporate brand—derives partly from its perceived willingness to speak out. Considered from this vantage point, *témoignage* moves from essential byproduct to strategic resource. Conversely, MSF's independence rests on its financial autonomy, and fundraising draws heavily on the group's medical profile and operational engagement. What matters most for MSF's image, then, is its continued projection of a sense of authenticity. To speak out on a particular issue might alienate part of the donor base, but to always keep silent would destroy MSF's claim to distinctive credibility. To simply become a rights organization, however, would threaten the group's core mission of medical humanitarianism.

Thus it is no surprise that the topic of witnessing has proved a continuing source of debate and commentary. Long-term members of the movement strive to be suspicious of their own ideology and to question any term that becomes too settled. When I interviewed him in 2003, the former president of MSF–France, Rony Brauman, expressed regret at having helped establish *témoignage* as a touchstone in the movement's collective vocabulary. In retrospect he felt that it had given rise to a great deal of misunderstanding, and he preferred to emphasize a more common sense of responsibility and a "refusal to be an instrument of political violence." Increasingly, he and others referenced public speech rather than the more amorphous action of *témoignage*. Another senior figure within the same section dismissed the tradition of witnessing as a *cache-sexe*, a fig leaf of activism used to cover the perpetual frustration of relative political impotence. And yet he, like most long-term members of the organization, also recognized the need to justify the obvious incompleteness of MSF's medical interventions with a sense of the wider effects of action. That MSF could never save the world through medical treatment alone remains quite clear to its most ardent constituents, even those most determined to preserve its field focus. As the legal counsel of MSF-France dryly summarized, "If they're massacring people, then there's no need to vaccinate."[31]

Nonetheless, by saving a few, however temporarily, the group might make a case against needless suffering. It likewise might potentially criticize and annoy others into greater action. In this light, one can understand why a member of MSF–Holland described the map of its projects to me in 2002 as "a very expensive pair of eyes." By intervening in desperate circumstances, with excellent communications technology and restricted political will, MSF had created a system for producing knowledge in the face of despair.

AN APPEAL OF WORDS, A POWER OF NUMBERS

The classic lineage of MSF's *témoignage* has remained an appeal of words. In practice this consists of a wide range of activities surrounding humanitarian action, extending beyond presence to quiet diplomacy and the transfer of information, on to public appeals and denunciation. On occasion, such speaking out has taken the form of strenuous accusation, often leading to the withdrawal of a mission. Common to all these gestures is an appeal to the morality of facts. Suffering itself is primary, and MSF's response to it is presumed to be direct, however strategic.

How, though, does one know when suffering is real? And how to make that ontological claim convincing to others? To establish its facts in any given setting, MSF commonly draws on two resources beyond its own direct observations. Accounts by victims and their relatives offer graphic testimony—personally situated and emotionally compelling—about painful events. For that reason the organization regularly features them in public documents alongside somber images of suffering and treatment. Statistical studies, on the other hand, offer a more collective measure of tragedy and lend an aura of dispassionate objectivity. Hence they more commonly appear in reports and other documents directed at a more professional audience. The group now regularly sponsors its own research, both in an effort to extend medical knowledge in areas relevant to humanitarian work and to strengthen a case for public appeal. Although this second practice might appear a departure from the tradition of public speech, in practice it complements the first and can even direct it. In this sense humanitarian appeals have acquired an intentionally scientific edge.

To illustrate MSF's particular combination of words and numbers I turn to a specific case. For humanitarians, the Democratic Republic of the Congo (formerly Zaire) has reprised its classic role as the heart of darkness. The country combines a long history of violence with a relative dearth of health data. It has hosted much of the recent serial conflict in Africa's Great Lakes region, and with it what is likely—in statistical estimates—the greatest loss of human life over the past few decades. In 2001 the Belgian section of the organization released an epidemiological report addressing issues of health and violence in the area, elements of which later found inclusion in an article for the journal *Disasters*.[32] On the basis of surveys conducted in five locations, the report concluded that mortality rates were disconcertingly high near the front lines of the conflict. Rates of infectious disease and malnutrition were likewise on the rise. After many pages delineating sampling methodology and providing results in the form of figures and tables, the article closes with a discussion of crisis in the country and MSF's actions to recognize and address its scope, aided by the specific results of this survey. It presents its fundamental finding in a distinctly dispassionate voice: "The medical and humanitarian situation remains acute across the country, particularly near the front line where mortality far exceeds alarm thresholds."[33]

Such conclusions are not intended to be surprising. Rather, the report sought to provide a small measure of precision within the statistical vacuum of political collapse, in order to lend scientific weight to its appeal on behalf of affected populations. Commenting on a similar study conducted in the Congo in 1997, an MSF author noted: "As a result of this survey, MSF was able to back up its *témoignage* with statistical proof of a kind that could justifiably be used to extrapolate evidence of the fate of tens of thousands of Rwandan refugees in the forest of Congo. This was especially important in view of the Congolese government's refusal to grant free access to refugees to a United Nations human rights investigation team."[34]

Here epidemiology is called upon to produce *motivated facts,* that is to say, a body of information that suggests the validity of probable truths already known in outline if not detail.[35] Their construction is partial both in the sense of being constrained by adverse conditions and in the sense of being directed by a guiding orientation that extends beyond the parameters of disinterest. The result is a most worldly conception of science in action: the production of "statistical proof" that could "justifiably be used to extrapolate evidence" in a setting where the norms of public health surveillance are lacking.[36]

Alongside this survey, the MSF-Belgium team also gathered first-person narratives of individuals who had suffered during the recent phases of the war. A selection found its way into a short book that appeared in French the following year. Entitled *Silence on meurt: Témoignages* (Quiet, We're Dying: Testimonies), elements of the work featured for a time on several of MSF's websites.[37] Like the epidemiological data set, the volume's narrative materials claim truth in their specificity. They do so passionately, however, striving to establish emotional connection through stories of individual loss: small, sharp markers of anguish that might reach deeper into empathy than generalized images or the abstraction of statistics. As the official description of the project proclaims, the goal is to "give voice to the Congolese, so that they might themselves present their unvarnished everyday reality."[38] Thus we are introduced to Samuel T., a fisherman, who speaks of lack of medicines and clinical care for his ten children. He resorts to traditional remedies and finally travels to a hospital only to watch his son die. Justine F., mother of seven, recalls losing a son and returning to find her house burned to the ground. Her husband is a teacher, she notes, and yet she faces the shame of being unable to clothe all her children. Mirielle K., a young single mother, recounts how she became separated from her child amid the panic of a rebel takeover of her town, and "only God knows" if the child lives or not or if they will be reunited. Several of these individuals comment on their own condition. Jean K., a sixty-nine-year-old teacher, can no longer look past the present: "We don't know if peace will last, so it is useless to think about the future." Or in the bitter analysis of François K. M., who has lost three children: "Laugh! Yes, we laugh because God created laughter as part of human nature, but inside we are eaten away as if by gangrene. It is with much emotion that I share my sorrow with the person to whom I am talking about my misfortune." Presented without embellishment and accompanied by images of distressed individuals in everyday settings, these narratives lend particularity to the mass experience of a suffering population. They also underscore that these are distinctly ordinary lives; their tragedies should resonate with anyone who has a child, or indeed with any "decent human being."

Together these overlapping projects share a common goal: to translate the suffering encountered by MSF's field missions in one of the world's most troubled areas into a collage of truth, one that will disturb and motivate reaction. The different numeric, narrative, and visual products seek to engage different audiences. Nonetheless, they all derive from specific engagements and claim authority on the ground of experience. Even when the results are effectively depoliticized in their generality—as in the perversely elegant images of nameless suffering, for example—they are potentially repoliticized through association with particular narratives and motivated statistics. The combination of words, images, and numbers evokes the collective violation within individual misfortune.

These efforts to represent suffering in the Congo share traits common to the much larger array of reports, articles, books, seminars, news conferences, workshops, films, and web postings that the greater federation of MSF produces on a continual basis. All seek to establish facts of suffering and thereby to make a moral claim. They rest their authority first and foremost on the organization's operational presence in the field. The entire logic of MSF's approach to aid revolves around this presence.[39] This is particularly the case for expatriate field workers, whose relatively expensive presence is frequently justified not only as expression of solidarity but also as a potential conduit to a wider circulatory network. At certain moments, some in MSF argue, it can be critical to have an outsider in place simply because that person can operate from a position of neutral ignorance, and—kidnappings aside—with a different degree of risk. The field simultaneously constitutes a primary site of self-formation for members of MSF. In order to speak with any measure of credibility within the organization one must have gone through an appropriate rite of passage on the front lines, preferably with scant material comforts and at least one bout of a debilitating disease.

Even reversals of official logic underscore the significance of being on site. In some cases medical care serves primarily as a justification for presence, allowing the organization to demonstrate solidarity even when its clinical work produces few results. MSF volunteers often become attached to particular mission sites, especially zones of chronic disaster, and collective experience over time in places like Afghanistan or Sudan has influenced organizational outlook. For many years Chechnya was one such area, and a senior figure within MSF-Holland described the impossibility of working in the ravaged shell of Grozny to illustrate a more general credo of "providing care as a protest." Acknowledging that the group's work there had little impact in a public health sense, he stressed the importance of remaining in place amid the destruction. MSF's mere presence, he felt, provided a physical and symbolic link to the outside world.[40] Individuals who have extensive field experience with MSF sometimes caution against abstract and dramatic conceptions of advocacy prevalent in the organization's offices. They emphasize that *témoignage* also involves an evaluation of what moments demand a public response, a sense of restraint that comes through exposure to comparable situations. As a head of mission in Uganda noted to me, "Information can kill other information." Rather than constantly talking about a situation, she stressed the importance of choosing a moment and having convincing arguments and figures at the ready in order to make an impact.

Members of MSF express discomfort with the idea of speaking out about things they or their patients have not directly witnessed.[41] Faced with highly scripted mediated representations of suffering (to which they regularly, if not always eagerly, contribute), they prize immediacy of contact and direct quotations. MSF documents intended for public circulation thus regularly feature the "voices" of those directly impacted, or, if unavailable, proxy testimony from those caring for them in the field. Translated and edited into manageable units, these statements emphasize individual experience in the hope of conveying a shared humanity across geographic and social distance. Amid the tradeoff between contextual detail and breadth of circulation common to such representation, we can also note a desire to defer authority away from the apparatus of dissemination.[42] A repeated theme in many of MSF's internal discussions is the importance of never losing sight of the victim. The act of testimony should not overshadow what it represents. Despite the obvious contradictions this ideal raises for activities such as fundraising—where the audience must not only be encouraged to recognize suffering, but also to donate to the organization—it nonetheless reflects the central altruistic claim of independent groups like MSF.

However, there remains an important qualification: for an NGO engaged in mobile testimony, presence on the ground derives from a desire to be there. Given that its charter dictates a commitment to engage with those in need, MSF's position resembles that of an advocate as much as that of a witness.[43] That this need might expand from physical care to representation only shifts the register from medicine to law. At the same time it reaffirms the fact that these are *anticipatory* actors, prepared to speak in general before any particularity of events requires it. The templates in the Dutch Advocacy Information Kit simply formalize a state of moral readiness and organizational destiny. Despite rhetorical emphasis on individual experience, the final voice of MSF takes collective form: moments of speech drawn together and disseminated by a large and quite professional media mechanism. Individual names fade behind that of the organization, the words of doctors, non-doctors, and victims alike folded under the mantle of medical concern.

The incorporation of epidemiology within MSF's project of public advocacy reflects a longer trend toward seeking professional respectability. In 1987, the French section launched a satellite organization called Epicentre to conduct epidemiological studies and assessments in field settings.[44] The goal in this entity's establishment was twofold. Having a separate research arm would assist MSF in generating an independent knowledge base, one specifically geared toward its needs. On a technical level Epicentre could evaluate health needs and assess the efficacy of field techniques according to a schedule determined by MSF. At the same time it could also provide the sort of data that might resonate in expert circles, enhancing the organization's credibility within a wider world of public health and improving its ability to "speak to the institution."[45] The desire for credibility was quite conscious following the tumult in Ethiopia. Reports from the era noted proudly that members of the group were studying in settings like Johns Hopkins, and protagonists I later interviewed recalled the initiative as part of a broad effort to boost MSF's technical capacity.[46] When engaged in controversy, it became all the more important to get facts straight and to project authority.

The existence of Epicentre serves two functions with respect to *témoignage,* its director explained to me in 2003. First, it provides a population-level perspective to balance the medical and moral impulses of clinicians responding to individual cases. Thus when a new strain of meningitis appears in Burkina Faso, Epicentre might caution MSF not to simply assume it will become a common problem. Or when members of the Access Campaign doubt malaria treatment protocols in Africa, MSF might sponsor its own review or clinical trial while embroiling itself in international debates. Second, it serves as a device to render suffering into the institutionally potent language of numbers, including publication in peer-reviewed journals. Beginning with a study of an overcrowded prison in Gitarama, Rwanda, in 1995, epidemiological reports have become part of a self-consciously "scientific" approach to the group's *témoignage.*[47] Having numbers—preferably good ones—offers another means to direct debate.

A nurse helping to coordinate MSF operations in Uganda expanded on these observations in 2004. Increasingly, she noted, the organization faced demands for information. Although enjoying its increased prominence, that and the emergence of an international court system opened new concerns about speaking beyond its actual knowledge or proper role. In her view, concentrating on testimony had pushed the group too far in the direction of Human Rights Watch. It was important to match advocacy with an explicitly *medical* perspective: "That's our greater responsibility; we need to use our own experience, own knowledge, own medical data. Whoever reads stories interprets them as they want. Our credibility comes from capturing statistics. As a medical organization, that's what we're trained for. I'm very critical of reports that don't use a combination of approaches."[48]

Like most issues in MSF, her opinion was not uncontested. The collection of emotional testimonials can prove more appropriate to certain patient groups as well as certain audiences. Late in the Bosnian crisis, for example, a former journalist told me how she found herself working with MSF amid a population of resettled refugees, "people who were not very sick, but so willing to speak." While the epidemiologists accompanying her struggled to find an adequate approach, she felt well equipped to record the refugees' suffering. Moreover, many members of the organization also remain deeply skeptical of the abstract nature of quantitative data on principle, particularly given the illusionary certainty it can project onto volatile field situations. MSF thus refuses to endorse the simple adoption of "evidence-based approaches."[49] Nonetheless, an internal analysis of MSF's public role suggests a growing shift from denunciation to description.[50] The emergence of the Access Campaign and the group's increased focus on specific diseases, trauma, and medical definitions of violence places greater emphasis on expert knowledge. The more MSF has sought to advocate for policy changes, lobby government agencies, or embarrass corporations, the higher the stakes have become for possessing authoritative facts.

THE PROBLEM OF NEUTRALITY

Throughout its long experiment with witnessing, MSF continued to retain a principle of neutrality in its charter. This observation begs discussion, given the apparent contradiction between a neutral stance and MSF's public expressions of outrage. How could any descendent of Zola appear neutral? Surely speaking out and taking a stand involves choosing sides. One response (by now conventional wisdom in the aid world) would be that humanitarian organizations view neutrality first and foremost as an operational concern, an elemental part of the politics of gaining access. Practitioners also often highlight impartiality, with its active assertion of equal treatment according to humanitarian need, over neutrality. Certainly both these points hold merit. The Red Cross was hardly blind to battlefield politics when it adopted a neutral stance and proclaimed discretion, and within medicine impartial care stands as a hallmark of professional ethics. Yet the issue, I suggest, may run deeper and prove more revealing. The dilemma of neutrality derives in part from conceiving of it as an abstract principle, one that represents an absolute condition. If approached as a historical practice, however, questions of consistency and completeness grow less significant than those of perception and effect.

Indeed, like *war, neutrality* may be an impossible word, one that appears sharp and sure on the surface but on close examination dissolves into a wide range of forms and events.[51] Most humanitarian accounts of neutrality start with the Red Cross moment of the nineteenth century. A slightly longer reach into European history indicates that neutrality emerged less as a principle than as a negotiated position. As Stephen Neff notes in his historical survey of the topic, "The law of neutrality, in short, was made not, as it were, from the top-down by scholars and commentators, but rather from the bottom-up by statesmen, generals, admirals and traders."[52] Neutral parties could be active as well as passive, and certainly self-interested. They hedged bets, conducted trade, and sometimes mediated. Moreover, theirs was hardly an absolute condition: a state of neutrality extended only to particular conflicts and to certain relationships within them. In this sense neutrality represented an effort to define parameters for situated action, always conducted without certain guarantee. Neutrality was a claim, one that might or might not prove possible to uphold. From the perspective of the present the historical record underscores a significant, often overlooked point: the refusal to take a political position not only has political effects, it is also a political strategy. Like any strategy, neutrality might or might not succeed in furthering specific aims under given circumstances.

Two additional historical observations also caution against taking a nineteenth-century principle as a timeless norm. Declarations of neutrality offered smaller powers a means to survive amid larger neighbors. By avoiding conflict they could assert independence and sometimes enjoy the prospect of profit. Their existence periodically served the commercial and diplomatic interests of their larger neighbors, even expansionist ones. Europe produced not only empires, after all, but also odd corners between them, minor countries able to present themselves as exceptional zones. Switzerland stands as a prominent example, one that evolved into a central ground for international affairs—including humanitarianism. Thus neutrality appears as much a strategic weapon of the weak as a hegemonic assumption of the powerful. Amid royal disputes waged by mercenary armies allegiances were fluid, and a measure of accommodation reigned in war as well as peace. Prior to the nineteenth century, degrees of "imperfect" or "partial" neutrality enjoyed some recognition; for example, states might continue to honor arrangements that predated the onset of hostilities.[53] The wider scope of total war, however, recast both conflict and neutrality in more absolute terms. As civilians and their livelihood began to play a larger role in military strategy, neutrality entered law as a more permanent and restrictive condition, and states such as Belgium were designated as being "perpetually" neutral to dampen potential conflict in the aftermath of the Napoleonic era. But conditions can change. Just as an image of warfare that presumes neatly arrayed, uniformed lines of troops no longer fits contemporary circumstances, a corresponding concept of inviolate neutrality may likewise clash with current practice. In this respect, our present may have more in common with earlier European experience than with the more immediate past.[54]

MSF's trajectory with regard to neutrality is only one variant in the broader field of humanitarian actors. Some groups overtly identify with religious inspiration. Others have gone much further in aligning themselves with political crusades or human rights ideals or, like CARE, have negotiated collaboration with military reconstruction with far fewer qualms. However, MSF inherited the ICRC tradition directly. It rebelled yet never fully left the fold. This elasticity may upset classificatory schemas of political science, in which MSF is only uncertainly "classical" (neutral) or "solidarist."[55] Nonetheless, recognizing such ambiguity helpfully returns topics like neutrality to the more fluid ground of actual practice. It also serves as a reminder that radical commitment to an overarching value, such as the minimization of suffering, may render other principles less absolute.

Given MSF's tradition of *témoignage* and the political complexity of many field situations, it is no surprise that neutrality has remained a topic of periodic concern in internal debates. One of the most astute analyses came in 2001 from Fiona Terry, then at MSF-France's research foundation. Raising the question of whether the principle of neutrality remains relevant to the organization, her position paper surveys the Red Cross history of the concept and its tensions with the practice of speaking out. On the basis of this last point she proposes that MSF acknowledge its history of engagement and adopt a pending motion to finally drop the principle from its charter. After all, she proclaims, "It is not possible to be a little bit neutral, or subscribe to a 'spirit of neutrality.'"[56] Following a year of extended discussion across the movement, however, the general assembly of MSF endorsed a statement in favor of retaining the term in the charter. The statement noted that neutrality continued to be associated with humanitarian action and did not impede the organization's ability to speak out. Indeed, formally dropping the principle might actually weaken MSF's position, particularly if it was already suspected of taking sides.[57] MSF would remain, as it were, a little bit neutral.

The resilience of this claim to neutrality reflects the organization's abiding pragmatism. When faced with contradictions in specific settings, it can adapt its principles to stay true to a greater good, much like a physician in a clinic. For example, MSF adheres strongly to impartiality, in the sense of providing aid "in proportion to need and without discrimination" and stressing financial independence to forestall undue political and economic influence on its decision-making.[58] Once put into practice, however, impartiality can carry its own risks and political complications. As Terry notes in her essay on neutrality, the needs of opposing sides are rarely equal from a medical perspective. By acting impartially one can thereby appear aligned, dispensing goods and services unequally between combatants. In the case of a particular conflict in Indonesia, the Christian population might most need assistance. "But as an essentially European NGO, MSF is perceived as being pro-Christian. Thus MSF is searching for ways to assist Muslim communities to avoid accusations of partiality in the conflict. The need to be perceived as neutral in order to remain present outweighs the importance of basing assistance on the greatest need."[59] Even *témoignage* might at times serve strategic ends, driven as much by field concerns as any moral effort to raise awareness. In an interview for an internal study about protection, the president of MSF-France responded to a question about Darfur by suggesting as much: "You have to create a relationship of power so that humanitarian action is respected, so that it is not co-opted. Your approach to your working environment has to be political and [speaking out] is one of the elements."[60]

Whether one considers neutrality as an imperfect claim or an absolute principle, its effectiveness ultimately depends on the perceptions of the actors involved, a former director of MSF-USA stressed to me. Most evidence indicates that people on the ground often have a hard time distinguishing between aid agencies or grasping the nuances of their ideological commitments.[61] Principles of neutrality, or impartiality for that matter, are likely less crucial than a positive reputation.

Given this, the strategic question for humanitarian organizations then becomes how best to influence perception to further their ideals. The classic Red Cross adherence to neutrality traded public silence for operational access and cast its moral appeal at the level of formal agreements and long-term influence. Its aura of authenticity thus relied on consistent adherence to principle and recognition by political powers. MSF modified this classic equation by claiming independence, adding public speech, and minimizing its patience for rights violations. Its moral authenticity therefore shifted to a more oppositional framing of virtue and a realist adjustment of principle to the humanitarian needs of the moment. Neither approach guarantees universal success in achieving humanitarian ends. But MSF's looser style reveals the political edge of a humanitarian ethic, as well as its strategic weakness. The organization's 2001 debate over neutrality occurred on the eve of the events of September 11, 2001. After subsequent shifts in U.S. foreign policy and a new scale of militarized action co-opting humanitarian rhetoric, the debate quietly subsided. Claiming neutrality clearly still had some uses.

SPECIFIC KNOWLEDGE, COLLECTIVE SPEECH

What then to say about MSF's evolving practice of playing a moral witness? Here I return to the medical persona of MSF and the question of whether the voice of a "decent human being" who speaks *as a doctor* carries any particular resonance. Not long after the group's emergence in France, Michel Foucault made a well-known distinction between what he called "universal intellectuals" and "specific intellectuals."[62] He posed this distinction as an analytic for understanding the history of political expression, suggesting divergent genealogies for points of authority within it. For Foucault, the universal intellectual represented a residual figure of leftist political imagination, the "master of truth and justice" who gives voice to the less articulate masses. He cast Voltaire as the prototype of this universal jurist, a great writer whose sharp pen could skewer falsehood and reveal injustice. By contrast, the specific intellectual represented a newer configuration between theory and practice, a distributed population of knowledge bearers defined by the precise conditions of their work. Foucault dated this latter form to the Second World War and named the Manhattan Project, and J. Robert Oppenheimer, as a key transition point. Thereafter, he suggested, a public person's knowledge could carry political weight due to specific expertise rather than general proclamations. The two examples contrasted centuries and national contexts as well as a man of letters and a man of numbers. According to Foucault, the emergence of the expert as a political figure placed a new premium on life itself within power: "He is no longer the rhapsodist of the eternal but the strategist of life and death."[63]

Foucault's distinction is of interest here for two reasons. First, it reveals key assumptions about who an intellectual might be, particularly the "public" intellectual repeatedly imagined and bemoaned in absentia.[64] Second, by contrasting this inherited dream with the less heroic figure of the located expert, Foucault recognizes the significance of science in contemporary truth claims, together with the limited revelation of specialized study. Moreover, he also suggests a central role for facts of life and death and the practice of medicine. Within a political regime that incorporates life into its regular accounting, the truth of a doctor carries particular weight. Thus the doctor can emerge as both ancestral prototype and key agent of the growing importance of life within politics.[65]

Foucault's specific intellectual remains an individual actor. However expert and defined by particular bodies of knowledge, this image now appears an antiquarian relic when compared to the dispersed mass collectives that author some scientific work. The issue is not simply one of allocating individual credit and recognition, but also one of the very identity of knowledge creation. Amid a large research or clinical trial, our inherited sense of the independent author misses the collective self at the very heart of key forms of contemporary truth making.[66] In order to extend Foucault's broad distinction to the world of humanitarian doctors, then, we should first complicate it by recalling the compound form of contemporary biomedicine. Even MSF's relatively simple procedures involve complex groupings of humans and equipment, not isolated subjects. To speak "as a doctor" is not quite the same as speaking "as a poet." Access to scientific truth more often requires sufficient apparatus and assumes an active network of colleagues.

Foucault was also writing and thinking in France of the 1970s. It was a context richly steeped in the tradition of public intellectuals but featuring few prominent nongovernmental organizations and a relatively modest, pre-internet capacity for the independent dissemination of pronouncements. While international NGOs and advocacy networks are by no means entirely new, their number and influence has increased dramatically over the past several decades.[67] Issues such as human rights, economic development, and environmentalism are now simultaneously defined and contested by groups large and small, such that the wider discourse would be unrecognizable without them. In an era when protests are scripted and organized and letters and petitions constitute an evolved and even automated genre, NGOs provide a counterpoint to Voltaire. Beyond heroic genius, beyond "specific intellectuals," we might consider "specific collectives"—entities that claim expertise on a group basis. Would-be public intellectuals now share the stage with cadres of experts and collective agents.[68] From this perspective MSF exemplifies the collective nature of contemporary claims on truth. Its evolving tradition of public speech, simultaneously moral and descriptive, appears less a shadow of Enlightenment glory than a sign of the political present.

Drawing more deeply from the history of science, we might also recall another legacy of Enlightenment objectivity alongside Voltaire: the image of the trustworthy, modest witness. Only a disinterested party could provide an account of nature that is both truthful and direct. In early modern England, that figure was a gentleman, perceived as sufficiently unencumbered by other gentlemen to serve as "a reliable spokesman of reality."[69] To achieve that affect, the person receded behind the facts. So too did other factors—dear to social analysts—that might compromise objectivity or imply interest: class position, gender, and race. Such a disappearing act was not equally available to all, a fact that suggests another politics of knowledge.[70]

MSF partly fits this lineage as well, asserting its independence as a source of veracity. Although fully committed to an equalitarian concept of the human, the organization nonetheless embodies an inherited politics of race, class, and citizenship. Its still largely European, professional expatriates disappear more easily as agents of truth, transmitting the less mobile voices of largely poor and non-European victims. At rhetorical moments the entire complex disappears into the nominal image of a doctor, historically not only white but also male. On the other hand the doctor, especially the displaced doctor of frontier medicine, was never quite a gentleman scientist. Far from removing itself from the world, MSF remains dedicated to the practice of a humanitarian form of medicine and the gritty particularities of suffering. Moreover, it adopts the immodest, oppositional stance of Voltaire or Zola, seeking to puncture the pieties of an established order. The knowledge the organization produces and circulates is thus undeniably motivated and built out of facts directly in the service of humane values. Collectively, then, MSF operates as a less modest witness, speaking not for discovery but "common decency."

Before this integration of human and professional integrity grows too comfortable, however, I will add two unsettling observations: Rudolf Ramm, a leading Nazi medical ethicist, once proclaimed, "Only a good person can be a good physician."[71] And as Rony Brauman himself caustically noted, were Auschwitz to happen today it would be called a "humanitarian crisis."[72]

Human Frontiers

We see you as money. Save the poor children, OK. God bless you. Maybe God blesses you too much.

PEN SELLER, UGANDA/KENYA BORDER, 2003

A TALE OF TWO BORDERS

On a visit to one MSF field site in Uganda, I had to travel in and out of the country to get there. The project, run by the Swiss section, was located in a relatively remote region on the Kenyan border, home to nomadic peoples considered quite wild by many in Kampala. Due to road and security concerns at the time, MSF vehicles regularly detoured through Kenya, favoring the known complications of the border over less predictable hazards. Their cars departed early, so on the appointed morning I set out in darkness to reach the meeting place in Kampala. Already the city was alive, the streets full of people walking, some returning from a long night, most setting out for the day. Children in bright uniforms begin to flow schoolward, small rivers of red, purple, green, while a few tired *boda-boda* drivers rested on their bikes in hopes of a fare. At the agency compound I waited with sleepy staff members until the clock struck 6:00 A.M. Then with admirable Swiss precision Martin, the driver, started the car and off we set with our load of supplies. As traffic thickened behind us on our drive out of the city, I noted more of the signs that make African vernacular advertising simultaneously original and poignant: "Lovesick Taxi" . . . "Classic Nursery" . . . "Good Daddy Primary School." An advertisement on the radio informed us that since "328 Ugandans a day die of malaria" the Standard Charter Bank and Chemical Company was pleased to sponsor bed nets. This first leg of the journey proved thoroughly routine, punctuated only by a brief encounter with a troop of baboons hoping for bananas. Otherwise our unmarked sedan sailed smoothly over asphalt, surrounded by ordinary vehicles and an unremarkable landscape.

The border itself proved surprisingly crowded, with long lines of trucks and people walking and cycling through the mud. A scent of business was in the air, though it was hard to determine how many of those milling and waiting had actual opportunities to match their hopes. While Martin dealt with paperwork for the supplies, I went to receive an exit stamp in my passport. A well-dressed young woman from the Ugandan ministry of tourism accosted me in the process, insisting I take a survey about my experience as visitor to the county. While I obediently complied, a race car from South Africa glided by on a carrier, along with its white-skinned crew of attendants, all sporting muscle shirts and close-cropped hair. A busload of European tourists followed close behind, their high, yellow-tented vehicle swaying as it edged around a clump of Red Cross trucks. Neither group, it appeared, planned to rate its experiences on a numeric scale.

Now officially out of Uganda, Martin and I approached Kenyan customs through a fenced strip of land. Here we parked again. Since Martin would remain in the country he dealt with customs while I waited in another line to receive a transit visa to cover the international segment of the trip. The request was an improvisation MSF had devised for this unusual supply route, wishing to minimize bureaucratic impediments and fees for a routine journey. As a staff member had warned me, the border officer behind the window looked noticeably exasperated by my request. "This is not a transit," he insisted, clearly annoyed by an appeal to that category for land travel. I assured him that my final destination indeed lay in Uganda. Several minutes of impasse ensued, before Martin arrived with documents and corroboration, after which the officer reluctantly issued the stamp with visible annoyance. He continued to frown and shake his head as he turned to the next case.

The border zone functioned as MSF's transfer point, the site where drivers met to exchange goods and passengers before returning to their respective bases. Martin and I now dutifully waited for the field vehicle to arrive and meet us, sitting together in the narrow shade of our car. By now the sun was high overhead and warm enough to drive most people under the building's overhang. Only the most intrepid among the vendors remained, hawking a remarkable array of goods large and small. On seeing my camera a large man wearing mirrored sunglasses and a dress shirt walked up and coldly warned me against taking photos. He demanded to know what was in the car, peering suspiciously through the window. Upon learning we were with MSF, however, he visibly relaxed and lost interest; this regular supply trip did not count as a threat. At long last our overdue partner vehicle pulled up. Unlike our nondescript sedan, this was a Toyota Land Cruiser, branded with full insignia and flying MSF's colors. In addition to the driver, it carried a Cameroonian doctor who had been on the project team and was now returning to the capital. Before transferring his luggage to Martin's car, he chatted amiably with our sunglassed security agent and another border guard, by now clearly on familiar terms with both. I moved my own bag the other way, and we all helped load the freight from Kampala into the Land Cruiser. Then after a series of handshakes, I climbed aboard next to the second driver, Elijah. As we traveled through the customs area officials checked our paperwork multiple times. The last guard leaned on the driver's window and asked whether we could give him some drugs, complaining that he was sick. After Elijah twice refused this request he reluctantly waved us through. The whole passage across the line had taken well over two hours.

We picked up speed as we set off through Kenya. Elijah kept an impatient eye on the road and muttered whenever traffic or a settlement slowed us; we were already behind schedule and he worried about arriving after nightfall. As the journey was all a novel adventure for me, I kept busy taking notes rather than recognizing landmarks and worrying about our time. In one town a storefront sign assured us that "the rich also cry." At another corner several boys ran beside us, thumbs up and hands out as they chanted "UN, UN!" We drove relentlessly onward, finally stopping in a major trading center to buy additional supplies. Elijah offered to leave me at a restaurant, a place where his passengers often dined, while he shopped. He looked visibly pleased when I told him I hadn't changed money and had no desire to add any delay. After a hasty snack of crackers we set off through the market vendors. His list was long, and not everything proved readily available. Moreover, our large, marked vehicle attracted attention, and people materialized with requests or propositions wherever we went. It thus felt doubly liberating to get back on our way. Soon settlements grew few and far between, and the road became rough as we wound up a plateau, a mixture of dirt tracks and dry gullies. Elijah knew the route well and navigated the obstacles with impressive ease and nonchalant speed. By now it was late afternoon and shadows grew around us. We roared by gazelle, sisal plants, and cattle herders standing with guns slung over their shoulders. Now and again we would briefly swing off our route to visit a police or other official outpost. To each we delivered a token tribute in the form of fresh newspapers from town. At one point we passed a small marker stone, half hidden behind a bush. Elijah casually waved at it, announcing that we were back in Uganda. On this lonely stretch of road there was nothing whatsoever to delay us. As the sun reddened we finally pulled into our destination, a small compound by the hospital that served as MSF's base. To Elijah's relief we had arrived before dark.

Several days later I returned to Kampala. Since MSF had rescheduled its ground transport I took a missionary plane, part of a network that quietly serves far-flung destinations across Africa. Following radio confirmation of its impending arrival, I rode out to the dirt airstrip with Elijah and the Swiss head of mission. While waiting we spotted another tourist adventure bus in the distance, trailing dust into the otherwise tranquil morning sky. At long last a distant speck appeared, grew into a small prop aircraft, lazily circled, and landed. The pilot cut the engine and clambered out to help unload several boxes of supplies, including blood. In exchange I climbed in with my bag, as well as a thick envelope destined for MSF-Switzerland's office in Kampala. Once resettled the pilot started the engine and bowed his head in prayer, asking a blessing on our flight and the larger endeavors it supported. Then we lumbered around and down the airstrip for takeoff. The plane climbed slowly, passing over the scattered thatched roofs of nearby villages and barely clearing the neighboring peaks. The small group of passengers—all members of religious institutions or aid organizations—sat quietly, one studying a well-thumbed Bible, others reading reports or dozing. The engine droned and the landscape slipped effortlessly underneath us. We passed the Nile and circled over Lake Victoria before banking toward the small grass airstrip. The journey had indeed proved quick and uneventful.

After arrival I waited at the tiny terminal building for a ride. Since I had not officially reentered Uganda after acquiring my Kenyan transit visa, I needed to acquire a proper reentry stamp to be a legal visitor. The small airfield where we had landed had no border outpost. For official evidence of arrival I had to visit the much larger international airport at Entebbe before returning to the MSF office in Kampala to deliver my package. At Entebbe I walked through the arrivals hall trying to find an appropriate official. Moving in reverse of the usual flow, I finally located a group of customs agents taking a tea break in one of the long lulls between scheduled flights. They asked me to repeat the name of the town where I had been several times, disagreeing among themselves about its location and openly bemused by my unusual request. At last deciding this was a harmless case, they issued me a stamp before returning to their tea, still shaking their heads and chuckling. Now formally back in the country, I could resume my way to the city and complete my courier duties.

RELATIVE MOTION

By recounting this travel story I seek to illustrate and complicate what movement entails at the level of practice. Borders take different forms, some of which require considerable negotiation to cross, others of which are easily ignored. On a well-paved and traveled main road, the gap between Uganda and Kenya stretches out in a complex barrier of buildings and barbed wire. To cross it you need the right story, supported by proper documents attesting to state sanction. By contrast, on a rutted dirt track in a region largely populated by nomadic groups, only an invisible line separates the two countries. People there move freely, without much regard for paperwork but with close attention to personal relations. To navigate both sorts of borders on a regular basis—like MSF does—requires a standing reserve of ingenuity. As an NGO MSF is a private entity and enjoys no diplomatic privilege. During its early, swashbuckling years the group could often rely on the legacies of colonial privilege, moral persuasion, and individual chutzpah to brush past barriers. In some settings the right passports and assumed wealth continue to permit considerable latitude. Increasingly, however, it has grown more difficult to move both people and goods. Between heightened security concerns and increased customs surveillance, international organizations now navigate less freely, even as their transport volume has greatly increased. Every experienced MSF logistician I talked to complained about the growing headaches of maintaining the group's mobility.

At the time of my trip the Swiss section of the organization was already considering whether to reorient future operations in this area to the Kenyan side of the border, a plan it subsequently followed. Neither the target diseases (visceral leishmaniasis and malaria) nor the nomadic population cared much about the border, and the tide of commerce pulled east toward Nairobi. At the time, however, the project fell into their Ugandan portfolio, and so they improvised the complex transit I have outlined. Even if a local border appeared relatively meaningless on the ground, the organization strove to remain within the boundaries of state law as defined by the capital. Thus when the Swiss administrator in Kampala cheerfully advised me to ask for a transit visa (a minor manipulation with monetary advantage), he also advised me to get a new entry stamp if I returned by air. Although he took care to note that ultimately it was my own affair in legal terms, the organization liked to maintain its regular procedures and would just as soon avoid any unnecessary problems.

An NGO such as MSF never operates in a vacuum. Even in settings of relative isolation, where the fabric of state institutions grows thin, the organization must engage with issues of political authority. Some routes stretch smoothly and between stamps and certificates, travel there feels largely routine. On others one encounters roadblocks and competing claims to power. There negotiation becomes a delicate and uncertain art, a matter of personal associations more than bureaucratic forms.[1] Neither of these alternatives is ever absolute, of course. Even in the most formal customs office it can matter who sits behind the window and what associations a given name, passport, or appearance might carry. Rules grow more or less flexible in their application according to a calculus of influence, will, and feeling. Conversely, even in the absence of state authority individuals can appeal to distant norms. A sense of "proper" procedure often lingers, like a half-forgotten rock signaling a borderline. But in any event the movement of people and things remains a profoundly public matter.

A traveling vehicle is also a container, the contents of which interest those it passes. Even when empty of cargo, the transport itself constitutes a treasure house of parts, fuel, and the potential for mobility. Large field vehicles incite particular interest, both because they are usually well marked with insignia and often flags, and because they often ply areas where travel is difficult. Like sailing ships or caravan camels, MSF's Land Cruisers lumber along through a relative void. To those who walk long roads by foot, they represent a point of stark contrast and a tantalizing potential resource. Even at its most crowded, people wedged in and spilling beyond the hard seats, MSF's mode of transport appears luxurious next to overloaded trucks or buses. Only the cars of less austere organizations—tinted windows rolled tight to seal in conditioned air—surpass its alluring possibilities. The mission teams I encountered would field regular requests for transport, most of which they denied out of concern for precedent and insurance. Vehicles were restricted to staff, patients, and authorized visitors. Their doors thus marked another border of sorts, a boundary that some crossed easily on a daily basis and others only when in a state of distress. In moments of medical concern teams bundled patients in, sometimes with accompanying caregivers. Those fortunate enough to regain their health, however, usually had to find their own way home.

MSF's field teams enjoyed permanent residence in this land of transport. They routinely used the vehicles for work and occasionally commandeered them for play. While on duty, and sometimes when not, they wore a T-shirt uniform featuring the organization's name and logo. Thus dressed they were readily identifiable, even to those who might not know them as individuals. They clearly belonged inside the vehicle. Who, then, qualified to become a member of the staff, to don the uniform and travel in style? MSF's project personnel included two groups. The smaller included foreigners of every stripe, collectively categorized as "expatriates" or "expats." The larger was comprised of Ugandans, considered "national staff" because they worked in their country of residence. Not all members of this second group were local in terms of a given project site; professionals in particular tended to have spent time in more urban contexts. None, however, had crossed a national boundary, and thus the organization considered them to be "at home." Within these two groupings a mix of different factors explained individual trajectories to a seat in the vehicle: qualifications, skills, experience, connections, and of course sheer availability of both person and seat. The most essential requirement for becoming and remaining a team member, however, was deceptively simple and yet pregnant with unexamined assumptions. To participate in a mission one had to be moveable, in both a social and geographic sense. Ultimately the person who best fit MSF's shirt was a being who could live a mobile life.

Relative mobility reveals a set of classically social as well as natural facts. Beyond questions of bodily health and psychological stability—neither insignificant in this context—a capacity to move involves other considerations. Could one afford to be absent, away from relatives and free of dependents? Could one live within the constraints of a modest stipend? Conversely, if receiving a payment that appeared a wage rather than a sacrifice, could one demonstrate the proper humanitarian motivations? Would pursuing humanitarianism as a career alter its alchemy of passion? Could one have stable relationships and children while constantly traveling? What if one was left aging and alone after a life of travel? Both expats and national staff faced dilemmas of attachment and detachment. What were the effects of moving alongside crisis when it came to fulfilling the terms of a "normal" life?

Such questions reveal the uncertain edges of the modern figure of the liberal individual. Common to much political and economic theory, where it thrives in a happy medium of abstraction, this figure assumes that humans operate as autonomous agents. Each unique subject makes independent choices through time and thereby pursues an individual career. If routinely presupposed in professional life, the individualist vision encounters regular turbulence in practice. This is particularly true when displacement reveals the connective tissue of human lives—perhaps nowhere more so than in the operation of nonprofit, voluntary organizations. When work involves values beyond labor, an economy of motion openly confronts economies of morality and affect. If acting in the name of an altruistic cause, one should not display the "selfishness" of personal interest or desire beyond a minimum of need. Yet in a world increasingly configured around consumption and individuated responsibility for the care of family members and the self, it is not easy to be a full-time volunteer. This is particularly true if coming from a context of poverty.

For the remainder of this chapter I will illustrate this point by exploring the relative motion of people through this global organization. I seek to outline MSF's mobile habits and their tensions. My goal is as much one of disruption as explanation, a recognition that even in its most mundane operations, MSF faces issues that resist easy solution.

"IN MY FORMER LIFE I WAS AN UNSHAVEN, CIGARETTE-SMOKING FRENCHMAN"

Like many nongovernmental organizations MSF emerged in the heat of a particular moment. The group's founders gave little thought to the future, assuming conditions would mirror their present. Because their vision emphasized professionals passionately volunteering for a part-time cause, the larger trajectory of an individual life played little role in their imaginations.[2] A few early members may have crossed the bounds of middle age but their collective sensibility was proudly young at heart and unfettered by family ties or social obligations. Moreover, at the time the medical profession largely remained the preserve of men. The women who made their way into emergency adventures were exceptions who mastered the rule; although accepted, no one expected them to be there. Despite the upheaval of decolonization, this was likewise an emphatically French and, later, European initiative, one that envisioned volunteers who traveled from metropolitan centers to serve the suffering, usually in former colonies. The possibility of other trajectories, and the implications of "volunteering" across unequal economies, simply did not arise.

Certainly in 1971 no one gave much heed to issues of retirement, or of placing couples—let alone children—in the field. Nor did they consider the inequities of highly qualified individuals facing limited prospects in their home country, or the problem of what to pay them if they expatriated. Instead MSF quickly produced a stereotype of its own self-image, one widely disseminated through other organizations. The essential *médecin sans frontières* was a cowboy doctor, tireless when fueled by alcohol, coffee, and tobacco, fiercely independent and loudly arrogant. Like most stereotypes, this one played on recognizable elements, and in this case one could find historical examples that came close to fulfilling the caricature. That said, the image largely distorts subsequent reality: in statistical terms MSF is no longer a collectivity of doctors, or an essentially masculine pursuit, or even really European.[3] Nonetheless, such a reputation dies hard; as an Asian American former volunteer once commented sardonically to me, surely in her former life she had been "an unshaven, cigarette-smoking Frenchman."

By the time I began my research this phantom past appeared largely in jokes and the memories of older veterans. However, it also lingered deep in the basic structure of the organization and its original emphasis on emergency. MSF's assumption at the outset was that its volunteers would be eagerly and effortlessly mobile. Unencumbered by social obligations at home, the medical humanitarian should likewise acquire few in the field, living lightly on the landscape and always ready to leave once urgency passed. The work might demand deep human passion and fundamental empathy, but its original form would permit few sustained engagements or long-term commitments. In this regard the colonial antecedent of such emergency aid work lay as much in the explorer or crusading adventurer as in the medical missionary. MSF's project sites represented temporary outposts— encampments rather than homesteads—and their relations with the surroundings potentially intense but categorically short-lived. Given such emphasis on transience in MSF's initial vision, it comes as no surprise that the strongest sense of family would emerge within the organization itself, amid its brotherhood of medical arms. In the casual classification of conversation, people became "MSF" or "not-MSF" and were further identified, if necessary, by their primary section lineage or loyalties. At the same time the emergency ethos distinguished sharply between mobile volunteers (whose presence would only last for the duration of the crisis) and the local population. Beyond the solidarity of their concerns and resources, the volunteers had little attachment to place or history. In conditions of conflict, moreover, they might claim greater freedom of movement and access precisely because they had no ties. Although MSF restructured itself as it grew, paying its volunteers a modest stipend and increasing professional standards, it retained a fundamental commitment to placing mobile personnel in the field.

At the same time, the organization's actual practice had evolved in ways that made matters of human connection and difference harder to ignore. MSF's missions now spanned a range of health issues beyond emergency care in refugee camps. Its volunteer staff included citizens of many countries, some retired and some with children. Many were women, a fact now registered in images used for public appeals, and quite a few were from nonmedical backgrounds. Some increasingly approached humanitarian work as a career in itself, bolstered by institutionalized training programs, degrees, and certificates. One could even chart a professional trajectory across organizations, moving from a shoestring startup to an established player like MSF and eventually graduating to the relative comfort of the Red Cross or UN agencies, with their better pay and benefits. Alternatively, one might remain within the larger MSF ensemble, shifting between sections and roles while accruing greater responsibility. If maintaining personal relationships or raising children, then those commitments grew increasingly significant when determining which posts to accept or pursue. Even for male doctors—the most direct inheritors of the original volunteer vision—continued involvement in humanitarian medicine could involve career decisions and the relative cost of living in their home country, alternatively casting an MSF post as a sacrifice or an opportunity.

The growth of MSF's operational capacity also meant that the group increasingly relied on local personnel for its labor needs. Recruited as employees rather than volunteers, these staff pursued their own career trajectories, often working for one aid organization after another. In settings with limited alternative forms of employment, such as a refugee camp, NGO positions represented the prospect of steady pay, at least while the project lasted. Although vital to day-to-day operations at mission sites, local support staff remained relatively invisible in the group's public profile. Whereas the international participants enjoyed ample media attention, their local counterparts hardly figured in the moral imagination surrounding this medical version of humanitarianism. This absence was not entirely surprising given MSF's historical and nominal focus on biomedical doctors and its moral calling to operate *sans frontières*. The respective official designations of the two groups as "national" and "expatriate" reflected the taxonomic power of the nation-state within this global ethic: only those who had crossed a national boundary could appear to be "without borders." By and large, staff hired locally filled support roles, serving as drivers, cooks, watchmen, interpreters, and assistants of all sorts. They were considered employees rather than volunteers, working as much for pay as out of moral commitment. Nonetheless, with MSF's metamorphosis into a relatively large and wealthy NGO, the sheer number of national staff proved increasingly hard to ignore. When noted, it often incited anxieties both inside and outside the organization about colonial legacies. If not always strictly accurate, these references reflected enough of a larger truth to prove discomforting.[4]

Most national staff remained relatively fixed in position, their contracts extending only through the duration of the project. On some occasions, however, local posts might lead to advancement within the organization. In MSF's case ascension required acquiring "expatriate" status though displacement to another country. To achieve this metamorphosis a national staff member had to demonstrate not only technical skills and a willingness to move, but also proper motivation. In MSF's moral sensibility, a humanitarian should appear a volunteer, not a mercenary. Human solidarity in the face of suffering, after all, was MSF's founding ethical principle. The fact that the organization had grown into a de facto employer of thousands worldwide was awkward enough. The possibility that someone might view it as a means to personal gain threatened its fundamental principles. Had MSF simply become a part of the charity business, shedding any pretext of its rebellious ethos? On the other hand, the organization's adherents were increasingly sensitive to the degree to which they replicated existing double standards, with privileged volunteers from rich countries directing less fortunate workers in poor countries. Had MSF simply devolved into a neocolonial enterprise? If so, how might it might it achieve "decolonization"?

THE GRAVITY OF LOCAL ATTACHMENT

My first visit to an MSF field site, as it happened, occurred entirely in the company of national staff. The project, the tail end of a long-running venture to combat sleeping sickness in the north of Uganda, had acquired research objectives that outlived its clinical justification. By the time I arrived, MSF's epidemiological subsidiary, Epicentre, was in charge and had relegated the remaining data collection to a Ugandan nurse and her driver, supported by a team of field assistants.

As the only non-Ugandan in the vehicle, I attracted the shouts of children ("Muzungu! Muzungu!") when we drove through remote hamlets, while the curious gaze of their elders was mixed with expectation: surely the white man in the white car would be in charge. The team's actual leader was Grace, an energetic Ugandan nurse who stoically negotiated the tensions of being a younger woman instructing older men. Originally from the area, she was intimately familiar with local languages and regional culture, a fact that she found a mixed blessing. She was glad at least to be working one district over from where most of her kin and classmates resided. Indeed, she eventually confided that her goal was one day to work for an NGO elsewhere—*anywhere* that was not a rural hospital in northwestern Uganda—since she found there were problems with operating locally: "I know the people here and they know me. They expect me to be just like them and to listen to their problems. At the same time the NGO wants you to perform a certain way. In town there would be nurses who were ahead of me; if I were in charge of them they wouldn't like it. It's much easier if you're from somewhere else and they don't know you."[5]

At first it had been difficult for Grace to take control of the remaining program. The staff, used to international leadership, failed to show up on time and ignored direction, to the extent that one driver had to be fired. By now she had garnered sufficient respect to exert authority but still found it a constant effort. Following this explanation I better understood her manner in wards and public settings like screenings, a forceful presence that I—used to a consumer-oriented model of health care, alternately obsequious or indifferent—found startlingly authoritarian. She spoke in commanding tones and frequently in English, the national language of education. Her dress was invariably "smart" in the British idiom. Like many Ugandans employed by MSF and other NGOS in positions of professional responsibility, she looked the part, in marked contrast to the casual camping aesthetic favored by international volunteers.

The driver—Mohammed the tire changer—had fewer qualms about his occupation or local status. Older than Grace, he remembered the Amin years fondly. After the fall of the regime he joined the exodus to Zaire (now the Democratic Republic of the Congo), where he translated his racing experience into another living behind the wheel, driving trucks and working for a large landowner. With the end of the Mobutu dictatorship he returned to Uganda, where he found a job as a replacement driver for MSF before moving to his present position. A big man with a self-assured manner, Mohammed easily filled the larger ambassadorial and guardian roles of his position. Fluent in multiple languages, he could gather information along with any necessities when we passed a small market outpost, or banter with patients and their relatives. He could also out-shout a woman who belligerently demanded a ride or simply lean protectively against the vehicle, keeping the overly inquisitive at a distance. He clearly enjoyed the authority that came with the driver's seat.

Nonetheless, Mohammed did have ambitions, as well as reservations about his current position. He outlined some to me one night over dinner in one of the two worn bars in town. Money was a constant concern; his five children, living in the regional center, stretched his salary thin. Being stationed in his home district, he no longer received a lunch allowance since the project had dwindled into its research phase, a fact that struck him as a significant injustice.[6] He was still driving long distances, after all. Did they expect him to drive home for lunch? He would happily work for MSF elsewhere, particularly back in the Congo. Mohammed doubted the organization would send him, however, as crossing the border in a professional capacity would reclassify him as a more expensive expatriate. He would be glad to travel further if the opportunity arose ("I'm a man of all weathers!" he proudly proclaimed). There had been one possibility to travel to New York, but the visa had not come through in time. His real dream, he confessed, was to work someplace like the United States, where he had heard a trucking company might pay as much as $5,000 a month. With such a sum he could purchase a small business like the one where we sat. Nothing special, perhaps, but an assurance for his future, a buffer against the prospect of old age.

Although both impressed me as exceptional individuals, neither Grace nor Mohammed was atypical of MSF's national staff. The conditions of relative autonomy they enjoyed hardly relieved the burden of expectations surrounding them. Indeed, in Grace's case it sometimes made her job harder. I later learned that she preferred not to have a key to the safe at the main office when back in the main town, as it only exposed her to potential demands and suspicions. Money was a continued source of tension from every direction. Another veteran driver told me how when he first started working for NGOs, some colleagues would habitually funnel off money at every refueling, even submitting receipts for quantities beyond the fuel tank's capacity. Now that MSF tracked all vehicle mileage religiously such irregular enterprise had vanished, to this individual's great relief. Suspicion, he feared, would have fallen indiscriminately on all of them.

Bernard, the expatriate director of MSF's garage in Kampala, recounted similar stories of unauthorized entrepreneurship. On one notorious occasion an employee for another aid organization had actually run a private bank with the group's funds, loaning them out at high interest. For years there had been a lucrative trade in used vehicles, and even now Bernard had to consider carefully how to sell or give away used parts, balancing things out so that no one felt slighted. A Frenchman enjoying an unusually long posting, he had nursed the workshop for years, felt deeply attached to Uganda, and held strong views about the need to understand a locale and its economy. He regularly trained mechanics who subsequently left for higher-paying jobs in commercial garages. He did not blame them, but rather advocated paying motivational bonuses to encourage and reward hard work. This suggestion, however, encountered resistance from his superiors, who felt it went against MSF's volunteer ethos. "Mechanics aren't here for humanitarianism," Bernard said brusquely. "They're here to make a living." Although passionately loyal to MSF as an organization, he disagreed with many of the group's employment policies, which he found willfully naive. Treating everyone equally only worked if conditions were equal; otherwise it simply distorted reality. In the past someone like Mohammed might quietly receive a posting in the Congo without being designated an expat. Now such a move would require raising his salary far beyond that of any of his peers. In Bernard's view individual good fortune would only inspire jealousy while further distorting the local economy and diverting funds from where they really should be directed. Noting that one former NGO "volunteer" had managed to build a three-story house in the city, he favored recognizing a scale between national economies. "A Ugandan in China—now that would be an expat!" he proclaimed. "He would deserve $1,000 a month. Or a doctor who's studied in Europe, who has skills . . . but a Ugandan driver in the Congo?" He shook his head.

Bernard's views about the crucial line of motivation dividing national and expatriate staff found an echo in an incident involving a Uganda nutritional project in 2006. When national medical staff at a therapeutic feeding center for malnourished children demanded better wages, MSF refused. The head of the Dutch mission wrote them a formal response, stating, "I would wish that MSF is not seen as an employer but rather as a movement and a nonprofit organization where we together as a team have a wish to assist others who are disadvantaged, living in distress, lacking a perspective."[7] When the staff subsequently went on strike, she fired them. As she later described the event to me:

> We had to terminate fifteen staff members. They were upset about conditions and went on strike. That was OK, but they actually let children die and threatened those who wanted to work. Now we have to refill all those positions, finding new clinical officers and counselors. MSF is looking at itself more critically as an employer. On a daily basis we confront corruption, theft, and threats. That makes it more difficult to empower national staff. It's especially hard in Uganda because national staff has all the training and ability you could ask for. . . . The main difficulty is having a trusting relationship.[8]

The key to such a trusting relationship, the administrator indicated, lay in a common commitment to humanitarian ideals. Providing care to suffering people should take precedence over any other motivations. When the strikers had reportedly allowed children to die, they had broken with MSF's fundamental rationale.

Demonstrating proper humanitarian commitment, then, came most naturally to those who could occupy the status of volunteers. "The real MSF," one veteran once said to me, "is people who give a lot to MSF and the mission and who don't expect a lot." He was speaking generally, not about national staff in particular. But differing economic facts of employment disrupted such a moral vision. To be a true member of the group one had to demonstrate passion, devotion, selflessness, and a rebellious spirit—all driven by a concern for others, not self-interest. Such dedication was doubly difficult for national staff to demonstrate, weighed down as they were by their local connections.

THE UNBEARABLE LIGHTNESS OF EXPATS

The only problem with MSF is the muzungus *[foreigners].*

JOKE AMONG NATIONAL STAFF IN UGANDA, RELATED BY AN EXPATRIATE

Beyond the sleeping sickness project, expatriates figured prominently in the MSF programs I subsequently visited. If outnumbered by their local colleagues, they occupied core positions in every project team; whether the mission responded to an emergency or a slower form of crisis, the organizational structure remained resolutely temporary. When not on duty the expats commonly congregated at the residence they collectively shared. Although hardly opulent when compared to some other agency outposts, these compounds were certainly at the higher end of any local comfort scale, with solid walls and a roof. The furniture ranged from monastic simplicity to flea market whimsy and included communal items such as hammocks or a sofa. If located in a settlement then there was usually more of it, as well as some means to play music and watch entertainment. The volunteers ate together and often spent what free time they had socializing with each other, collectively or in small groups. Personal property varied but dress was invariably casual, starting with the field uniform of white T-shirts featuring the organization's logo.

Such details acquire greater significance when placed in relation to MSF's larger problem of fostering a temporary, mobile form of community. As a guidebook issued by MSF-France's human resources department suggests, "In the particular context of missions, behavior that would normally seem insignificant can in fact have consequences for the unity of the group and how the team functions."[9] Volunteers therefore should be considerate when it came to such habits as smoking, playing music, shopping, and venturing out on the weekends. They should also watch their choice of language, for while it might be normal to lapse into a native tongue after a day of laboring in a foreign one, it remained imperative that every member of the group feel included in the team. The guide likewise encouraged rest and recuperation in order to stay "in good physical and mental shape"—observing time off on weekends and taking a week away every three or four months, preferably in country so as to learn more about the mission setting. At the same time, volunteers should keep mission objectives in mind and minimize contact with family and friends at home, effectively cutting "the 'umbilical' telephone/internet cord." Instead the goal was "to get to know and understand the values of the people around you," not only to ensure a more fulfilling personal experience, but also to further the mission and its security. Good relations with local people often proved crucial in a crisis, the booklet noted, and required adapting individual behavior to the surrounding environment.[10]

The concern about local knowledge expressed in the guidebook reflected a growing realization of cultural errors present and past. Like other international NGOs the group had weathered its share of minor as well as major embarrassments, recounted in conversation by people inside and outside the group with either regret or glee. As a consequence MSF had produced a longer line of briefing documents, such as one from the 1990s I found in MSF's New York office offering advice to American volunteers departing for Africa (under women's dresses: "something your grandmother likes!"). Two additional developments also affected the connection between expats and their field environment. Changes in communications technology meant that teams were now far less isolated than they had been in the past. Whereas a posting had once meant a year over the horizon, people now expected computer and phone links, both to the organization and to their nearest and dearest. As the head of logistics at MSF's Brussels office told me in 2003: "The new generation of volunteers in Europe is used to having constant connection to GSM [mobile phones], email, and so forth and aren't always happy to have to go through a communal communication system. We have to explain again and again that the picture from Grandma is too large and can become a problem."

The larger communications problem was not limited to clogged lines (significant as that could be) or even disconnection from the locale itself. It could also affect the operation of a mission itself. As he subsequently observed, "With the radio system you get one message, from the head of mission. With mobile phones you get multiple messages, multiple updates, multiple chains that spread quickly and can create confusion." Along with new technology, the growth of both MSF and the general humanitarian milieu had produced a daunting array of protocols and restrictions. Many reflected heightened anxieties over security and consequently restricted the movement of expat staff in settings where they might be vulnerable to attack or kidnapping. As a result the organization began to worry anew about the connection of its field teams to their locale.

The various tensions related to expat disconnection converged into the term *proximity*. The Dutch section held a workshop on the theme in 2002, which included a quiz featuring questions like "How much do tomatoes cost at the local market?" and "Who is the most popular local musician in the country?" Most members of the group with whom I discussed the term—even in Holland—quickly pointed out its awkward fit with experiential reality. As one noted, proximity was surely more a relational challenge than a defined thing: "In Sudan you are an extraterrestrial, what to do with them? Go to a bar?" Another called the term "jargonizing and lexicalizing," dismissively suggesting, "What it really means is being a fucking human being." To emphasize his point he told me a joke about the international aid worker who finally climbs out of a hulking, air-conditioned vehicle, prompting one local to comment to another, "I didn't know those people had legs." In contrast, this veteran made a point of taking time to talk to people in and outside of his work, sharing pictures of his own life and family so that communication would be a two-way street. Such gestures might hardly compensate for inequality, but at least they recognized potential exchange. Older members of all sections tended to rail against bureaucracy and new security concerns, fondly recalling the years of improvisation and casually taking local transport. Relative isolation from headquarters had fostered both independence and greater interaction with the locale.

Clumsy as the term *proximity* might be, it named a fundamental problem for any humanitarian organization that prized mobility. How to demonstrate common human feeling—let alone achieve any sort of solidarity—when people were always coming and going? Compared to national staff, expat members of MSF floated free. They would arrive in a flurry of eager energy and new ideas, carrying a delicate web of connections beyond the horizon. They lived their lives only partly in place, and then they were gone like butterflies, leaving behind a thin residue of artifacts and memories. Their departure might be quietly mourned or celebrated by those who remained behind (who in either case invariably marked the occasion with a ritual party). But as projects opened and closed they built few monuments or lasting legacies in the countries where they worked. Moreover, their foreign status partly insulated them from the outcome of both local politics and individual risk; in the event of direct threat or personal emergency they would be evacuated.

Mobility also held consequences for the flow of knowledge within the organization. The state of disconnection that allowed expats to stand strategically outside local alliances also assured a degree of ignorance about the settings in which they operated. Beyond a rapid briefing, few arrived equipped with much historical background on a project, and fewer still spoke anything other than international languages. This was hardly a personal failing; in a place like Uganda, with mutually unintelligible vernaculars at different project sites, the difficulty of working across even one country grew abundantly clear. However, in practice it placed a premium on translation and the mediating skills of local (and not just national) staff. The steady stream of new expats likewise assured a need for constant orientation. While effectively guarding against stasis and ossification, the turnover rate also assured an overabundance of new initiatives. As Bernard observed, "The biggest problem is new expats: each one wants to change everything. Either the house has to be changed, or the office, or some procedure." Consequently he, like the national staff, greeted the new arrivals with some trepidation ("It's like the lottery, you never win" went one joke). Some personalities were wonderful, others disastrous, but all had ideas. The French head of mission at the time recognized this problem of overpollination and sought to alleviate it by involving the national team more in turnover and briefings. "They have to adapt themselves to us and that is not very good," she noted. "Rather the reverse would be better, but it's not always easy to achieve."[11] Indeed, in most meetings I observed that expats spoke freely, whereas national staff rarely said a word unless directly queried.

The problem of proximity only grew more acute as MSF expanded its portfolio beyond emergency missions. Whereas emergency medicine and surgery emphasized speed and distanced technique, other forms of medical care presumed a slower and deeper relationship between doctor and patient. Treating a chronic condition such as HIV/AIDS required more stability and intimacy than responding to a gunshot wound. In such cases the mediating role played by members of the national staff took on new importance; counselors and clinical officers equipped with requisite language skills and a greater measure of cultural familiarity shouldered much of the work. As with emergencies, recruitment of personnel who combined professional certification with true local knowledge, however, was not always simple.[12]

Longer-term missions also permitted greater variation within expat life. Even as amplified technology and heightened security concerns further distanced the expatriate experience, some volunteers developed attachments to particular countries, returning for another tour with a different section or taking a job with another organization to remain in place. A few married, acquiring the geographic obligations of kin ties. A larger number fostered less formal alliances, not all centered on sexual desire. Perhaps the most poignant I observed took the form of quietly paying school fees for individual Ugandan children. This last gesture—a hallmark of particularistic charity rather than rebellious humanitarianism—at least offered the solace of human connection.

DISCOVERING GENDER AND AGE

The significance of basic forms of human difference grew more apparent as the pool of MSF's recruits broadened. Somewhat in spite of itself, the organization slowly recognized that gender and age might matter. By the start of its fourth decade the group counted many more women within the ranks of its volunteers. Informal estimates put doctors and administrative personnel at around gender parity, with female nurses outnumbering their male counterparts. Women even appeared in logistics posts, long a bastion of the most grizzled male volunteers. This partly reflected a larger generational shift. In place of the working-class adventurer who might wander into a mission while, say, riding a motorcycle across Africa and subsequently display a talent for improvised repairs, the new breed of logistician could wave a résumé full of certified training. The new logs conceived of themselves as professionals choosing a career path from among many options. Nothing, however, disrupted the logistics stereotype more directly than the appearance of female technicians. The two women I met performing this role in the field both came from backgrounds in engineering and business. Each had decided to take a break from a conventionally successful career to pursue something more "meaningful"; whether as sabbatical or redirection remained unclear. Their mere presence, however, provided a sharp contrast to the machismo associated with logistics.

The situation among the national staff, however, remained far less fluid in terms of gender. Hired as local employees, they filled established available slots just as they would elsewhere in the regional labor market. Men served as drivers and guards; women cooked and cleaned. Among those playing more professional

roles, gender varied to a greater degree. I met both male and female administrators and medical personnel, although women were more commonly nurses than
doctors or clinical officers. For certain posts such as counseling, gender became a
factor in selection; MSF maintained the standard therapeutic logic that women or
girls might respond better when discussing sensitive issues with another woman.
Informal patronage might at times promote exceptional individuals (Grace's
trajectory, outlined above, owed something to support from expats, including
women in leadership positions). However, there was no coordinated policy to alter
gender roles directly at any field site. Rather than seeking to promote social
change, the organization simply evolved through its milieu.

MSF's discovery of gender was hardly quick or spontaneous. One could trace
a line of exception stretching back to the group's early days, where a few women
did appear among the men. However, senior women I queried recalled the 1990s
as a time of real transition, when norms began to alter through the sheer mass of
accumulated numbers. The change was uneven across the organization. Although
the French could point to prominent pioneers, other sections surpassed them
when it came to women in leadership roles. Francesca, an Italian nurse who had
worked for several sections before filling a post for MSF-Switzerland in Uganda,
described the group's shifting dynamics in the following way in 2003:

> Gender was a big issue; for a long time you wouldn't speak about it or you'd be la-
> beled feminist. But I think that's finally over. . . . People with children are an issue.
> Women have kids; the question is, can you manage both? The field does have con-
> straints. In some ways having a child here [in Kampala] is much easier than at
> home, as it's easy to get assistance. Headquarters is different. How many young
> mothers come back from pregnancy leave? You have to work 20 hours a day, smoke,
> and drink coffee through the weekend to live up to the image. Plus there's breast-
> feeding and all that. There's no clear better or worse, but it wouldn't be true to say
> it's not an issue . . . Even our medical approach has begun to recognize gender. With
> gender people think of women. That's no surprise, but it annoys me when people
> think it's a women's issue that people are victims of horrible abuse, AIDS, rape, and
> so on. And then in a country like this you have high maternal mortality. It's not
> seen as an emergency, but for me that's an emergency too.

Francesca had spent time as a single mother and was acutely aware of the difference it had made to her mobility. Now part of a happy couple with another MSF
volunteer, she considered future postings with an eye for potential joint appointments in more child-friendly environments. Outspoken and opinionated, she also
expressed strong commitment to initiatives focusing on gender violence and
longer-term, disease-specific projects, hoping that the NGO would continue to
expand its work in those directions.

Francesca's interests were far from idiosyncratic. The organization's gradual
feminization coincided with a dawning recognition that its patients might also be

differentiated by gender and that associated physical and psychological suffering could constitute a legitimate medical concern. A 2005 issue of MSF-France's
house journal *Messages* included reflections on the group's changing attitudes
toward pain as well as sexual violence and abortion. Once viewed as something
of a luxury and an afterthought, pain management had transformed into a part
of standard procedure "that no one was against." The fact that as recently as
2000 the group had dispatched only ten ampoules of morphine to the field now
appeared scandalous, particularly next to the fact that a woman in France
would receive up to six ampoules following a Caesarian delivery. Meanwhile
sexual violence had emerged as a matter of medical responsibility as well as
personal commitment for doctors certifying its physical reality.[13] Likewise abortion now appeared a legitimate if ever troubling concern. The subject of one
article summarized this change in response to her interviewer's query: "Before,
we did not perform abortions. We did not listen to women's requests, we did not
consider it a medical priority and did not provide the means to carry out the intervention. When I was on my first mission in Afghanistan even I, an obstetrician/
gynaecologist, did not give the issue any thought. Everything changed when we
started to address the specific issue of women's health and medical staff were faced
with cases where abortion was an integral part of the healthcare to be provided
(rape, fistula . . .)."[14]

Around poles of reproduction and violence, gender grew visible at both ends
of the medical encounter. From the perspective of a humanitarian organization,
the lives of caregiver and patient alike now extended beyond isolated bodies.

Francesca's family situation was far from unique. While in Uganda I met other
couples with children, with one or both parents working for MSF. Most were
based in Kampala, though for a period a pair of French doctors ran the organization's HIV/AIDS program together in a regional town. By and large these families
lived far more modestly than foreign aid personnel who received international
salaries but well above the standard of the majority of Ugandans. They faced continuing issues of proximity through questions of childcare and, as their children
grew, education. What school to select? In what language? How long could—or
should—they maintain a nomadic lifestyle? MSF's tradition of continued mobility
limited the period they could spend in any one setting. At the same time their
range of destinations remained restricted. Both organizational policy and parental choice opposed bringing children on an emergency mission; only relatively
stable field settings were a possibility. In this sense Francesca's interest in longer-
term projects fit with her parental status.

Other factors of human difference also mattered when it came to placement.
The head of the French section's mission in Uganda (herself a woman) noted that
gender and citizenship could also play a role under conditions of heightened risk
for the volunteer and for the team in general. In crisis zones like Sierra Leone and

Afghanistan, for example, the organization only sent women who had extensive field experience (those "known to be OK"), otherwise favoring men. Following September 11, 2001, it appeared riskier to include Americans on teams operating in Islamic parts of the world. As a consequence many ended up in calmer destinations like Uganda. In general the organization faced an experience deficit; while regularly receiving many times the number of new applicants that it could accept, retaining proven veterans was more of a problem. People burned out or moved on.

Questions of the future weighed heavily even on those expats without children. Would aid work grow into a career, not simply a passion? And if so, would MSF be the best venue in which to pursue it? After acquiring experience as a volunteer, adherents could advance to a range of coordination posts as salaried employees. These positions were generally not highly paid—a moderate increase from the expat volunteer's stipend—and all were held on a term basis. Although details varied across the wider organization, MSF prided itself on retaining a modest salary ratio (the president of the French section, for example, earned only three times as much as the lowest-paid employee). As a consequence some people would eventually move to other organizations that offered better pay and benefits. Discussing the topic in 2003, the communications director of MSF-France observed dryly that the group "should send bills to WHO, ICRC, UNICEF, and so on, for all the training we do." The problem of retention involved more than simply money, however; it also required a commitment to aid work beyond youthful adventure. In a generational compensation of sorts, the organization had begun to receive older recruits, including youthful retirees and inquisitive individuals whose children had grown. While they might not resolve problems of continuity and institutional memory, they introduced a different dynamic in team composition.

During the course of its fourth decade, MSF-France also started to celebrate its own first retirements. When people began to age they also began to worry more about job benefits and the prospect of living on a pension. The coordinator of a Swiss mission put it bluntly: "What happens when you arrive at 60 with kids and nothing? What am I supposed to do then? Kill myself?" A cartoon in a 2001 issue of MSF-Belgium's journal *Contact* reflected a similar anxiety, portraying a couple in the year 2025, walking past a homeless MSF veteran begging outside a metro station. An accompanying image showed a figure reading an applicant's curriculum vitae and commenting, "Make a career out of MSF? Possible, but not *at* MSF." The background featured portraits of the surprising number of luminaries like Kouchner who had left the group to pursue political careers.[15] These concerns might appear exaggerated in the context of European welfare states. Nonetheless they highlight the fact that a humanitarian organization is hardly an ordinary employer and that the legacy of rebellion included little consideration of old age. Moreover, as MSF welcomed recruits from an ever-widening circle beyond Europe, the larger problem of benefits and care only grew more pressing. In some cases volunteers also faced the prospect of their own medical or psychological treatment well before retirement. Others found themselves responsible for older relatives, which likewise affected their priorities and limited their movement.

Staying with the organization took more than just the right humanitarian spirit; it also required an ability to accept a lifetime of displacement.[16] Jacques, a field coordinator in Uganda for MSF-Spain originally from Canada, put it to me eloquently in 2006:

> Only in MSF did I not feel like a stranger or, to use my own term, an extraterrestrial. I feel at home here. So it's not about reintegrating, but integrating. My family is not so much biological as one I've constructed around me. They're scattered all over the world, and I may only see them every few years. But they're closer to me than people in my own city. What I fear the most is trying to go back to Quebec to reintegrate, so to speak. But I don't feel trapped in MSF. Even if I'm not earning much, I don't feel the need to go outside of MSF. I'm constantly arguing with one of my friends, she's a social worker, who says MSF is not real life. But I ask, what is real life? We are always changing, but we are always in places of transition. I don't feel labeled as strange here. I am a foreigner, but not a stranger. In MSF the best thing I know is how to lead a team. Not because I am charismatic or have ambition to become a head of mission or director general. But I have found my place as a field coordinator. I work with people to solve problems, to build teams. I begin with what others abandon, feel comfortable where others do not. In fuzzy situations, crisis situations, I feel comfortable. In places that are ordered I have no place.

Not all shared Jacques's equanimity in embracing a state of perpetual crisis. Many of the veterans I talked to complained about the life of suitcases and short-term abodes. A head of the Dutch mission in Uganda, Isolda, expressed a more general concern in 2004:

> I have given up my life, the last few years of my life. Is that a good thing for me? If not then I wouldn't feel satisfied. We're asking for super people: highly professional and highly voluntary. Those two things are almost inherently [mutually] exclusive. We want to increase retention while we want to decrease operation costs. We're not paying enough attention to why people stay. Some do because they have no other life. It can become a prison . . . if it does, how do you help them keep their mental health? But it becomes emotional blackmail. . . . If you are the person with the right motivations it's impossible . . . to leave if there's no one else. You're better than nothing. That puts you in a terrible position. . . . For me that's the biggest dilemma of the organization: asking the impossible of people. Every now and then life comes back to you. I haven't called my friends in over six months. So then I think, I'd better get out of this before I get in too deep. You have to know when the moment is to step out, or you'll be lost, a lost cause for MSF and for yourself.

Originally from Spain and fluent in multiple languages, Isolda wandered into MSF from a background studying politics. Despite her continuing commitment to the humanitarian cause, after her fifth mission she felt herself to be at a cross-roads. Would this become her life? The prospect gave her pause.[17]

Medical personnel faced a similar choice, if amid different considerations. A senior doctor within MSF-France told me about having made a conscious decision to stay with humanitarian medicine in the late 1980s, realizing that he was committing to different diseases and forms of specialization than would be the case in a European suburb. Although he had gone on to leave a significant mark on the organization, it was the "end of his professional life in France." Isolda reached a similar conclusion from the opposite perspective when recalling the advantages of her own experience:

> The doctor on my mission is bored with scabies and doesn't want to go to Iraq. It's a medical organization, but in many ways the nonmedics are driving things. A doctor in the West can't afford to spend a whole life in MSF. Nonmedical people can. . . . With ten years of experience in foreign affairs, management skills, I'm not doing my career a disservice by staying in MSF. For doctors it's different. Other than AIDS work they aren't getting anything professionally useful out of it. At the same time, it's harder for us nonmedical people to get into MSF.

Although doctors continued to fill the top ceremonial posts across the organization and medical schools produced a surplus of fresh recruits with reliable regularity, the organization had begun to worry that it might lose its distinctive profile.[18] In professional terms the organization offered doctors and surgeons from wealthy countries a vivid and highly moralized experience of practicing in poor ones. Extending that experience into a career, however, held varying costs, depending on one's country of origin. Bernard, the garage director, once told me how he had lived in the same house with a Russian, a French, and an American doctor. The last was there for just three months, and when his French colleague challenged the brevity of such a stay, the American answered that given his medical school debt it was all he could afford. The others, who had enjoyed state-subsidized training, listened in silence.

LA MANCHA AND PROBLEMS OF "DECOLONIZATION"

Are we the churches of neocolonialism now?

SPEAKER AT MSF-USA GENERAL ASSEMBLY, 2003

In 2005 the different sections of MSF convened a once-in-a-decade meeting to take stock of their shared dilemmas and discuss a common path forward. Whereas earlier iterations had followed periods of intense internal conflict, this time relations were comparative peaceful across the wider movement. Entitled "La Mancha" in a tongue-in-cheek reference to *Don Quixote,* the event mixed serious reflection with a more festive effort to inspire a renewed sense of purpose and community. In addition to gathering position papers from former and current members of MSF and outside commentators, the group also encouraged discussion among its field staff in the run-up to the meeting. The larger goal was to produce a new common accord that would "clarify MSF's role and limits" while improving governance.[19]

The status of national staff had emerged as a major issue well before La Mancha. Two years earlier, when I attended a national assembly of adherents to the American section held in New York City, the topic had already been the object of heated debate. One speaker denounced the perceived "colonialistic attitude" of some expats—a phrase that "covers lots of things so I don't have to be specific"—and called for including national staff within each team, while encouraging promotion and expatriation. Another argued that the term *neocolonial* was really the one to use, since the problem lay in the present, not the past. Yet another responded that he hoped there weren't too many actual neocolonists associated with MSF, "as to me it's a strong term, like *pedophile*." He urged making a distinction between "culturally unaware, eyes-closed behavior" and intentional domination. The colonial reference clearly disturbed some participants and also defied easy resolution, beyond advocating an enhanced role for national staff in the organization's work.

Indeed, the pages of MSF's various newsletters recounted a number of awkward incidents and denunciations attesting to the larger problems of history and perceptions of human difference. For example, in 1998, MSF-Norway launched a publicity campaign under the eye-opening slogan "Africa needs more white men." When MSF-France protested, the director defended the decision by countering that the French failed to grasp the Norwegian context and were themselves thus guilty of cultural imperialism. "Better to be a neo-con than an old-style colonialist," he retorted.[20] Beyond matters of representation, the larger questions of decision-making and motivation weighed heavily. Should national staff be involved more directly in decisions? If working for money, would they still exhibit the right humanitarian motivations? Conversely, of course, one could ask similar questions about expat volunteers themselves, as several of them pointed out to me. In response to the term *colonialism* Francesca launched into the following reflection about race and gender:

> Of course there's an exotic thrill of being white, having a status of authority you could never have in your own country, at least not at that age. There's a status of color in much of Africa, your authority and knowledge are rarely questioned when you're white. That can lead people into despotic behavior, particularly if they're insecure. The thrill of bossing your father around. And you do have money relative to people around you, plus enormous access to very beautiful, very young women. I don't see it as a moral thing, but some just can't handle it. But then that whole age is changing. People are coming for other things, people with more experience.

There's not so much of that "movie in the head" anymore. Now you have people who've learned how to manage themselves, people who can travel. It's still easier for young men. The male stereotype of free travel, versus women being asked about marriage, children, unless put into a religious box as a nun.[21]

Similar points were made by Ruth, a Ugandan doctor who had worked for MSF on several missions elsewhere in the 1990s before returning home to a post with a development organization. During that time she found MSF's recruitment of expatriate European staff woefully lax. Although Ruth considered the medical people very professional, the administrators struck her as "more half-baked," particularly the French, who sometimes made her wonder whether they had been simply taken "just off the streets of Paris." In particular she resented the Europeans' accusations of national staff when money had gone missing from a safe, and inappropriate design of buildings by arrogant amateurs who ignored local advice. Such incidents struck her as racist, with an unpleasant whiff of colonial prejudice. She thought MSF could learn more of the "soft skills" of people management. Again, she particularly accused the French, who she felt gave preferential treatment to Africans who spoke their language as opposed to English: "The French think, 'We invented culture.' I said, 'What did cave men do until France was invented?' They would have meetings from 8:00 to 1:00 AM, with lots of wine, cheese, and olives, where everyone wants to talk. After all they did invent it. In the end it was just lots of disorganization. What did we say? Get out of it? Nothing!"[22]

Unlike Francesca, Ruth felt her status as a woman had made relatively little difference. Indeed, she found even the MSF of that earlier period relatively "gender sensitive" once she had established her professional credibility. As for children, the European perception of mothering as a full-time role was the main stumbling block. In a country like Uganda, she pointed out, all kinds of relatives participate in child-rearing. If they were not available then you could easily hire someone. "This is," she observed, "a very child-friendly place." She felt her racial status had weighed far more heavily on her trajectory through the aid world and therefore favored more "South to South" connections like those her current employer sought to foster.

The varying geography of the vaguely defined "Global South," however, presented its own conundrums. During the time I was visiting MSF missions in Uganda it had become relatively common to encounter expats arriving from countries well beyond Europe, not all of them rich. I met volunteers not only from Japan and Australia, but also such places as Cameroon, the Philippines, Ethiopia, Malawi, Croatia, Kenya, Tanzania, and Argentina. Each one told an individual story of displacement: the man from Malawi, for example, had been a national staff member for an MSF project and married a Greek expatriate. Together they had proceeded to Ethiopia before moving to Greece. Unable to find much employment there, he continued to undertake missions to earn a living. The Cameroonian doctor likewise maintained a family from abroad, regularly sending remittances home. The Croatian one, by contrast, was on a youthful adventure. All, however, could translate MSF's stipend—modest by Western European standards—into a relatively sufficient wage. Did they continue to embody the proper MSF spirit amid this circulation? Bernard had his doubts, calling it "completely crazy" to send Cameroonian doctors to Uganda while simultaneously sending French doctors to Cameroon. Moreover, there were long-standing concerns about encouraging a "brain drain" exodus of professionals from the places that sorely needed them. And yet in its most literal sense, the phrase *sans frontières* inspired a vision of precisely such human mobility. If only some were free to travel, then the maps of aid organizations would all the more uncomfortably resemble those of empires.

These examples suggest the breadth of associations conjured up by references to colonial history. For MSF it was not only a question of specific pasts and their aftermaths—the legacy of the Belgian Congo for the section based in Brussels, for example, or even the complex web of connections between France and French-speaking populations elsewhere. Rather, it was the larger problem of the foreigner cast in the role of expert rather than guest or traveler. Whether obnoxious or sympathetic, the MSF expat was ever an outsider who exerted control. Moreover, the shadow of race loomed large. This was particularly true in an African context, where the heart of MSF's operations and the eye of its imagery firmly rested. There physical appearance sharply distinguished the majority of expats from the surrounding population. Any hint of paternalism or cultural arrogance threatened to open old scars.

Within this charged symbolic terrain, the real issue confronting the organization was the status of national staff and their relation to the larger enterprise. The byproduct of MSF's commitment to running mobile emergency programs—simultaneously operational, directly controlled, and temporary in form—this category of personnel had once appeared so natural as to not merit statistical mention. Now, however, the organization perceived it as a problem. A small cartoon in MSF's official internal newsletter from the La Mancha conference summarized this realization. Beneath the bold pronouncement that "90% of all staff are national staff" a white figure responded nervously, fingers in his mouth: "You're telling me that almost all MSF people are black?" The crux of the problem lay not with color, however, but rather with the confession of a deeper ignorance, as the accompanying text makes clear. Although the organization generated data about its expatriate volunteers, the national staff remained an embarrassing cipher: "We have never tried to understand who they are and the nature of their relationship with MSF."[23] The motivation behind this sudden curiosity grew clear at the end of a list of draft points for discussion a few pages later. Here, under the heading "Diversity and Inclusion," the organization acknowledged that national staff actually performed the majority of "acts of humanitarianism" and recognized that it might have failed to provide equal opportunity "based on individual competence and commitment rather than mode of entry."[24] The document proposed urgent efforts at engagement while still preserving the "spirit of volunteerism." The group should encourage national staff to seek membership in MSF's formal association, and if launching new sections, focus on "underrepresented" regions, in other words, not Europe or other rich quadrants of the globe.

MSF's newfound desire for diversity encountered little resistance. The organization was enjoying a period of relative harmony between sections, and unlike in previous years the question of its greater cohesion and international cooperation provoked few squabbles or suspicions. Moreover, ideals of equality and reflexive anticolonialism were, if anything, moral norms both within the organization and across its intellectual milieu. Ultimately MSF considered itself to be an association, or set of associations, composed of individuals dedicated to a common cause. The only real requirement for membership was experience with the organization; otherwise everything should be *sans frontières*. Thus agreement was easy in principle.

In practice, however, the matter of altering the status of national staff proved more difficult. Only a year after the La Mancha meeting, a senior member of MSF professed disappointment to me. He feared that momentum was fading, and that the initiative—like so many within MSF—would ultimately generate far more talk than action. On the ground in Uganda, efforts to further engage national staff met with little response. Although exceptional individuals like Grace might hope to expatriate, few national staff showed any interest in pursuing the association membership now open to them. Out of the handful who had, a member of the Swiss team told me with regret, two already thought of leaving. They saw no particular benefit in it, especially if they eventually went on to work for other organizations.[25]

MSF did achieve tangible progress in some areas of reconceiving its staff as a singular category.[26] Belated efforts to improve health benefits for national staff finally corrected what many members of the group had recognized as a scandal: that one might work for a medical organization now committed to combating AIDS and still not automatically receive treatment. The sections also agreed to work toward standardizing their stipend and pay scales to address imbalances between them. But they could not overcome the fundamental divide between traveling expatriates and the much larger pool of workers circulating through a local job market. Even if both occupied temporary posts, they traveled through different expectations and possibilities beyond the borders of the organization. Since MSF came and went, so did its national staff, not always in the same rhythm. To retain them permanently would require a fundamental reorientation away from mobility. It would also entail embracing humanitarianism as a routine enterprise rather than an exceptional act of volunteerism. The more MSF defined itself as an employer—even a good one—the less it stood apart from any other business operating at a global scale.

DOUBLE BINDS OF MOBILITY

In the middle of the twentieth century, the eclectic anthropologist Gregory Bateson introduced a novel theory about schizophrenia. Suggesting that the condition derived from communicative breakdown, Bateson and his associates posited a scenario in which a "victim" repeatedly faced contradictory injunctions posed by a valued interlocutor, neither of which could be satisfied without failing at the other. Calling this impossible position a "double bind", they linked it to the schizophrenic's psychotic inability to process conventional order in the world.[27] Double-bind theory has enjoyed an extended life well beyond mental illness. Here I will deploy it as a final point of reference for considering MSF's travails over human mobility.

The specter of colonialism that MSF confronted at La Mancha stemmed from world history. Nonetheless, there is a sense in which it also arose from within the organization, as a byproduct of its very existence. To operate "without borders" implies a movement of equipment, funds, and personnel. But as people cross borders they expose the differences between parts of the globe and tensions between them. The very quality of distance that might allow an outsider to operate more freely or serve as a recognized witness simultaneously created a need for proximity. The very ties that rendered a local knowledgeable, or a politically appropriate representative of certain interests, could also make it difficult for that person to move or manage. When these abstract qualities took shape in settings haunted by past exploitation—Africa, in particular, where the bulk of the organization's projects unfolded—they conjured colonial imagery.

In attempting to "decolonize," MSF faced contradictory demands and a series of questions it struggled to answer. If providing its volunteers with a stipend, how large should it be? Should it matter where the volunteers came from, or the economic landscape their relations inhabited? To what extent should MSF accommodate the personal lives of its personnel? ("I thought working overseas would teach me how little I need," an American friend once told me ruefully in Kampala. "Instead it taught me how much.") What sort of salary and benefits should it offer its veteran staff? If too small they would have difficulty remaining, if too large it would appear unseemly. How much should it pay support staff it hired for mission sites? A large gap between national and international personnel would simply replicate existing inequities. Yet when NGOs pay excessive wages it can distort the local economy, making it harder to build alternative institutions. Moreover, if people took up humanitarian work as a long-term livelihood, what effect did that have on its moral purpose? Encouraging motivated national staff to expatriate might help alleviate some of MSF's cosmopolitan parochialism, but it hardly erased the larger imbalance it reflected.

I allude to Bateson here loosely, translating across conceptual terrains in order to underscore one aspect of the original theory, sometimes overlooked. A double bind entraps its victim precisely because he or she wishes to answer *correctly* to each injunction. Threats of punishment or withdrawal of love prove most daunting when one cares about the relationship and wishes to do the right thing. The anxieties of a transnational organization are hardly identical to those of a psychiatric patient. But as MSF confronts its own turbulent array of exhortations and prohibitions, it shares this predicament of caring with Bateson's communicative victim. As a collective entity it wishes to behave ethically, to "do the right thing" in response to each injunction about people and money. Its resulting failure might not produce schizophrenia, but it contributes to continuing discontent. Lurking just beneath lies the unsettling realization that goodwill itself offers no sure remedy.

PART THREE

Testing Limits

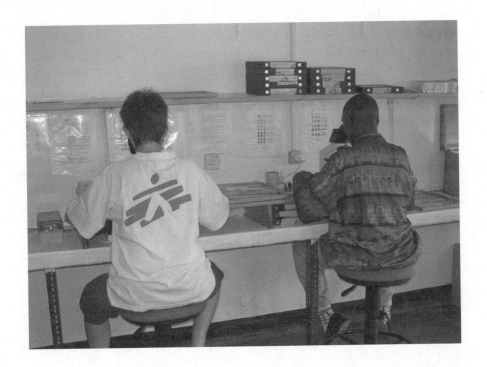

The Problem of Triage

One life today cannot be measured by its value tomorrow: and the relief of suffering "here," cannot legitimize the abandoning of relief "over there." The limitation of means naturally must mean the making of choice, but the context and the constraints of action do not alter the fundamentals of this humanitarian vision. It is a vision that by definition must ignore political choices.

MSF, NOBEL PEACE PRIZE ACCEPTANCE SPEECH, 1999

What place might death have within an ethic of life? Among secular inheritors of religious tradition the answer is not always clear, given that funerary rites, afterlife, and relations with ancestors all fall within the personal realm of belief rather than public action. Working across lines of culture and language only increases the uncertainty; once life stops, assumptions about human commonality grow harder to sustain. When Henry Dunant offered succor to wounded soldiers, it included the act of accompanying the dying as an expression of Christian duty and love. If largely forgotten in later retellings of Red Cross mythology, the moment stands in contrast to present aid sensibilities, where death signifies failure rather than an expected passage. This is particularly true for a medical organization confronting the results of curable conditions and human cruelty. Like any doctor, MSF can accept death as an eventual outcome. But however peaceful, a patient's demise does not really stand as a satisfying result; emergency medicine is not hospice care. Mortality may be a given, but it remains apart from the current vocation of medical humanitarianism, particularly in secular form. Beyond situational fears of contagion, biomedicine has little to say with regard to final rites, leaving that to cultural preference and religious tradition. It has no designated role to perform, no action beyond determining cause. To sit with the dying or care for a corpse would be a human gesture, nothing more. The doctor could display no particular expertise.

The possibility of actively choosing death, however—of killing, selecting who might die, or even justifying death for some greater good—deeply troubles the humanitarian mind. Like many other aid groups, MSF leans on the general Hippocratic precept of avoiding harm. The possibility of iatrogenic injury, the fear of producing negative as well as positive effects, regularly features as a topic of debate in aid circles, albeit within a framework defined around action. The organization has already made a general commitment in favor of intervention of a biomedical, clinical variety. Therefore suggestions, say, that a public health emphasis on infrastructure or hygiene might ultimately have greater effect than doctors or nurses ultimately carry little weight.[1] While attentive to outcomes and measuring effects, and regularly deploying the results of epidemiological studies, MSF's humanitarianism operates under the clinical logic of "one patient at a time," seeking to treat "the patient before us" (to quote two common lines from the group's literature). In many projects it advocates hygiene and practices health education, quite in keeping with the larger tradition of public health. But it is not about to accept the certain loss of the few while doing so, even to save the larger group. Like a good shepherd, it seeks to secure each and every member of its conceptual human flock. If practicing a minimalist form of biopolitics, it remains in the mode of pastoral power, the legacy of a religious politics of care.[2]

DEATH AMID LIFE

The tradition was that people died. That in itself was a coping.
MSF HUMANITARIAN AFFAIRS OFFICER, AMSTERDAM, 2002

In the modest but growing genre of humanitarian memoirs, even an ordinary death can loom large. Consider the following account from a young Canadian doctor in Sudan:

> No death is easy. If it starts to become that way I'll change my profession. But this one is more difficult than most. . . . I leave the room and walk down the hallway. The baby is lying on the bed, where we left him, crying. I push through the curtain and a man with wide, wet eyes looks at mine, and knows. "Malesh," I said. I'm sorry. Sorry I can't speak Arabic or Dinka. Sorry about the intravenous and the baby and your wife and the fifteen minutes and the no more. He tells me, through one of our nurses, that he wants transport to the graveyard. I tell him we don't do that, we can't. We couldn't save his wife, and we can't move her body. He asks, What am I to do, hire a car, where, the market, where? I don't know. Malesh. Sorry.[3]

Beyond its evocative portrayal of an individual moment of professional defeat, the passage describes a limit of biomedical expertise, and consequently the compassion of an organization. MSF's vehicles are ambulances, not hearses. They transport the living, and only exceptionally the dead. This stems not from a lack of feeling, but from a categorical definition of priorities and relations, and the understanding of life that informs them. Medicine—particularly emergency medicine—finds an impassable border in death, beyond which it cannot reach. The body returns not just to a state of nature, but also culture, the particularity of a locale and its traditions of grief.

The humanitarian discomfort with death only grows in exceptional circumstances. For disorders where medical science offers no remedy and risk of infection runs high, the tensions surrounding the purpose and mode of intervention become apparent to participants. A discussion on the theme "Justice and MSF Operational Choices" sponsored by MSF-Holland in 2001 addressed a recent outbreak of the Ebola virus in Uganda. As the summary noted, with such deadly diseases the organization could not simply claim saving lives as its justification for intervention:

> Motivation and justification are two different words. The motivation behind MSF's intervention in Ebola might have been a genuine epidemiological concern to know about the disease. The justification might be that it is an immediate public health threat, also of concern for the population. . . . Viral haemorrhagic fever epidemics do not happen that often; there are three organizations now with field experience on how to deal with them—CDC, WHO and MSF. They have accumulated experience through the last four or five epidemics and there are not many others who can do it. When the team was going into Gulu, all the other international and national organizations were running the other way. This population was left completely alone because of the fear of this epidemic. The public health response was probably being dealt with in the traditional (local) way by shutting people away in the barn and not feeding them or looking after them. Such a response traditionally would probably have broken the epidemic as quickly as anything we did, but the motivation for MSF was the alleviation of individual suffering. Alleviation of suffering and dying with dignity was enormously important. We know we saved very few lives.[4]

Faced with suffering it could not cure and dealing with abandoned patients, the organization found itself in a similar position to that of Dunant on the battlefield of Solferino. The palliative care of relieving pain and offering comfort was all it could realistically achieve. At the same time MSF reluctantly recognized that a well-contained death might help end the outbreak: it had to include mortality in its pursuit of living. Or as a member of MSF-Holland's Humanitarian Affairs Department once bluntly observed with regard to a different situation in Afghanistan, "The tradition was that people died. That in itself was a coping." In such cases the group had to acknowledge not only the general fact of human mortality, but its potential effects. Moreover, the quest to relieve suffering here translated into seeking a good death, not a preservation of life.

Unlike the devout Dunant, however, MSF felt ill equipped for this terminal bedside role. At the general assembly of MSF-France in 2005, members of the association debated issues of medical responsibility. A report on the event described particular concerns related to an outbreak of Marburg virus in Angola:

The highly lethal nature of this viral hemorrhagic fever meant that the teams had to work wearing special protective clothing, similar to those worn by cosmonauts. In the town of Uige, MSF set up an isolation and treatment centre for patients, which led one volunteer to comment "We're asking them to come here and throw themselves straight into the grave." A member of the audience described that we were reduced to "health police," while another expressed regret concerning the remote, paranoiac attitude of the majority of caregivers, increasing the gap that already exists between doctor and patient. Most ultimately agreed that the brutality of the operation was regrettable, and concluded that in future anthropologists and psychologists should be involved to a greater degree in such circumstances, since caregivers' actions consist here in particular of supporting the patients and their loved ones through the dying process.[5]

In treating a deadly contagious disease, health care workers needed to protect themselves. Yet doing so left them feeling not just medically impotent, but also potentially inhuman. This particular edge of suffering required other expertise—which secular imagination here identified with relevant branches of social science rather than religious figures. Comfort would be given to the living, including those in the dying "process" as well as those they would leave behind. Beyond that MSF could not reach.

Although accepting the fact that life ends, contemporary medicine remains uneasy about mercy in the form of killing. Euthanasia discloses a gray area in liberal ethics, a potential limit to individual choice. A choice of death likewise creates disturbance for humanitarians, appearing pathological in all but extreme final circumstances. The question is not solely confined to suicide. The prospect that some might prefer death to a debilitating cure likewise reveals a limit to medical reason. For doctors there are few prospects worse than dying, a view not always shared by their patients. Speaking before the Carnegie Council in 2001, MSF-France's former president Rony Brauman described a particularly troubling case:

> During the war in Mogadishu—the last time I personally was confronted with this problem—we obviously had to treat many bullet wounds, and in a number of cases we had to amputate because of massive infections that could not be treated properly. In our experience, the decision to amputate was a medical, technical diagnosis, which doesn't incur any criticism because it poses a solution to a life-and-death situation. Thus we were surprised to find that most of the young people we wanted to operate on refused to be amputated. They preferred—and this took us some time to understand—to die with their entire body than to live with a visible mutilation. It was quite difficult for the surgeons, the anesthesiologists, and the surgical teams to accept this because it seemed to violate their raison d'être—if you cannot amputate in a war situation, your role is severely diminished. As a result, many of us felt seriously conflicted. And some of the surgeons ironically found themselves in a life-and-death situation. Their lives were threatened because of their attempts to convince the wounded that it was in their best interests to be amputated. From the point

of view of the Somali people, their interest was not to be amputated; their interest was not to remain alive at any cost. That is a rather stark illustration of a clash in values over health and what is important in life. Our technical approach, which to us seemed irrefutable, was scorned by the very people whose lives were in danger.[6]

It is important to emphasize that this experience—like the treatment of rare viruses such as Ebola or Marburg—constitutes an exceptional example. The norm for MSF's work remains a problem of responding to an overwhelming surplus of people seeking treatment, not to the few refusing it. Moreover, most of the group's work focuses on relatively simple, eminently curable conditions. Nonetheless this resistance to amputation serves to recall that surgery is a form of controlled violence and that its effects can be severe. To save lives, the practice of medicine involves tradeoffs and imperfections.

As an organization MSF remains fundamentally committed to a medical perspective. The question of preserving life, however, extends well beyond humanitarian health care. Under the twin terms of *security* and *protection,* the aid world now grapples with the larger question of protecting the healthy, not just the ill. To what extent should aid workers risk their own lives while seeking to preserve those of others? To what extent should humanitarianism focus on general safety alongside the delivery of assistance? Such questions hold both theoretical and practical implications for an entity like MSF. Over the four decades of its existence, the group has had an evolving sense of how far its responsibilities might extend and how best to define its nonmedical role.

The spectacular rise of security concerns since the 1990s, whether or not it reflects any increased threats or changes in statistical risk, has altered expectations.[7] Unlike many other organizations, MSF may not have added designated "protection officers" to its staff. Nonetheless, as an extensive review of the topic by Judith Soussan suggests, the group now thinks through that idiom: "The word protection is in fact spontaneously associated with the concept of témoignage (thus suggesting that care-témoignage is MSF's term-by-term equivalent of the assistance-protection combination)."[8] At the same time, she notes that the organization has moved away from earlier moments of bravado in which it viewed itself as a sentinel for human rights or imagined it might protect populations by speaking out. Instead it pursues a more limited ambition of ensuring the delivery of aid. Past experience, growth, and shifting external factors have combined to puncture illusions about what an unarmed medical NGO can achieve in the face of violence. At the same time a sense of threatened security has pervaded many aid organizations in recent years and altered their perception of risk. Many older members of MSF regularly express disgust at new travel restrictions that they view as unnecessary and counterproductive. Others worry about a related retreat from *témoignage.* In actual practice, Soussan notes, the question of protection remains deeply troubling, and far from closed.[9]

SECURITY AND "HUMANITARIAN SPACE"

One evening when in northern Uganda I attended an MSF staff security meeting. The project was relatively new and the situation in flux; consequently the team had accumulated few traditions or local ties. At the same time, it was imperative to plan for disruption or sudden departure, even if nobody knew how much longer this particular site might stay in operation. We sat on mismatched furniture in the project's main building; outside the light quickly faded as the field coordinator, Bruce, ran through a series of essential points. Communication was critical, he stressed. At the moment the mission had a shortage of working radios, so it was important to keep in mind where they were at any point. After dark staff should only move when with a handset. In the event of a threat, people staying in the smaller annex should come to the main building. He stressed a "three-minute rule" of readiness: everyone should have a small bag containing valuables and a change of clothes either packed in advance or near ready. Should armed men appear at the house, the goal was to deal with them as calmly as possible. Under no circumstances should anyone attempt anything rash or become belligerent. "No superheroes," Bruce said firmly. If violence, rape, or theft seemed possible, opt for the least bad option; it was better to lose things than people. Male staff would take the lead in negotiation, ideally keeping guns outside the door. If the house itself became "compromised," then staff should rendezvous at an agreed meeting point. Everyone should also be aware of the hierarchy of command within the team for any decisions related to evacuation. Given sufficient time, team members would bring expensive equipment and files with them, remove insignia, and put everything else into storage. The priority, however, remained human life.

Before closing his remarks, Bruce reminded everyone that good communication with camp residents was vital to staying on top of local mood and rumor. Even so, team members should avoid discussing anything that might suggest the project's value as a target. In general staff should avoid mentioning money and only engage in financial discussions when inside MSF buildings. Also, he cautioned, the group should reduce talk of nationality. Although not a secret and often the basis for friendly conversation, it would be good to keep it at a minimum. Sometimes people had an exaggerated sense regarding the relative worth of different passports and fantastic expectations about ransom or rescue. Bruce then opened the floor for discussion. A visiting MSF veteran with frontline experience made additional suggestions, such as preassigning tasks and the best way to order vehicles for a convoy. An expatriate woman objected to the proposed distribution of people in the house, feeling it might foreclose escape. It had been a long day, however, and most people seemed ready to defer discussion to the next meeting. During all this talk of threat, packing, and sudden flight, the national staff sat quietly. It was not at all clear whether they would be going anywhere.

The Ugandan project's security concerns were not unwarranted. The surrounding conflict merited the description "low-intensity" given its sporadic flareups of small-scale attacks. Still, the line between rebel threats and army warnings felt thin. A combination of fear and government policy had driven a remarkable number of people into displacement camps, and most aid organizations traveled with military escorts—MSF and ICRC being the exception. In the year that followed, several NGOs found themselves under attack, setting off a new wave of tension in area. Moreover, the organization was also acutely aware of its status as a target worldwide. Earlier that spring, a Dutch volunteer for MSF-Switzerland named Arjan Erkel had finally gained release after nearly two years of captivity in the volatile Caucasus region. A few weeks after my security meeting, five members of MSF-Holland were ambushed and killed in Afghanistan, prompting the organization to withdraw from the country.

The case of Arjan Erkel became a major issue as his imprisonment dragged on and on. Although debating which strategy to pursue, the different sections of MSF rallied around the general effort to free him. They eventually engaged in a fervent public campaign to rally support, hoping to increase political pressure on European states to work for his release via the Russian government. His ultimate freedom came through the classic mechanism of a ransom paid to his kidnappers by the Dutch state. It provoked a secondary controversy of its own when the Dutch unsuccessfully sued MSF-Switzerland for reimbursement. The case thus inadvertently revealed the potential value of such kidnappings in embarrassingly precise terms, in addition to confirming the general inequality of human lives.[10] It also underscored the lengths to which MSF was willing to go to save a single individual, particularly one of its own. Erkel's symbolic significance derived not from any particular facts of his identity—such as the intriguing detail that he had studied cultural anthropology and joined the group after conducting a research project in refugee camps in Uganda commissioned by MSF-Holland. Nor did it matter that he had been in Dagestan or that his abduction coincided with the release of another colleague. To MSF he was simply "a dedicated, honest and hardworking colleague. Not exactly an idealist, but certainly someone with his heart in the right place."[11] Visiting the organization's offices during his captivity, I was struck by the heartfelt display of concern about his fate. Beyond the innumerable variations on the theme "Free Arjan!" displayed on every open space, updates on his fate met with a visible display of concern and commitment. As an American country coordinator told me in Paris in 2004: "It's important . . . that people don't give up. Looking at the [rescue] effort in terms of work/time economy would be very interesting. In my estimation it's [been] the biggest project in New York for the last eighteen months. It feels very comforting to know the level of commitment made to every single volunteer; it's good for all 2,500 people out there. It's a big organization, but with a feeling of solidarity behind you." Whatever else, the

case made it very clear that MSF would not accept aid work as a form of martyrdom. The one could never be offered up on behalf of the many.

Humanitarian security is not simply a matter of individual safety, however.
Rather, it reflects a fundamental precondition for aid delivery. Instead of advocating any right to intervene or duty to interfere, MSF's rhetoric over the past two
decades has actually focused on what it calls "humanitarian space."[12] This abstract
formulation refers to the ability of humanitarians to work freely in a given set of
circumstances. In effect, it seeks to define the situation so that medical practice
will stand apart as a recognized exception. In this sense it follows the historical
strategy of the larger concept of neutrality, defining a limited relationship outside
conflict that permits the pursuit of another interest. At the same time the spatial
metaphor suggests a mobile variant of religious sanctuary, in which certain
ground grants immunity from profane conflict.[13] Like the work of the Red Cross,
this assertion ultimately relies on moral suasion. Although sometimes referenced
against legal precept, its real calibration stems from practice and the reiterative
normalization of humanitarian action.

Like most aid agencies, MSF seeks to signal its distinctive status—an active
claim to operational neutrality and impartiality—through the form and content
of its missions. Starting with the uniform T-shirts and the ubiquitous white vehicles, every object associated with the organization normally carries its logo,
signaling a status that is at once distinctive and recognizably generic. Vehicles and
key buildings also commonly carry a no-weapons logo to indicate MSF's refusal
of arms. Moreover, the group takes every opportunity to remind all actors on the
ground of its medical focus, and it underscores the noncommercial and professional nature of its involvement by offering its treatments free of charge, under
criteria it defines as medical need. In this sense it asserts humanitarian space by
occupying it. Although claiming international humanitarian law as an authorizing precedent, as an independent NGO MSF depends less on treaties than on
personalities and a fragile web of local agreements. Whenever possible, mission
field coordinators take care to pay regular respects to all local potentates, with
ritual visits a recognized part of operational routine.

Humanitarian space remains a fragile fiction easily disrupted by state strategy
or violence. When military forces undertake missions pursuing humanitarian
goals, the humanitarian space demarcated by MSF blurs back into a larger con-
tinuum of conflict. The case of Afghanistan proves instructive in this regard. Following the romantic adventure in the early 1980s, MSF spent another two decades
in the country, staying on and on through dark days of civil war and Taliban rule.
The organization protested against food drops by U.S. forces during the 2001
campaign and sought to distance itself from state-sponsored reconstruction efforts. Nonetheless, MSF—like all foreign agencies—became increasingly identified with the American effort.[14] After the murder of five team members in 2004

the group abruptly withdrew. Those deaths, together with the absence of a meaningful state response, effectively collapsed MSF's definition of the situation.

The precise balance between MSF's conception of humanitarian space and its practice of speaking out remains unclear. Public speech certainly breaks with medical and humanitarian traditions of discreet silence and stands in implied contradiction to strict neutrality. In historical terms most of the prominent instances of public speech have involved moments of major humanitarian disaster and operational frustration or collapse.[15] At the same time instances of kidnapping or murder affecting members of the organization's staff trigger particularly passionate and loud responses, even as they reveal uncomfortable inequities between the relative worth of particular lives. Under extreme conditions the group has few strategic options available to it other than withdrawal and denunciation. As it agonized over its public response during the Rwandan genocide and issued frantic declarations, MSF also removed its own compromised insignia and worked under the flag of the ICRC.[16] In retrospect none of these actions proved that salutary or provided much satisfaction.

In abstract terms, humanitarian space is a space of life. Within it all other considerations take a secondary role, suspended for the duration of extreme need. It is a conceptual, floating hospital of sorts, an update on the medieval European convention of standing *hors de combat* or the Red Cross protection of the wounded. However concrete and tied to specific conditions MSF might seek to be, humanitarian space nevertheless displays inflationary pressures. One could always spare more, extend greater mercy, and further expand the scope of aid. To illustrate this deep tension within MSF's work, I turn to a theme introduced by one of its members, namely that humanitarianism works "against" sacrifice. The author's immediate concern was the cynical willingness of the international political order to accept that certain populations may die. The expansive terms through which he made his case, however, prove particularly revealing. Thus I take this claim quite seriously while extending its logic.

A REFUSAL OF SACRIFICE

Then you find yourself asking: "Why go to the right, when there are all these men on the left who will die without a word of kindness or comfort, without so much as a glass of water to quench their burning thirst?"

HENRY DUNANT, *A MEMORY OF SOLFERINO*

In 2003–2004, MSF released another volume in its irregular book series on the theme "populations in danger." Titled *In the Shadow of "Just Wars,"* the collection positioned itself against warfare justified by humanitarian goals.[17] Jean-Hervé Bradol, then president of the French section of MSF, provided the introduction. In it he denounces what he described as "the sacrificial international order," a political logic that inevitably produces victims in its quest for stability and a "better world."[18] While recognizing that legal efforts to "humanize" warfare might offer tempting situational benefits, he stresses that humanitarianism's investment in law must remain opportunistic. If law itself becomes a form of violence, then anyone fully committed to relieving suffering must oppose it. In this sense, Bradol suggests, his organization remains fundamentally oppositional: "Humanitarian action, as we understand it, directly challenges the logic that justifies the premature and avoidable death of a part of humanity in the name of a hypothetical collective good. 'Are all these deaths really necessary?' is the question we systematically address to political powers. Why? Because we have taken the arbitrary and radical decision to help the people society has decided to sacrifice. . . . Consequently, if humanitarian action is to be consistent, it will inevitably clash with the established order."[19] The humanitarian spirit, according to this rendering, rejects both *Realpolitik* and political utopianism, to the extent that either might justify human misery.

Couched in grander terms than most aid writing, Bradol's allusion to sacrifice helpfully displays the full extent of MSF's moral ambition. In place of the superficial vision of redemption through self-sacrifice that is often projected onto humanitarianism, it suggests a more absolute and obstinate commitment to defend existing life. The sacrifice that Bradol expressly refuses appears in examples of callous extermination or thoughtless neglect. Beyond the immediate victims of political conflict, he cites AIDS patients lacking drugs, North Korean refugees, and famine victims in Angola. To pursue a "just war" while overlooking any of these suffering populations would surely violate a fundamental humanitarian principle. All who are currently living deserve attention. No death should be justified for other ends. In this sense Bradol's proclamation indeed represents a categorical moral claim, even as it rejects both utopian illusions and realist cynicism. It also breaks with the larger pattern of behaviors that anthropology has categorized as ritual sacrifice.

In 1898 Henri Hubert and Marcel Mauss authored a defining study of the topic entitled *Sacrifice: Its Nature and Functions*. In it they examined a wide range of rites before finally providing a definition focused on the relational and transformative significance of destruction.[20] In this functionalist schema, the sacrificial victim serves as a conduit between the profane world of ordinary existence and the realm of sacred value. A victim is chosen and offered up with the expectation of a return. For Hubert and Mauss, struggling to encapsulate a broad swath of human traditions, ritual acts are necessarily significant in social terms. In this sense the loss involved in sacrifice is never absolute but always relational and ultimately generative. These are deaths that inherently matter. No victim dies in vain, given that the act itself reinforces social bonds for those participating and believing in the rite. Moreover, classic ritual sacrifice stems from willful action, not carelessness or oversight. The thing lost necessarily commands value. Whatever sacrifice has been in various times and places, they suggest, it has always entailed signification extending beyond the being or thing sacrificed. And like any ritual, it would implicate other times than the current moment of action: a past to be taken as precedent and a future to be taken as a promised return. Refusing sacrifice, then, would constitute a radical insistence on the present, disrupting any cyclical renewal of social bonds. It would, as Bradol suggests, be a fundamentally oppositional act, valuing life above all else.

When Bradol refers to a "sacrificial" international order, however, he means something both more and less than traditional sacrifice. The far-flung victims he cites are not all intentional ones, let alone carefully selected to represent an offering. Some are casualties of active devaluation, others of passive neglect. What they share are the fact of their destruction and the suggestion that their lives are expendable, mattering little if at all. The scope of this sacrifice is thus quite expansive, and its significance relatively weak. At the same time the collective good putatively achieved in exchange—political order—remains at best a limited and relatively profane variant of the sacred.[21] Moreover, Bradol implicates a wide range of actors of a greater aid system within the logic that would submit humanitarian concerns to political interests.[22] Many of these actors (such as UN agencies and NGOs) share MSF's concern for life, and the system as a whole presents itself as alleviating suffering. His humanitarian position is thus hardly external to the international order, however oppositional it may strive to be.

What then to make of Bradol's refusal of sacrifice with respect to politics? Humanitarianism lies symbolically embedded in a landscape of altruism and giving. Popular imagination positions the humanitarian worker as a figure of virtuous self-denial engaged in good works. Yet humanitarian morality cannot sanction the loss of human life or dignity or yield them up in a ceremony of destruction. Classic ritual sacrifice would be unthinkable for a proper humanitarian, as would any rite involving physical pain. Secular understandings of life limit appeals to spiritual redemption or public forms of religious ritual.[23] The justification of suffering for utopian ends—a common feature of political ideology—is likewise unavailable. Indeed, any life-threatening political action remains suspect. Whether political powers intervene militarily, pursue political involvement, or abstain completely, their response to a crisis inevitably involves a logic that can justify death, dividing those who may live from those who must die. Humanitarian action, Bradol believes, must fundamentally "refuse to collaborate with this fatal selection process."[24] Faced with multiple outrages and the suffering they generate, MSF and similar organizations seek to reclaim the value of life by loudly defending human "dignity." In this context dignity stands in as a baseline of value inherent in human existence. By appealing to it, even deaths otherwise without weight can be rendered sacred again, "sacrificed" in the etymological sense of the term. For humanitarian thought does not permit the possibility of truly *meaning-less* suffering, only "stupid" deaths that should not occur.

Humanitarian action thus represents a complicated reworking of sacrifice, one extending beyond a gift economy or a volunteer ethos. On the one hand, humanitarians resist the practice of destruction inherent to sacrificial rites, re-fusing any exchange whatsoever for life. On the other hand, they resist the de-valuation of life by others, and, in that resistance, effectively reconsecrate nonsacrificial killing by recasting it as tragic destruction. This double logic be-comes apparent in the enumeration of victims, a practice in which humanitarians routinely engage even while resisting its potential dehumanization.[25] Counting bodies to measure suffering, they simultaneously demand that each death register as a categorical loss, all equally precious. On such grounds an organization like MSF could reject the logic of "just wars" due to the suffering they would entail. At a rhetorical level the significance of death remains incalculable even when it is used to enumerate. At an experiential level, however, the problem proves more complicated and unsettling.

Didier Fassin engages Bradol's theme within a persuasive formal analysis.[26] The humanitarian encounter, Fassin suggests, can indeed be read in terms of sacrifice, though its terms are less starkly Manichean than those of Bradol's call to arms. Rather, the gap between those "society has decided to sacrifice" and those who seek to help them illustrates what Fassin terms the "politics of life"—the dif-ferential value of ordinary lives and the stakes revealed between them. Even when humanitarians seek to oppose such distinctions and insist on the categorical equality of all human existence, their own actions ultimately reveal the disturbing depth of human inequality. Fassin provides several illustrations for this general point, most dramatically the decision by MSF-France to stay in Bagdad during the outset of the 2003 Iraq War, and then subsequently to withdraw after several team members were kidnapped. Beyond the specific failure of the mission, Fassin suggests, the equation between lives never balanced, either in philosophical or practical terms. The position of those who freely risked their lives remained fun-damentally distinct from those who stood in danger of sacrifice, divided by the possibility of action and an unreturned gift. Not only was MSF unable to save lives, it was also ultimately unwilling to risk them. Nor could the organization come to terms with the depth of inequity separating national staff and expatriate volunteers. Thus the problem with the humanitarian stance on the sanctity of all life, Fassin astutely observes, is that "this equality does not long withstand the test of the facts."[27]

Fassin's analysis exposes a deep fault line in humanitarian reason. In the end, MSF participates in a greater logic of sacrifice whether it wants to or not. It can protest but not escape the politics that surround it, including the inequities of life. To the extent that it engages with actual problems, it encounters the effects of sovereign choices regarding life and death, the very "fatal selection" that Bradol denounces. Some things are given up and exchanged, even by MSF. In this sense its refusal to "collaborate" clearly fails before it even begins. The only return comes in the form of protest, exposing again the deeper architecture of inequality and injustice.

Still the attempted refusal itself remains provocative as well as poignant. How can one resist the imperative to choose amid crisis, particularly when operating independently in the name of conscience? Or rather, how to select even as one "refuses" to choose? If MSF follows an ethic of action as well as refusal, then it must engage, under protest as it were, but also in a manner that appears to favor the good.[28] This problem of picking without discriminating is a constant one, not simply an aberration of exceptional circumstances like those in Iraq. Moreover, it applies not only across the yawning inequities between human groups but also between those at relatively the same level. Actual interventions undertaken in the name of humanitarianism face an inherent problem of selection. Amid a landscape of disaster, where should aid be provided, and to whom? Who stands first in line and who must wait? To address this second problem I turn to the medical tradition of triage.

TRIAGE AND THE IMPERATIVE TO CHOOSE

Instead of dwelling on morality, let us confine ourselves to ethics. Practical ethics. Decision-making ethics. Pragmatic ethics. Which, by definition, are never fixed. There are no ends, only means.
MSF DOCTOR MILTON TECTONIDIS, *MESSAGES*, 2005

Alongside categorical denunciations of suffering, groups like MSF must continually decide how to allocate their resources. Here we encounter the dilemma of selection in an everyday as well as an exceptional form. To examine the larger problem of choice involved, I turn to the medical practice of sorting known as triage. Like modern humanitarianism of MSF's variety, triage derives from the experience of war and a medical logic of crisis. The term *triage* derives from the French verb *trier* (to pick or cull) and now applies to a wider set of methodical procedures for establishing treatment priority in medical settings. Historians canonically extend its historical lineage—again like that of the ambulance and the associated logic of emergency care—to the chief surgeon in Napoleon's army, Dominique-Jean Larrey. He recognized the importance of battlefield evaluations and categorization of wounded soldiers by severity of their condition rather than social status or familiarity: "Those who are dangerously wounded should receive the first attention, without regard to rank or distinction. They who are injured in a less degree may wait until their brethren in arms, who are badly mutilated, have been operated on and dressed, otherwise the latter would not survive many hours;

rarely, until the succeeding day."[29] Appraising the mass of wounded with a medical eye, war surgeons should see only bodies, not the insignia on the uniform.

By the First World War the practice of triage had become a norm of military medicine. Along the way two other potential criteria for selection appeared: the pragmatic principle of favoring the salvageable over those clearly dying, and the utilitarian one of determining what might serve the greatest good for the greatest number.[30] This latter principle included emphasizing war priorities and military interests rather than those of the patient. Thus the needs of battle could come first. When the new wonder drug penicillin arrived in North Africa in 1943, U.S. physicians prioritized soldiers with venereal disease over those with severe wounds, on the logic that the former might return to duty sooner. With the rise of emergency medicine in the second half of the twentieth century, triage grew into a routine feature of hospital admissions. Following the emergence of new technologies it also became a reference in ethical debates about allocation of medical care.[31]

Triage can emphasize survival, prioritizing those who have a chance to live when others will not. Alternatively it can emphasize severity of need, prioritizing those who need immediate attention. In contexts of relative abundance, it assumes that all will eventually receive care. The most routine variation of triage describes the daily sorting of any hospital emergency room, whereby a heart attack patient would receive treatment before someone with a minor laceration. Less familiar and more disturbing variations of triage apply to contexts of severe lack: disaster settings or the distribution of any limited medical good amid a condition of relative scarcity. While a popular source for conundrums in ethical philosophy, this latter version proves distressing to health care providers, humanitarians, and anthropologists alike. Writing about access to AIDS treatment in West Africa, for example, Vinh-Kim Nguyen situates the stark results of inadequate supply in a longer history of cruelly selective care.[32]

When prioritization becomes a matter of life and death, health care delivery can resemble sovereign choice. In the color-coded system recommended by the World Medical Association, a black label represents "expectant" status—those who cannot be saved and thus no longer have any claim to priority. However painful such a determination might be for health care workers, when facing mass casualties with few resources, the fate of others may depend on it. From the perspective of emergency medicine, undue attention to one patient would be an "unethical" squandering of resources. Inactive contemplation would prove even less defensible: "Failing to act due to moral uncertainty is unacceptable, however, since inaction is often the worst of the available options."[33]

Here I use the term *triage* to gloss the general problem of humanitarian prioritization. I also stress the potential significance of Larrey's ethical innovation—that the tradition of triage assigns value on the basis of immediate bodily states.

However passionate the moment, it expects the exercise of dispassionate, professional judgment. The medical gaze thus discriminates in the name of bodily egalitarianism. Larrey himself noted that officers who had horses could transport themselves to hospital care.[34] His system of "methodical succor" opposed waste, including that produced by relying on happenstance to produce patients or simply accepting them on a first-come first-served basis. Instead, Larrey sought to institute a more systemic approach based on explicitly medical criteria. In the broadest sense, triage represents a system of selection based on the facts of suffering themselves. As such, it rejects all other claims to value, disengaging with social, political, or religious criteria that might distinguish one victim from another. When asserted in emergency settings it suspends other liberal norms that usually govern medical practice: autonomy, fidelity, even ownership. In their place triage favors life, health, efficiency, and fairness, the last understood as a procedural and distributive good.[35]

Unlike sacrifice, triage is not about symbolic exchange, political strategy, or social connection with people or deities. Rather, the practice maintains a pragmatic focus on immediate action in response to physical condition. In this sense it offers a widely relevant point of reference for considering the problem of humanitarian selection, particularly in crisis settings. Humanitarians may, as Bradol has it, refuse the greater justificatory language of sacrifice. They cannot, however, avoid the responsibility of choice. Their vision might resemble that of a public hospital—a global waiting room, for instance, like the one featured in MSF's inaugural publicity campaign in the 1970s, an open venue where all can eventually find care. Their practice, however, involves selection, and selection necessarily entails loss. In the face of overwhelming demand, the need to put some things first entails giving up others. Moments of triage thus confront humanitarians with a potential conundrum of designating their own "sacrifice" of sorts, even while opposing the sacrifices of others. The widening field of concerns addressed by organizations like MSF, combined with the global scope of contemporary media and humanitarian action, only exacerbates the problem of selection. Although the potential range for action has expanded, the duration of media attention has not, blurring different crises into a single form. The more humanitarians respond to enduring conditions like AIDS or sexual violence or recognize root problems like poverty, the more they confront a problem of sorting and choosing, particularly if operating worldwide.

Aid agencies rarely refer to triage except as a technical term. However, they increasingly deploy techniques that mobilize its larger logic, and perhaps none do it more continuously or pervasively than MSF. Because the organization has achieved a degree of financial independence while claiming to impartially treat the entire world, it shoulders a particular burden of responsibility for how it expends its resources. Working on crisis issues "without borders" entails constant mobility and hence constant selection. This process of selection is rarely clear and remains open to continual questioning. It also epitomizes the humanitarian problem of emphasizing the present. "Of course we think about change," one person put it to me near the outset of my research, in a phrasing later echoed by many others, "but at *this moment* what do you do?" The question is quite real when one is faced with a potential crisis and equipped with the wherewithal to respond. "Do you start to prepare supplies for 100,000 displaced people before anything happens," an operational director for MSF–Holland asked rhetorically, regarding Macedonia in the summer of 2001, "or wait until they actually are displaced? There will be criticism either way." He noted that even less overtly political crises such as flooding in India and Pakistan raised the fundamental quandary of scale: "We could put all the budget of the whole movement toward it, but even that couldn't do much." Given that it could rarely offer a solution on its own, even for the shortest of terms, what should MSF do?

If operating as minimal biopolitics, the logic of humanitarianism is ever inflationary. Humanitarianism cannot sanction allowing death, only fostering life. If the goal is to alleviate suffering, then why should cause matter? Surely an AIDS patient deserves care as much as a war victim, as many in the organization had come to believe by the turn of the millennium. An expanding range of potential duties, however, only further complicates the essential problem of which to actualize. Even as the group's assets and organizational capacity continue to grow, they remain finite. A few of the many potential patients can be treated, but the vast majority must continue to wait. Thus humanitarian practice involves selection, in effect giving up those not chosen by leaving them to their fate. Such is the discomfort of putting "ideals into practice," as one of the group's recruitment slogans has it.

To address the difficult matter of operational choice, MSF filters decisions away from the field and through its various section headquarters. There an upper echelon of administrators sifts and weighs the relative value of existing projects as well as potential new ones. Particularly difficult matters and long-range planning involve officeholders and governing boards, both elected by members of MSF's associations. Coordination units within each section seek to standardize medical and logistical approaches, while the international office struggles to keep the different sections more or less aligned. The details of this greater architecture have varied over time, as have the particular structures maintained at different operational centers. Over the course of my visits, office staff discussed the relative merits of different systems for project oversight, ranging from the relatively more vertical "desk" approach epitomized by the French (often described as particularly controlling by members of other sections) to the relatively shorter "chain" of the Dutch section, which sought to amplify field perspectives. Nonetheless, I found the general similarities of practice far more striking than variations in their respective flow charts. Throughout MSF personnel constantly rotate through posts, a practice meant to guard against institutional sclerosis. All branches of the organization fear excessive planning and fret over complacency. MSF's project portfolios remain structured around the geography of nation-states, only sporadically addressing issues regionally. And at every stage personalities loom large and discussions can grow heated.

The logic of this general approach derives from MSF's commitments to emergency and mobility and the inherently nomadic perspective they foster. However deleterious to institutional memory, the constant turnover of personnel guards against developing an overriding attachment to any one geographic location or a superficial sense of expertise. "Ignorance not a problem," one senior administrator even assured me in Amsterdam in 2002. "Indeed, it's perhaps an advantage." He explained that a degree of ignorance encouraged questioning and a constant return to fundamental principles. One should always ask if a mission had become a part of "the system" rather than remaining focused on patients. Limiting the stay of the heads of missions for each country, he maintained, created "constantly reinforced ignorance" of this sort. At a higher level the organization likewise guarded against developing undue regional focus. Rather than following the conventions of area studies or dividing the globe into contiguous slivers, the administrative systems incorporated a hodgepodge of countries under each desk or operational director. The goal was to protect against balkanization while encouraging comparative thinking and cross-fertilization. Even in field-friendly Amsterdam, headquarters kept a sharp and comparative eye on every site, as another administrator there explained in 2006:

> Each operations director covers part of Africa and one other region. MSF-Holland feels everyone should be exposed to Africa, since it's the core of crisis, but not only Africa. That way we're forced to create a balance within each portfolio and avoid a fight between Africa and Latin America. Uganda could go with Sudan or Congo more naturally than with Colombia, but those are big problem regions so [it was] added to us instead. Comparison helps us look beyond simple needs. Although suffering is absolute, it is also relative. Otherwise we would throw everything into Darfur, or at least everything into Africa. MSF-Holland also tries to maintain a focus on conflict, that's why we went into Iraq, even if we weren't as clear about our role in terms of needs. Needs of a different kind are always hard to judge.

Such structural safeguards notwithstanding, patterns still developed. As a number of people observed, projects in Latin American—by and large less focused on emergency—more often incorporated an intercultural dimension and leaned toward political engagement. Conversely MSF often struggled to find its footing in heavily bureaucratized settings such as China or the former Soviet Union, where its impatient habits ran into a wall of forms and regulations. ("In a way, working in a collapsed state has its advantages for an NGO like us," another member of the Amsterdam office noted candidly). Geographic patterns also extended beneath the national level. When the organization either stayed in or returned repeatedly to any given country, it also acquired a tradition there, as was the case for the French and Dutch sections in Uganda. Within countries particular regions grew familiar, and familiarity could in turn make it more likely that the group would work there again. As a Canadian administrator for MSF-Holland acknowledged in 2002, "The world is full of inequities. Even choosing village X to work in creates inequity ten kilometers away. A minor inequity, yes but on a micro level it mimics larger ones. On a micro level we do contribute to inequities." She found the thought troubling, and yet moved on; the key was to identify the worst places, where the organization could have the greatest impact. Such settings, she added, offered the inspiration of seeing just how strong and resilient people could be; she confessed that she herself "would have been a statistic if born in Africa." A Spanish colleague of hers observed that at a certain level, such selection was ultimately arbitrary: "In the Congo throw a dart at the map; we can work anywhere." He too stressed deep admiration for people in dire circumstances "who go on, surviving, even enjoying something in life."

The French director for communications later confirmed that realities of publicity and fundraising likewise shaped choice: "It's true that if there's a major crisis MSF needs to be in on it. It's what we're supposed to do, in both our own eyes and those of our supporters." On occasion the group would attempt to alter this equation, such as when it suspended fundraising in the wake of the Indian Ocean tsunami. In this sense a claim to triage could operate at a more general level, with the group championing "underreported" crises overshadowed by those in the news. The tsunami was a case in point, not due to any exaggeration, but rather because the sheer scale of the disaster dwarfed any reasonable claim MSF might make to expertise. The communications director offered this frank assessment:

> With such a catastrophe, the first three days are all about life saving, so that's mostly local people who are on the spot. By week three or four you'll have more therapists than patients, otherwise it's all post-emergency work, and that's slow and takes a lot of time. Yes, there is a need for mental health, mental health is important. But it's not life saving in the direct sense. Reconstruction, something like the Marshall Plan in Europe after World War II, that wasn't NGOs—most of it will have to be state to state. If the west coast of France were suddenly hit by something like that we wouldn't be waiting for NGOs, but for something like the U.S. military. The scale is just different. We were out of our depth; it's really the responsibility of the state. But it became this big fiesta of aid world fundraising, and we opposed that. I mean, forty million euros in ten days, what we spend for a whole year in Darfur. Niger will be financed with un-earmarked tsunami money. Ten million euros can save 25,000

children. But we can't pretend we need to keep raising money for the tsunami it-self. . . . You can do things with NGOs and be effective, but not total reconstruction of a large area.[36]

At the same time, the presence of other actors in settings like the tsunami zone could make it easier to leave or take a stronger stance. "Decisions are often made in relation to other organizations," the director of MSF-USA noted in 2007. "Certain big decisions (such as withdrawing from camps) might be different if no one else was there. Every organization is aware of other ones." Choice also depended on individuals, as stressed by an administrator in Geneva in 2004. "One of the most interesting aspects of MSF is that someone can make a change in the operational program. A single person, that's all it takes. You must be convincing, but that's it. The harder issue is maintaining a global view, a sense of proportion so as not to intervene every time." Action invariably took place within a larger ecology, where both MSF and its various members often saw the ethical problem as "choosing the least bad option."

At times the parameters of such choices grow not only restrictive but also emotionally wrenching. A German woman overseeing MSF-Holland's missions in Uganda bluntly framed the burden of responsibility that could accompany offering care, explicitly referencing triage:

> It's a painful issue having to accept limitations and accept a different level of care between places like Berlin and here. But as an aid worker you have to or you can't continue. I always compare it a bit with the triage system, where, say you have forty victims and have to decide which ones to treat. I remember having to do this in Chechnya in 1995 after the bombing. It was hard, but then if I was not there and acting no one would have any care at all. I think about this when making decisions. I'm a nurse, and perhaps there's a difference in having medical training. It's difficult to admit that we choose, that we make decisions, that we decide.

She paused and then added softly: "Today is a historical date. I was in Srebrenica with an MSF team, and we had to choose who would stay and who would go. The young men went and it's hard now, knowing what happened." She fell silent again, staring into the distance.

Such decisions prove no easier amid an immediate drama of life and death. In a memoir recounting his own humanitarian journey, former MSF international president James Orbinski describes a particularly harrowing moment of selection amid the genocide of Rwanda:

> There were so many and they kept coming. Patients were taped with a 1, 2 or 3 on their foreheads: 1 meant treat now, 2 meant treat within twenty-four hours, and 3 meant irretrievable. The 3s were moved to the small hill by the roadside opposite the emergency room and left to die in as much comfort as could be mustered for them. They were covered with blankets to stay warm, and given water and whatever

morphine we had. The 1s were carried by stretcher to the emergency room or to the entrance area around it. The 2s were placed in groups behind the 1s. We were overwhelmed. The dead could not be moved fast enough. The wounded could not easily be carried over the dead bodies to the ER, the operating rooms or the wards.[37]

The procedure may have been crude, but it was a classic attempt to achieve some sort of medical rationality amid an incomprehensible welter of suffering. As a doctor, what else could one do? The individuals who experienced such choice, however, seem clearly haunted by it, if sometimes finding inspiration in the strength of those who suffered. For his part Orbinski recounts the words of a horribly disfigured woman amid this tragic queue who, noting his distress, whispered for him to take courage and attend to others. At the very moment of despair one might find resolve for further action.

On occasion, however, medical rationality encounters the challenge of an alternative logic. Rony Brauman describes a different troubling scenario of selection, this one in northeastern Uganda, where the preferences of aid workers clashed with those of the people they sought to help. In the early 1980s, amid the chaos of the organization's first famine project in Karamoja, MSF struggled to distribute insufficient food supplies. Following medical perceptions of risk and aid tradition, the team focused on small children. However, team members soon faced an unexpected form of culture shock:

> We very quickly observed that the food was being taken away from the so-called target population of children under five and pregnant women to be given to the elders in these villages. For us, there is a very direct moral value attached to pregnant women and to children—they are innocent, they are the future, and these are both important values (not for me any longer, I want to be precise, but it was at the time, and I can see that it is still a very commonly shared perception). But for the Karamojong, which was the dominant group in this part of Uganda, maintaining their elders was of supreme importance for reasons that may be obvious even in the West: social coherence, social authority, and decent social standards. Whereas the kids—of course, the death of a kid is always painful, wherever one goes in the world—can be replaced easily. An elder cannot be replaced. That is an obvious yet painful observation. So who was right; who was wrong? Were we right to try to reach these populations that we'd decided were the target groups; or were the Ugandan people right to give a sort of privilege to the elders and to sacrifice the under-fives? The question is of course meaningless. Nobody was right; nobody was wrong.[38]

From a humanitarian perspective the only solution was to attempt to increase food aid to alleviate the need for such a "dire choice," something MSF struggled to do. Some on the team tried to ignore the uncomfortable issue, while others denounced what they perceived as injustice. Even if the incident ultimately exceeded simple moral evaluation, as Brauman suggests, it produced "very intense and emotional discussions." Children lay at the very heart of humanitarian sensibilities, as attested by MSF's fundraising motifs. To select against them would be the most distressing sacrifice of all.[39]

THE ORDINARY PATHOS OF CLOSURE

MSF opens and closes a number of individual projects each year, responding to acute crises, handing over projects to other actors, and always monitoring and remaining flexible to the changing needs of patients within a given location.

MSF ACTIVITY REPORT 2005–2006

Triage of the battlefield variety remains a rarity, even in humanitarian contexts. A far more ordinary problem of choice arises for MSF when contemplating whether or not to leave a given field site. Unsurprisingly, the organization's focus tends to rest on initiating projects rather than closing them. The practice of any sort of selection disrupts the categorical moral logic usually deployed by humanitarianism by distinguishing among victims. Even if neglect and suffering remain the responsibility of political actors, as Bradol suggests, it is not difficult to hear an echo of sacrificial logic when a group dedicated to action chooses to withdraw or declines to intervene. MSF may strive to maintain a realist sensibility about what it can and cannot actually accomplish. It may favor a medical rationale over a political one. But its actions still involve uncomfortable tasks of selection and prioritization, the act of deciding what to do at any given moment.

Members of the organization recognize this continual predicament. "Closing down a project is very difficult," an administrator told me emphatically at the outset of my research, an assessment I would hear repeated many times. As teams in the field often grow attached to a place and its people, the burden of decision usually falls to heads of mission and staff in the sponsoring headquarters. Weighing pros and cons, they assess whether or not the project has met its initial objections and if the situation has sufficiently stabilized to merit the designation of being "post-crisis." Mission creep remains a constant concern given the inviting array of health problems in many locations. Ideally MSF would transfer its projects to state services or other organizations better suited to long-term interventions. In practice, however, all too often this does not happen. Governments lack capacity, other organizations are unavailable or overextended, and MSF itself often fails to adequately plan for its departure. "It's always gratifying to have a team that recognizes its ability and plans for withdrawal," an administrator noted approvingly in New York in 2006, describing a happy exception. The organization's emergency ethos and its focus on present problems, however, leave little time for such planning. Although a predictable eventuality, closure is never the primary concern.

My own initial encounter with a field project—the French section's long-running sleeping sickness program in northwestern Uganda—occurred during its final phase of withdrawal. A sense of loss hung in the air throughout my conversations with local health authorities and the remaining personnel. MSF had not only provided services but also employment and a sense of bustling activity no one expected the government to match. By chance I shared a return journey with the new head of mission who had suggested and authorized my trip. "We know how to open, but we still don't know how to close," she acknowledged as we traveled back to Kampala together. In her view things should be done step by step in order to minimize the impact of the group's departure . Still, that was not always simple to achieve, particularly for an organization weaned on emergency. Later she elaborated: "We close a lot of projects not because they are finished—this work is never finished—but to hand them over because we have limits. It's not [about] objectives, but means and strategy that we can put in place. We can still make an assessment and hand [them over] to others. For example in the north of Uganda we make a big deal of food, but that's not our thing. It may be the same with social issues. We touch on mental health, try to understand culture, but I'm not sure we're that good at counseling. It's not bad to have limits."

This theme of limits arises frequently when MSF discusses closure or decisions not to intervene. From a realist perspective the group's actual capacity stands in contrast to its expansive rhetoric. Even a relatively rich organization cannot treat a whole country, and in seeking to work worldwide its coverage grows painfully thin. Moreover, like all aid organizations, MSF operates within a wider political and economic context, the same that produces and reproduces international order. Likewise, humanitarian action depends heavily on a media presence, given that private funds derive from public sentiment. In this sense, aid agencies remain ever partial and limited in their ability to choose a constant course of action, let alone care for populations. Where need greatly exceeds resources some form of choice proves inevitable, as revealed in moments when the group draws a line.

During a discussion about medical responsibility sponsored by MSF-France, a deputy program manager in the Democratic Republic of the Congo stressed the group's restricted reach and the resulting temporary nature of its programs: "I prefer to talk about the limits. To meet our goals, our intervention must be defined in space and time. In the DRC, we are creating access to care that often did not exist before and which will not exist afterward." His colleague added, "Whether you like it or not, it's parenthetical!" In such a relative "health desert" care could only prove partial, the two asserted: "If our decisions to step in were based solely on epidemiological criteria, particularly in terms of emergency thresholds and death rates, we should be opening projects everywhere in the DRC. It is therefore essential to define the humanitarian problems to which we decide to respond." In practice, however, this perspective proved hard to translate to local communities.

At one project site, the two administrators reported, responses went from an initial "Don't bother—we're already dead!" to protests against the group's departure. They acknowledged that it was hard to respond to a mother who asked, "My kid, who's going to take care of my kid when you leave?"[40] Nonetheless, since the center of conflict had migrated, so too should the organization. To open elsewhere it had to close, and in opening, recognize that any project had a finite lifespan.

The basis of objectives is not always obvious to those inside the organization either and remains a topic of frequent discussion. As an epidemiologist working for MSF in Uganda pointed out in 2004, "What is aid: more years of life or guaranteeing health?" From his perspective the organization should stick to the more modest goal of limited relative improvement, rather than pretending to anything greater: "Why go if it's not going to last? The Americans and Brits come in talking about sustainability, but when they go things still collapse. But then some people had a few more years of life. The gap between Africa and the rest of the world is getting bigger every day. With all the books and so on written about it, it's still a complete disaster. When MSF does a program, the idea is to do a program well and then go. We don't believe much in sustainability."

Noting that poor countries continued to grow poorer, he insisted that only increased expenditure through political action and economic activity held out any hope of improving the greater health picture. MSF's role should be to show what could be possible, no more or less. Personally invested in living in Africa, he also cautioned against overemphasizing the "disaster" of health at the expense of recognizing the potential "beauty" of life even amid hardship: "Here people keep hold of something basically human." Life, in other words, was about living, not only survival.

For many within MSF recognizing and abiding by such limits proves easier said than done. Closure remains a predictable challenge, frequently tinged with nagging doubt as well as a sense of loss. Any longtime observer of the group's actions could point to counterexamples for every stand taken in the name of principle, suggesting that coherence arrived as much in retrospect as in the heat of any given moment. An administrator in Amsterdam recognized as much in 2006: "We have lots of principles to rationalize at the end of the day. But there comes a time when a decision has to be taken. I may sound cynical, but I think that our rationale often occurs after our decision. I don't mean that I think everything is Machiavellian, but that in hindsight things grow clear. Even with efforts to engage in careful reasoning, MSF remains decision driven." Decisions to leave, however, often expose personal investments in the collective ethical stakes. The very organizational openness that allows for individual initiative also expands the burden of responsibility. The closer one gets to the field program, however, or the deeper one's attachment to the project type, the harder it is to maintain any sense of proportion or "global view."

Like death, the demise of programs proves unsettling to humanitarian sensibilities. The medical rationality of triage can resolve action but rarely emotion. Along the edge of crisis the decisions MSF makes regularly disturb the fundamental humanitarian values of its members. When a situation drags on it must determine what constitutes an acceptable "normal" state in this setting and the limits of its own operation. It must decide whether to withdraw, even if other nonemergency health problems remain. Such a decision is rarely easy. As a lawyer working for MSF-Holland told me, "How do you argue against human suffering? If you really want to keep a project going, you say, 'Are you going to let those people die?'" And yet here concern for life confronts the organization's practical constraints and global commitment, its mobility and independence. MSF continually must choose amid its array of programs, acknowledging in pragmatic terms the larger frame of inequality that surrounds each crisis and the fact that lives have quite different values in ordinary times. Alongside its minimal biopolitics it thereby engages in what Didier Fassin calls a politics of life, "making a selection of which existences it is possible or legitimate to save."[41] Such a selection stands in contrast to MSF's vision of radical moral equality at the level of life, in which one existence should never balance against another. But in the absence of a clear emergency, the choices that the group makes take into account the work of other organizations and the larger realities of poverty and inequality, as well as its own relentless need to move on. Having proclaimed itself "without borders," MSF struggles to define its limits. This problem remains a human one: messy, uncertain, and fully charged with feeling.

The *Longue Durée* of Disease

At first the focus is not to die. Then come other questions of living.
MSF FIELD COORDINATOR, AIDS PROGRAM, UGANDA, 2004

A HUMAN QUESTION

The patient is an older man, skin taught across his skull, eyes darting here and there. He wears a light-colored dress shirt, frayed but clean and carefully buttoned. We are sitting in a small room—too small now with my extra chair wedged into it—at MSF's AIDS clinic in the northwest of Uganda. Together we wait for the French doctor in charge to return. It is a busy day at the clinic, full of interruptions, and staff members are juggling several different demands and a full waiting room. The patient's eyes turn to me. He has been told that he indeed has the deadly virus, and that the results of his tests qualify him for antiretroviral treatment, the scarce wonder medicine of the moment. Nonetheless, he seems uncertain. "Is there a cure?" he asks, seeking a second opinion. I am somewhat disconcerted by the question. Despite its simplicity it hangs heavily, weighted with expectation as well as the residue of rumors and suspicions. I have no expert opinion to offer, only a general knowledge of the disease, and exposure to the world of people seeking to combat it. My official role is that of observer rather than participant. Moreover, my presence in this particular room is an unexpected development of the day, the result of local expectations rather than my own. I have not planned for it. But for a patient in a crowded Ugandan hospital, what are such qualms but an irrelevant luxury? I am there. Judging from my skin tone and clothing I have obviously arrived from the wider world beyond. He knows me to be a university professor, and whatever he might make of that fact, I indeed enjoy easy access to information. His eyes rest on me, searching. He has asked a question.

So I tell him what I can: that this is not a cure, but odds are good his health should show improvement. However, he will potentially have to take these drugs for life. "For life?" We go over this several times. Then we circle back to the question of whether or not this is a cure. He seems to hope I will say something else. The doctor returns and resumes his place. The patient expresses surprise when told he will not receive drugs today and furthermore must return regularly to renew his prescription. He lives at some distance, and transportation promises to be difficult and expensive. Could he not have a larger supply? The doctor, growing impatient, repeats again that he must return with a caretaker who can monitor his treatment, and moreover that they both need to speak with a trained counselor who knows his language. Treatment cannot begin until after those conditions have been met. He then must take the drugs carefully and properly if he wants to live. Standing up, the doctor finally indicates the visit is over. It has already run over the allotted time, and we hear rustling outside in the hall; many others sit waiting, part of the afternoon's endless stream. The man, still looking uncertain, reluctantly rises and slowly heads out the door. As the doctor waves the next case in, the patient turns one last time and gives me a last searching look. I do my best to smile encouragingly. Then he is gone.

I encountered many memorable individuals that particular day, all dressed with cautious dignity for their clinic visit. An elderly woman laughed and laughed when offered a condom, saying her husband had died years ago. An elderly man stoutly protested the need to apply an ointment to his ears, as he found it turned them blue (after some banter the medical team suggested he wear a hat). A youth minister informed us that his general advice to his flock was to "add medicine on top of God as you're praying." A girl, tragically young to have the AIDS virus, sat silently during her consultation with a Ugandan clinical officer until he recognized her linguistic limitations. ("She speaks only one language, can you imagine?" he wondered aloud, looking for an appropriate interpreter.) But the patient I would recall most sharply was the man with needy, skeptical eyes, the one who unexpectedly sought my advice. The moment felt distinctly human in the humanitarian sense. His entreaty recalled the essence of MSF's appeal in the force of its simplicity. He was a stranger and remained so; I did not record his name. Yet for a brief moment he involved me in concern for his life and death. He asked a question and I answered—the smallest of actions, without even the benefit of expertise, but an engagement nonetheless. The appeal was personal and direct, lacking the buffer of other considerations, and I responded in kind. It was the human thing to do.

CRISIS BEYOND EMERGENCIES

The fact that my minor humanitarian moment occurred during a routine clinical visit, not the frantic aftermath of a disaster, indicates the expansive horizon of human suffering. It also illustrates the extent of MSF's organizational evolution.

What had been an endeavor focused on emergency in the form of disaster and conflict now recognized a much wider field of crisis, including AIDS. At the level of practice this was not entirely new. Indeed, it reflected an enduring tension. Only a year after its birth, recall, MSF placed volunteers on longer projects and was already deliberating its duty with regard to "chronic emergency."[1] Even in the 1980s the Belgian and French sections both sponsored small missions within Europe focused on "social exclusion," and the larger record of the group over the decades included a number of efforts aimed at offering clinical treatment to poor, underserved populations in different locations worldwide—indigenous people and street children being two popular categories.[2] Moreover, it had also expanded beyond physical care to offer psychological services. HIV/AIDS, however, was front and center in a more general transformation, one that deeply challenged the group's self-conception and historic limits.

At the time of my first encounter with its Ugandan clinic in 2003, MSF had undergone what its international president recognized as a "paradigm shift" in the treatment of certain infectious diseases:

> Humanitarian action is called for in silent wars as well. The death toll caused by treatable infectious diseases such as HIV/AIDS, malaria and tuberculosis (TB) remains staggering, especially in the poorest countries. During the past few years there has been a paradigm shift in the "accepted" thinking on infectious diseases. Patient treatment is becoming the focus as opposed to economic or public health mores. The World Health Organization (WHO) and many governments and donor agencies now agree with MSF that it is unethical to keep giving chloroquine to patients suffering from highly resistant strains of malaria. In the same way, it is no longer considered ethical to allow the 30 million people currently infected with HIV/AIDS to die due to lack of treatment.[3]

MSF went from being a relative bystander in the swirl of activity surrounding the pandemic to a significant participant. The shift of focus from prevention to treatment provided the group with both a platform and a rationale for its involvement. Beginning with a handful of programs to offer free antiretroviral (ARV) drugs to poor populations in 2001, most notably in Thailand and South Africa, the project quickly scaled up. Between 2002 and 2004 patient numbers jumped from 1,500 in ten countries to over 13,000 in twenty-five. The project continued to expand exponentially, and by the end of the decade the organization had over 160,000 HIV/AIDS patients under care worldwide.[4] In simple numerical terms, the program could claim considerable success: lives were indubitably being saved.

At a conceptual level the project had also achieved several major goals. Part of a much larger wave of determined efforts and converging interests, it had helped transform the landscape of AIDS care and the assumptions surrounding it. The sky-high pharmaceutical prices that once highlighted the medical injustice of inequality had fallen. An alliance of activists, generic manufacturers, and middle-income governments like those of Brazil and South Africa had—in the short run at least—triumphed over entrenched corporations and national patent interests. Where conventional wisdom had held that poor people, particularly in remote rural areas, would never adhere to a strict drug regime, many now clearly did. Alongside others, MSF had helped pioneer a model for treatment. Imperfect and difficult as it might be, one could treat HIV/AIDS in almost any setting.

Questions still lingered, however, within this happy story of relative success. No matter how large it might grow, MSF could hardly sustain a program to treat more than a small fraction of those suffering from AIDS worldwide. More directly, it was not clear whether it could ever hand over many of the patients it had amassed to a reliable alternative source of care. Both national governments and international organizations appeared to be falling short of their goals. The ambitious rollouts of the early years of the decade had only partly materialized. MSF might be a wealthy NGO able to independently underwrite an ARV program. But once in, it was not clear there would be a sure way out, even as the continuing commitment hampered its mobility. At the same time new trade agreements and shifting patterns of drug resistance threatened the future of inexpensive medication. The organization thus found itself with additional worries, many well beyond its accustomed niche of expertise.

Most fundamentally, AIDS did not constitute an emergency in MSF's operational sense of the term. Rather, it constituted a slower moving crisis: the HIV virus could lurk for years before precipitating a decline, and even after the onset of AIDS the timeline of care was hardly sudden. For those patients who responded to ARV treatment, the disease became a chronic condition, something to monitor and manage for a lifetime. For MSF, then, the AIDS experience proved a watershed in defining its humanitarianism. To fulfill its new vision, the group would need to recognize "silent" crises in addition to obvious disasters. If MSF was no longer accepting economic and public health limitations in addressing infectious disease, it would need to bypass the frailty of infrastructure to deliver these services as well, testing the limits of its kit system. It would have to address the larger economic questions surrounding drug prices and structural issues affecting pharmaceutical supply. Moreover, it would need to continually rethink which problems it addressed and which it ignored. If treating AIDS, what about TB, with which it was often linked? What about malaria, and more "neglected" diseases like sleeping sickness, with which MSF had a long history? AIDS enjoyed the spotlight but hardly exhausted the wide range of ways to expire amid poverty.

"In terms of the destruction of human life," the president of MSF-France wrote in 2004, "what difference is there between the wartime bombing of a civilian population and the distribution of ineffective medications during a pandemic that is killing millions of people?"[5] From this perspective, MSF's self-imposed policy of providing only emergency response gradually proved porous. The same logic that opened the door to AIDS also admitted other potential humanitarian concerns. Matters of life and suffering, after all, extend well beyond basic health care in refugee camps. By the group's fourth tumultuous decade, then, MSF faced a widened range of possible concerns. Issues of "social exclusion" and lack of treatment access appeared periodically in MSF's portfolio. Things that MSF had once famously dismissed, such as mental health, reemerged as legitimate humanitarian concerns. Each new problem area had its own history, and once visible, it altered the boundaries of normal procedure. Here I focus on Uganda and AIDS, an approach that both simplifies and complicates the chronology of MSF's programmatic expansion while clarifying the stakes involved in the humanitarian alternative to public health.

By the end of the twentieth century, HIV/AIDS had emerged as the signature disease of medical morality, one of intense interest to doctors, activists, governments, and anthropologists alike.[6] The former fulcrum for anxieties about perceived social deviance in North America and Europe had gone global, acquiring a new aura of urgency in the process. AIDS stood for life and death. It revealed stark contradictions, the fragility of established human solidarities, and the injustice of inequality. Consequently it also mobilized people into new alliances and associations. With the development of a relatively successful treatment regime, these grew into practical arbiters of health care and medical forms of citizenship. Sub-Saharan Africa stood at the epicenter of both the pandemic and its response, just as it did with humanitarian emergencies. There, health care and medical research filtered through abiding tensions tied to race and colonial legacies of mistreatment and misrule. The result proved epic, tragic, and unsettling, all on a numbingly vast scale. It was also clearly compelling, as an extraordinary array of entities rushed to respond in various ways. MSF, however, initially resisted engagement. Only when AIDS treatment became a battle line did it fully embrace the problem as its own. Once involved, the organization found its sense of time stretched and extended, the clear limits of emergency falling away. This crisis had no obvious end.

A STUDY IN SLEEPING SICKNESS

Before AIDS there was sleeping sickness. This is true for both MSF and for Uganda, as a mission site and as a onetime colony. Sleeping sickness—or, in its less evocative official name, human African trypanosomiasis (HAT)—provided a precedent at several levels, both for the experience of a complex epidemic disease and for the practice of another form of medical humanitarianism. Most immediately it offered a ready template for an alternative type of MSF mission, one adjusted to a slower rhythm of response and concerned with drug availability, medical protocols, and the products of research. For nearly two decades MSF sponsored an evolving program in Uganda focused on sleeping sickness. At the outset it was a relative anomaly within the group's assorted projects, with AIDS not even on the humanitarian horizon. By the time it closed the situation had dramatically altered, and a gleaming new clinic dedicated to ARV treatment was rising in its place. The connection between the two was not simply geographic.

Sleeping sickness once inspired its own health panic. Between 1900 and 1905 an epidemic swept through the area, then a British protectorate. Perhaps a quarter of a million people died, arousing considerable concern among colonial authorities. The Royal Society dispatched a research team to investigate, and in October of 1902 it identified a "fish-like parasite" in a blood sample, matching the trypanosome discovery made in Ghana less than a year before.[7] Although accounts of a distinctive "African lethargy" had appeared centuries earlier, sometimes credited with emptying whole villages, this was the critical moment in the biomedical definition of the disease. Having linked the pathology with a parasitic infection, researchers subsequently identified the tsetse fly as the insect vector of transmission. Over the ensuing years further scientific research revealed an increasingly complex picture of sleeping sickness, which came in several forms affecting both humans and livestock. The human varieties were hard to detect without screening. If left untreated, however, the infection would ultimately move beyond the lymph nodes and across the blood-brain barrier. Sleeping sickness thus proved a fearsomely fatal disease. Researchers gradually came to realize that its prevalence, however, depended on a relatively delicate balance between parasite, fly vector, environment, and human host. Only under certain conditions—within a certain temperature range, at particular intervals of feeding—could the parasite develop in the fly's gut and subsequently infect its human host. By and large, the collapse of stable settlements offered ideal opportunities for the spread of the pathogen. At the same time it could not spread indefinitely or range far from its regional habitat. Both Europe and India, it turned out, were safe from this African scourge. Most Africans were safe as well, as long as they inhabited stably settled and well-cleared land. Ecologically constricted and yet potentially mortal, sleeping sickness proved a quintessentially colonial condition.[8]

As it became clear that the insect vector remained regionally confined, initial fears of a wider threat subsided and focus turned to effective governance. From the perspective of colonial administrators, both human and animal forms of sleeping sickness constituted a threat to their rule. Like other colonial powers, the British subsequently sought to control the prevalence of the disease, if opting for more of an ecological approach than the medical one of their French rivals. In a telling irony of history, their wider activities likely contributed to both cause and cure as they regulated outbreaks in part induced by the larger disruption of imperial expansion. Some early researchers recognized that the shift of sleeping sickness from endemic to epidemic owed much to the disruptive effects of population migrations and invasive expeditions.[9] In this sense control of the disease was ultimately a question of political stability, and not simply efforts to treat humans or eradicate flies.

Sleeping sickness reemerged as a problem during Uganda's upheaval in the early 1980s. With the movement of refugees in both directions across the border with Sudan, the collapse of control programs and other health infrastructure, and the decline in land cultivation, the country faced another epidemic. Tsetse flies, it turned out, also thrived on civil war.[10] In 1986–1987, MSF was still relatively small and almost entirely focused on projects providing basic health care in crisis settings. Although their Belgian rivals displayed a willingness to engage beyond emergency, the ancestral French section maintained a strong aversion to longer missions. In Uganda, the French had been running refugee projects in both the north and the south of the country. The political situation slowly stabilized after the victory of now-president Yoweri Museveni's forces, and MSF closed the southern mission. The northern part of the country, however, posed more of a dilemma for the group. There the health infrastructure lay in ruins, and the new government—based in the south—displayed little urgency in reconstructing it. "Everything was destroyed," one of the MSF protagonists recalled in 2003, describing the moment to me in his office in Paris. "Uganda had achieved a certain level in the sixties and seventies. So the north had once had hospitals, the whole system." Moreover, while refugees streamed back from Sudan, the group realized that rates of sleeping sickness were reaching epidemic proportions. As it happened, a key doctor on the field team had written his medical thesis on the disease. Given this state of collapse combined with outbreak, my Parisian veteran noted, MSF faced a fundamental question: "Did we have a place after the war?" MSF decided to stay, both to combat the disease and to monitor the situation. "At the time no one knew much about sleeping sickness except a few British researchers in universities. . . . There was no government, so why not see what happens, work with the epidemic and returning refugees?"

Beyond the contingent facts of this immediate context, MSF's decision to launch a sleeping sickness project also recalled the pioneering efforts of Eugène Jamot. A doctor in the French colonial medical service, Jamot's legacy inspired the early generation of French humanitarians.[11] In contrast to the British emphasis on fly habitats, he established a more medically oriented approach to the disease, one focused on mass treatment. Rather than relying on the incidental observations of existing health personnel, he established a vertical organization with trained teams dedicated to screening the population and tracking down cases in areas of high incidence. To the extent that it followed a similar logic and schema,

MSF's effort quite literally reanimated this colonial antecedent. A classic menace required a classic response: in the words of an MSF author, "the return of Dr. Jamot."[12]

The resulting project lasted far longer than anyone initially anticipated, evolving through a series of different sites in the same general region. It also came to incorporate a research element alongside its clinical practice. In both these respects it contrasted with MSF's emergency missions and at times even resembled efforts at community health development, a form of engagement from which the organization (and especially the French section) generally distanced itself. As the Ugandan Ministry of Health slowly revived, the group saw itself working in partnership, contributing one element to a more comprehensive effort to combat the disease. By training a network of personnel it might also aid the larger cause of rebuilding the country's health infrastructure.

Sleeping sickness proved an elusive and entangling disease. When the prevalence rate fell in one locality, MSF teams would find a fresh trove of cases in a neighboring one. The work thus had no quick and clear end. In addition, by focusing on this specific disease, the group became increasingly aware that the prevailing medical protocol itself was a problem. The second, deadly stage of the disease that followed the parasite's entry into the brain was the point where symptoms grew debilitating and even the most reluctant sought medical care. It also proved difficult and hazardous to treat. The primary medication in use was an arsenic derivative known as melarsoprol, discovered in 1949 and substituted for an earlier related compound, atoxyl. Although melarsoprol could cross the blood-brain barrier, it had painful side effects. Moreover, not only did melarsoprol fail to work in over a quarter of the cases, it also ended up killing some 5 percent or more of those treated.[13] Unfortunately, few alternatives had appeared in the pharmaceutical pipeline. As a vector-driven disease confined to marginal habitats, sleeping sickness almost exclusively afflicted poor populations. It thus offered little prospect for profit and was of little interest to commercial drug companies engaged in the risky and expensive endeavor of testing new substances. Laboring in the fields of frontline medicine, MSF stumbled into a fundamental weakness in the infrastructure of international health.

To the extent that "no one" beyond a few researchers knew much about sleeping sickness at the outset of this particular endeavor, the organization found itself needing to develop expertise. It began in a statistical desert, ferreting out facts bit by bit on the ground. With the creation of its epidemiological subsidiary, Epicentre, MSF acquired the means for better organization and analysis. Epicentre developed an electronic database in 1994.[14] Conducting studies and comparing protocols, it grew deeply involved in the sleeping sickness program, even administering a final follow-up phase after the clinical work finally ended in 2002. By this point the French project was hardly alone, and the larger MSF collective, equipped with data and eager to innovate, had established itself as something of an authority on the disease and its treatment. It was also facing a different plague, one far better publicized and far more geographically promiscuous than sleeping sickness, with Africa again cast in a leading role.

AIDS: TRADITION BEFORE TREATMENT

As the notoriety of the Amin era began to fade, Uganda became known for HIV/ AIDS. This new, rapidly globalizing disease also flourished during civil war and emerged as a full-blown problem for the country in its aftermath. Early action by the Museveni government drew international acclaim, as well as producing a well-known and intensely debated model for public health response, the ABC program (abstain, be faithful, use condoms). At the same time citizen organizations like TASO (The AIDS Support Organization) and NACWOLA (National Community of Women Living with HIV/AIDS) emerged to offer support to those infected, combating stigma and providing inspiring examples of civil society action recognized far beyond the country's borders. Uganda also became a favored site for medical research on the disease, with numerous international institutes and experts setting up shop and conducting studies. The government appeared to cooperate with medical research and development projects, shifting away from Marxist rhetoric to increasingly invite international assistance from Europe and the United States.[15] The country had a ready supply of patients and sufficient health infrastructure to locate needy populations, if not always to care for them.

Up to this point MSF had generally avoided involving itself in AIDS work. In the days before antiretroviral drugs redefined treatment, many in the organization saw little they could do where the disease was concerned. The group's expertise, they felt, lay in emergency response, not prevention or health education or extended hospice care. Besides, the scale was daunting and the condition already commanded considerable attention, to which the contribution of outsiders would be superficial, if not neocolonial. Others could and should take the lead. Although sections of the larger collective might make tentative steps toward engagement— the French sent a delegate to the Montreal AIDS conference in 1989, for example, fiercely debating the resulting report, while the Belgians opened a free screening center in Brussels—advocates of greater involvement remained a distinct, if passionate, minority.[16] As one advocate later phrased it with emphatic simplicity, at the time AIDS was *"not MSF."*

Nonetheless, this resistance slowly eroded. Advocates of treatment remained vocal and active, keeping AIDS a topic of discussion. They also managed to create a number of HIV projects, largely with backing from headquarters other than Paris.[17] Uganda was one such exception. There the small Swiss branch of the organization sponsored a couple of early ventures, unusual not only in their existence but also their form. An annual report from 1997 provides the following retrospective synopsis:

> When the Swiss section of MSF arrived in Uganda in 1988, AIDS had reached nearly a third of the urban population and approximately 10% of the people in rural zones, more than a million and a half people out of a total of 17 million inhabitants. . . . In a country where a large number of NGOs are helping to fight AIDS, MSF operates in areas where help is scarce or nonexistent. In 1991 and 1992, MSF started two projects. The first, Moyo AIDS Control Initiative (MACI), is a prevention project in the district of Moyo in the north of the country where MSF has its help program for Sudanese refugees. The second, Traditional and Modern Health Practitioners Together Against AIDS (THETA) is focused on a collaboration between traditional healers and health workers to define new strategies of prevention and care. . . . These two projects, MACI (1991) and THETA (1992) have now been formed into Ugandan NGOs which, with the help of MSF, are on their way to becoming autonomous.[18]

The report glosses over the resistance these projects faced at their outset from within the larger organization. Like the sleeping sickness program, they owed their existence in no small part to the force of will of those who established and defended them, as well as the organization's loose structure and tolerance for contradiction. (As a member of MSF Belgium put it bluntly, with reference to a later, famous AIDS project in South Africa, "A crazy guy . . . can push and push and build a program.")[19] While stretching the limits of MSF's self-conceptualization, these Ugandan projects grew into separate entities cast at a national, rather than international, scale. Neither redefined the group's general approach to the disease, and so they would be largely forgotten following the embrace of an antiretroviral response.

Nonetheless, the THETA project proved particularly interesting and long lasting. MSF had already created a number of spinoff entities by that point, but these generally conformed to conventional biomedical understandings of health. Forms of care now described as "traditional healing" fell far beyond such parameters. Their slow timeline and extra-somatic logic contrasted sharply with the sensibility of emergency medicine, which emphasized speed and physical intervention with a delimited body. The medical profession at large remained dismissive of alternative approaches, and individual doctors—particularly those working in marginal locations—were often nervous about being associated with them. In addition to concerns about professional reputation, Uganda had an anti-witchcraft law on the books. Nonetheless, there was the unavoidable fact that health care outside of cities clearly involved traditional healers. The founders of THETA recognized this reality and sought to mobilize this other network in the greater cause. As one of them stressed to me, "access was the point" in venturing beyond biomedicine, even if the parent organization did not yet recognize this.

THETA emerged as an offshoot of MSF's MACI project in Moyo district. It involved two team members from that effort in collaboration with a physician from the Ugandan group TASO, with early financial assistance from the Rockefeller Foundation. The Swiss section agreed to support THETA as long as additional funds were raised, and it provided a basic template for operational details. "Toshiba laptops, Toyota Land Cruisers, positions like doctor, admin, log," another founder recalled, "that was what we knew." In key conceptual respects, however, the new venture deviated sharply: "We had just been in Kigali, where Belgians were running the hospital, very colonial. So we were trying to imagine how it might be different if run by Rwandans." Even if THETA's roots lay partly in European humanitarianism, it should grow firmly in Ugandan soil. To this end, the initial vision explicitly departed from the emergency tradition:

> For years MSF secluded itself from the aid business via emergency medicine.... Like a chair with one leg, always unstable. How to build something more durable? Ninety-five percent of MSF projects don't survive MSF. Either you say I'm here to do this or you don't do it right. Individuals may benefit, yes, or learn. But what about communities or countries? We haven't left behind structures, except [the] transient ones of MSF itself. It's like saying, "Here I come. I want to teach you how to drive my car but never let you sit in my seat. We stay in that car for a year and then my brother comes to teach you again."[20]

The Swiss venture in AIDS was thus a doubly radical effort. Despite the fact that the French sleeping sickness program had been long-term and achieved medical success, it remained an international project that would wither quickly after MSF's departure. Most of the Ugandans it trained would wait in vain for an equally reliable employer. THETA, by contrast, would seek to settle in place and time, fitting a particular milieu. To do that it would become a separate entity.

The new organization undertook two briefs: conducting outreach and training with traditional healers and running clinical trials to evaluate traditional therapies. The former endeavor concentrated on building a network of healers who could function as volunteer community counselors, while the latter focused on materials used to treat secondary opportunistic infections associated with AIDS.[21] Funding remained tight, coming in fits and starts from a variety of international donors. Nonetheless, by the time MSF withdrew its last support in 2000, the organization that remained had acquired its own building and vehicles, as well as a distinctly Ugandan staff. It would indeed survive the separation.[22]

Near the end of 2004, I participated in a THETA venture in public relations. The guest list reflected the heightened reach of AIDS as a public issue as it included not only the Centers for Disease Control's country director and the American ambassador, but also two stars from the reality television show *Survivor*. After a presentation at the organization's office, we were driven to visit a traditional healer in the greater Kampala area. That visit did not go smoothly, running late and featuring elements that the more impatient guests found extraneous, such as lengthy ritual speeches of welcome at the community site. The ambassador applauded heartily, as befit his role, but indicated afterward that he remained a skeptic. Nonetheless, the fact that the event occurred at all implied a coming of age for both the organization and the disease that animated it. The guests who undertook this particular pilgrimage, removing their shoes to enter the dim interior of the healer's shrine, displayed considerable faith in the greater cause.

By that point the terrain around AIDS had shifted considerably. Treatment had displaced prevention as the keyword of response, and controversy swirling around the South African president's resistance to antiretroviral drugs had tarnished the reputation of alternative approaches. In THETA's presentation the speakers took pains to emphasize their recognition of biomedical expertise and their desire to fulfill a complementary role. Even the representative healer, speaking in translation, referenced terms common to public health like "transmission rates" and "discordant couples." AIDS had become a new language of exchange.

Meanwhile MSF itself had pivoted from aversion to full embrace of the disease. The appearance of antiretroviral medications in the mid-1990s served as a catalyst, reorienting the horizon of AIDS work from prevention to treatment. Alongside ad hoc provision to people infected with HIV through personal networks, ARVs entered an MSF kit for accidental exposure. By the end of the decade they became a mission rationale of their own.[23] Pursuing a program that a member of the Brussels office described as "well thought-out disobedience," the organization launched a series of projects to deliver the new drugs and joined the larger advocacy campaign to lower their prices. Its involvement at an operational level propelled the group into new legal and economic arenas, while questions of pharmaceutical procurement and distribution—such as the use of Brazilian drugs in South Africa—acquired political significance. This AIDS adventure also displayed explicitly global ambition. Thus even as the final phase of the sleeping sickness project in Uganda wound down, a new program geared up in the nearby town of Arua. Its location derived from a perception of the area's relative neglect, but also from the organization's history in that corner of the country. The French section established a clinic in the main hospital to care for AIDS patients and administer antiretrovirals to those who needed them. Although a simple structure, compared to the rest of the worn buildings it gleamed clean and new, emitting an aura of confidence and urgency. Treatment had arrived.

ARVS AND "OTHER QUESTIONS OF LIVING"

While visiting MSF's AIDS clinic in Uganda, I found myself spending an unexpected amount of time with patients as well as with project staff. This stemmed largely from the initiative of the staff, who assumed this was what all visitors should be doing, and to a lesser extent the patients themselves, some of whom had avidly embraced a spokesperson role. By this point in time such programs in Uganda experienced a small but steady stream of guests, including journalists, medical and foundation professionals, and political sponsors. The highlight of most trips was the testimonial encounter, where patients of ARV medication would recount their miraculous recovery in personal terms. Although the pattern quickly grew familiar, it remained riveting when told by a protagonist as a fundamental tale of survival. Health professionals assured me that this type of encounter was highly effective in converting skeptics to the power of the pharmaceutical approach. AIDS, it turned out, was a disease conducive to such interaction and patient self-representation. However much people might suffer they retained their faculties, unlike those in the later stage of sleeping sickness. Both decline and treatment of AIDS were a drawn-out affairs, unlike the rapid demise caused by cholera. Moreover, by the time MSF entered the fray the condition had acquired a moral aura as well as activist expectations about a need to speak.[24] It also had become the subject of considerable anthropological inquiry, key insights of which I would find amply borne out.

Since the project team was invariably busy, many encounters occurred while I dutifully followed them in their daily practice. Crowded into the corner of cramped consultation rooms or ducking in and out of dank concrete wards, I met a stream of the afflicted, each carrying one of the faded exercise books that served as their medical records. Even in a relatively well-funded program like this, the experience was a world removed from similar venues in the United States, particularly with regard to assumptions about service and privacy. Hospital staff issued orders, not requests. Patients and attending family members waited quietly, and then waited some more, often with only the benefit of thin walls or a periodic language barrier to separate them from their neighbors. In such a setting it was painfully obvious that access and survival outweighed legal self-determination on the list of daily concerns. Those who sought treatment could hardly expect the luxury of anonymity. MSF may have renovated the building used as the AIDS clinic into a gleaming oasis and carefully trained its counselors, but it could not alter the larger landscape. Outside the clinic, at the hospital gate, and along the surrounding roads there stretched a regular gauntlet of eyes.

On my second visit to the project in 2004 I met a patient wearing a worn but still impressive suit fashioned from purple corduroy. His face was similarly lined, and he projected a gentle air of dignified suffering. We sat together with a counselor, who queried him about his recent health. As he spoke no English she occasionally translated for my benefit, recounting details of his Lazarus-like recovery thanks to ARV therapy. Partway through this litany, however, he realized that I understood French and switched into that language. Like quite a few in the region, he had crossed the border and was now "staying" in the Congo, as the expression went. Ignoring the counselor (who could no longer follow the conversation and began to look annoyed), he told me proudly that he was a businessman. Now that he felt relatively recovered, he hoped to renew commercial activities and asked for my phone number on the chance he might have the opportunity to contact me in the future. He then proceeded to complain about the difficulty of getting from his real home in the Congo to Arua town, the only place where he could receive treatment. Although he had managed to reestablish enough of a Ugandan profile to qualify for MSF's program, it took a considerable investment of time and funds to keep his appointments. He spent a few minutes enlarging upon these concerns, becoming more and more animated. At last the counselor had had enough. She cut him off by handing him forms for new medications and showing him the door. As he left, he seemed to sink back into himself, his face settling into its earlier aspect.

Our exchange was brief and I never met him again. Nonetheless, the memory stayed with me as the man in the purple suit began to embody a central contrast I noted among the AIDS patients. At the moment of medical encounter most were quiet and attentive to the point of subservience, focused on receiving the promised treatment and quickly promising to observe proper procedures. When opportunity presented itself, however, they quickly and volubly detailed the larger panorama of their daily problems: the many dependents and obligations, the odyssey that even minor travel entailed, and the endless difficulties in scratching out a livelihood. Members of the MSF team were clearly aware of these issues. They discussed ways to modify their work, such as creating satellite clinics to ease access, a step they would later take. Nonetheless, the greater problems of poverty lay beyond their project capacity and medical expertise. They could only do so much. Although this tension between health and poverty will be broadly familiar to anyone immersed in the narrative arc of the AIDS pandemic, the particular dilemma of MSF within it proves acute: how does an emergency organization treat a chronic condition?

One morning I had a formal interview with Joyce, a long-term member of the Arua branch of the national women's support group NACWOLA. A vivacious woman, bright eyed with high cheekbones, she wore a violet dress and seemed full of life. Although only in her early forties, she was relatively old in this setting, and beneath her bold front her body appeared frail. The staff member who introduced me to her spent several minutes joking about how much weight she had gained. Together they examined her still-thin arm, recalling how sticklike it once had been before breaking into happy laughter. Her health confirmed, she sat and proceeded to tell me her life story. She had clearly done this many times before and was comfortable with the medical phrasings of her condition as well as the terminology of NGOs. Although such language fell incongruously on my ear, it quite precisely represented the experience that she wished to recount.

Joyce had been born in Arua, though she had gone to secondary school in another town, and lived for a year in the Congo during the war in the 1980s. A primary school teacher, she had two children of her own. Their father died in 1994, the same year that NACWOLA came to Arua. She joined the group for "psycho-social" support, in this case a matter of home visits, small packages of soap and sugar, and discussion groups. NACWOLA's signature activity—a memory project to document family history—was particularly meaningful for her, as it offered a way for her children to come to terms with their parents' condition. For many women, the action of compiling family accounts offered a way to break the news gently. Joyce went public even before her husband died, and her children were not happy. As she noted, "Going public means bringing your whole family to go public." Creating a memory book helped, and since she was a teacher she soon found herself assisting others who were illiterate, helping them to assemble nice legacies for their children. The group grew from four to over 300 members and established an office. At the same time, however, her own health began to deteriorate. She came down with TB and experienced hallucinations and nightmares as her body wasted away. Soon she was a near skeleton, unable to walk unassisted. The new drug program arrived just in time, and as she saw it, because she "came out early" the MSF staff worked especially hard to save her life.

Now that she felt stronger again, Joyce had resumed her prominent role in the support group. In addition to holding monthly meetings, NACWOLA gardened, kept rabbits, and dreamt of establishing a larger resource center. They also sponsored a "Saturday club" for children, providing space for play, the expression of feelings, health education, and general encouragement to pursue schooling. "We try to look on children as the continuity of our lives," Joyce said. "Education will help them when their parents are not there." At the same time, in her view the club also served as a refuge from the shadow of the disease, allowing a semblance of ordinary pleasures and emotional stability. "AIDS or no AIDS," she emphasized, "life must continue." She felt strongly that having aided her dying husband helped her own survival. "I know that the fact that I looked after him gave me energy to continue. If I had not I would have been haunted. To be able to forgive and look at him as a human being was very important."

NACWOLA had many plans and was actively seeking sponsorship. They had considered starting demonstration plots, to learn "more scientific ways of farming." They also hoped to expand their center, move sewing machines there and expand craft production to foster income for their members. But they faced a number of significant challenges. Not only was their property several kilometers out of town, which posed transportation problems for many women, but it also lacked electricity and water. Security was also an issue, and the women wanted a fence and a guard. Even as they imagined adding carousels and swings, they feared that the children's toys they did have would be stolen. They also felt a need for technical staff, particularly a secretary and craft instructors. But in order to achieve any part of their vision they needed to find additional funding. MSF had provided them with the equivalent of US$5,000, Joyce noted appreciatively, but wanted them to look elsewhere. For a while Save the Children UK had given money to protect children's rights following reports of abuse among AIDS families. But that money ran out, and most of it was earmarked for education. They had also received some German money to train children in carpentry, but not all the children had understood their community obligations and some had disappeared. Even getting those women who could sew to train others could be difficult. "Many support us but few are committed," Joyce sighed. Having juggled being a teacher as well as a mother and patient she understood the difficulties faced by many of her fellow members first hand. Indeed, she saw herself as luckier than most, who were illiterate and lived hand to mouth. They couldn't be expected to give much time to the organization, particularly on a volunteer basis.

With the arrival of ARVs, Joyce sensed there was now more focus on medical issues in foreign funding. Although the seeds of Arua's AIDS network came from Uganda's most famous citizens' organization, TASO, the Arua group realized it needed a different strategy "because of donor fatigue." However, amid all the shifting priorities it was hard to keep up. Furthermore, some things were always difficult to support. "Many organizations don't want to give money for salaries, just activities," Joyce astutely observed. "But then how to motivate people as workers? That has been a challenge for us. Food is the first medicine, and without food there is always a problem." Moreover, most grants had relatively short funding cycles and offered no standing guarantees, as "no donor comes and stays forever." Even the MSF project was officially on a five-year plan. What, she wondered, would happen after the five years were up? Joyce had little confidence that the Ugandan Ministry of Health would be able to take over the project successfully. "They are overwhelmed," she said simply. "We will have to plan carefully and think independently."

Later on the same day, I met Andrew, a founding member of the considerably smaller men's support organization known as ADMACHA (Arua District Male Community Living with HIV/AIDS). A tall, thin, older man with a wispy beard, only the slowness of his gait hinted at illness beneath his air of dignity. Like Joyce, Andrew came from Arua and had spent a period of youthful exile in the Congo in the early 1980s. He also was a teacher. However, since his schooling ended prematurely he could only teach as an unqualified primary teacher. Drama and debate had always been his favorite subjects. As he noted with some pride, he could talk to anyone, for he had "a convincing tongue." In 1996 his wife died while they were living in another town, and as they had no children he found himself alone. When he began feeling sick himself he returned to Arua. Although his body flashed hot and cold, at the time he had not yet been tested and did not realize his condition. "There was no one to tell me," he said, "and my brain could not think alone." As his illness progressed he lost the factory job he had briefly found and was admitted to the hospital for TB. While there he met women from NACWOLA, including some relatives, who convinced him to be tested in 2000. Although the MSF program had not yet started and ARVs were beyond his reach, he found solace in associating with NACWOLA and participating in their dramas. That helped "rebuild his self-esteem," particularly as he realized he was good at this genre of public speech.

Inspired by NACWOLA, Andrew and several associates had recently founded a parallel support group for men, christening it with an equally impressive acronym. Neither group was exclusive, he explained, as men could belong to the women's group and vice versa. Although the two organizations collaborated extensively, each had its proper sphere. ADMACHA targeted males, particularly those "difficult men" who avoided treatment and refused responsibility. Andrew felt much of their reluctance stemmed from their "negative attitude" and fear. Men were likely to claim that they didn't care and to worry about losing both their livelihood and ability to attract women if they admitted even the possibility of their infection. Some of them, he added, were "just stubborn."

ADMACHA remained a fledgling organization. Newly equipped with a constitution and a post office box, it now sought funding beyond its modest membership fees. Thus far MSF had not offered material support, though Andrew hoped there would soon be a discussion of it. He asked my advice on finding additional donors, as he understood that funding for AIDS circulated well beyond the hospital walls. Money was the central concern for his organization, and a theme he returned to repeatedly: "Sincerely, the group I'm with has shown activity; if we can find financial backing we have the motivation. Most of us are jobless, and that can easily discourage." Even some modest employment, craft work, or part-time paid counseling would help. Perhaps they could found a CBO, he added hopefully, using the aid acronym for community-based organization. They had recently received an invitation to a workshop on "capacity building" and that was a good sign.

As well as the continual problem of resources, the return to life brought other concerns, including reawakening desires for sex, companionship, and offspring. "Loneliness," Andrew observed, "is a terrible thing." He himself had an HIV-positive partner and planned to stay faithful, but he feared that over time others would lapse without support and guidance. Beyond satisfying physical desire, companionship held pragmatic benefits, especially for men. "The gender roles of household tasks," he said, "are a challenge to us." In a setting where kin ties played a crucial role in daily affairs, reproduction was also a concern. Some men, he told me, were wondering whether they might risk fathering children now that their health had returned. He himself was considering raising the possibility as a discussion topic and hoped to receive further guidance from MSF staff. Andrew had great faith in the organization, he told me, having seen it operate across the border in the Congo during the West Nile wars. Once MSF arrived in Arua, he knew he might have "access" and so hoped to live again. He was quite disturbed, however, to think that MSF might eventually seek to hand the project over and leave. In particular he worried about drug security, doubting that the district government could provide it.

Discrimination against AIDS patients had ebbed in recent years, but Andrew recalled painful examples of "stigma." The experience of people looking at him as if he were an outcast, the sight of people recoiling from infected friends and relatives and refusing to touch them, even going so far as to throw them food, had left its mark. Although the situation was now much better, the very existence of treatment and support for the disease ironically produced another backlash:

> We face jealousy when put in a ward for intensive treatment. We are given enough medicine, so there is jealousy. The others wish MSF doctors would treat them. They think it's discrimination or sectarian when they only attend to HIV cases. If it were possible, it would be nice to have a small ward just for HIV cases. The way that ordinary people look at you when you're feeble, you need privacy. It would be nice to be attended to without interacting with others. Sometimes when we were issued food support they felt we were favored by being given free food. So a feeling [arose of] "I wish I had HIV so that I would get the food." With ARVs HIV is no longer quite the same threat. A good many are saying now, "There's medicine." Even if we try to explain with drama that the virus is not quite killed but dormant, many are now thinking it's more a disease like malaria.[25]

It was precisely this sort of attitude that ADMACHA hoped to combat through a steady stream of testimonials and educational dramas. As our allotted time came to an end, Andrew again underscored his group's gratitude to MSF, particularly for choosing a poor and rural area of the country for its AIDS program, and expressed hope for his own organization's future. In response to his queries, I did my best to explain grant writing and suggest ways he might approach international NGOs and other potential donors.

Both Joyce and Andrew were Ugandan citizens with ties across the border to the neighboring Congo. As AIDS patients, however, they were also caught up in another forms of quasi-citizenship, forms predicated on their condition.[26] Both displayed ready familiarity with the favored terms and acronyms used by aid organizations, sprinkling their sentences with expressions like "stigma" and "psycho-social support." They also revealed an astute grasp of what donor organizations might generally favor, even if they were not always certain about the particulars of accessing assistance. Literate English speakers with prior pedagogical experience, they had emerged as leading figures in their respective organizations. Now they sought support for themselves and their communities from the most likely economic source available to them: the myriad of governmental and nongovernmental agencies seeking to assist people like themselves.

Unsurprisingly, Joyce and Andrew expressed gratitude when speaking about MSF's AIDS program, and apprehension at the thought that the organization might leave. Beyond the concern that a sudden vacuum would leave them without care, they were uncertain about who might prove a reliable successor to MSF. Neither had much faith that Uganda's Ministry of Health could run the program as effectively as MSF, even if it were somehow supplied with funds. They associated the state with corruption and inefficiency, suspecting that someone would siphon off goods before they were delivered. Theirs was a world in which NGOs were not only a natural part of the political and economic landscape but the preferred conduits for employment, patronage, and redistribution.

CARING FOR LIFE

Tensions about the limits of MSF's AIDS program and its relation to the government health system were as evident to those providing care as to those receiving it. Over the course of the same visit in 2004 I had several conversations with Amélie, the French doctor who served as the field coordinator for the Arua project. Thin, thoughtful, and intense, she also looked irrevocably tired. She had come to Uganda from a similar project in Kenya, and the constant effort to meet the vast need was clearly wearing. In medical terms the ARV program had proved largely successful to this point, with some 85 percent of the initial patients still alive and under treatment. But as the numbers continued to expand, program management and longevity were growing issues.

"I think we have an obligation to care for AIDS patients and of course you want to treat more," she said. "But here in Arua we are overwhelmed." She explained that the problem was not simply the scale and intensity of the work itself, but also the challenge of trying to root the project in local soil so it would prove a healthy transplant: "If we want to do it all tomorrow we can do it with MSF, eventually with more staff. But if we want it to last long that won't work." As she saw it, expansion was as much a matter of personnel as patient load: "We need to take care of the team; we're burning out some people as we're asking a lot. Most of the team is leaving in a month. Why do we leave? I'm exhausted. I will tell you that very honestly. How to keep this going? It's not an emergency project, but most days we work at this speed. You can't make people work like on an emergency for years . . . and HIV/AIDS means care for *life*."

While the MSF program had forged ahead quickly, the Ugandan Ministry of Health's own effort had yet to materialize. Yet MSF had no authority over ministry staff or policies and sought to support rather than supplant them. This structural imbalance led to awkward moments of friction. "Do we do it for them," Amélie mused, "or do we do it with them?" In her initial meetings with officials, she sensed they hoped the former; health care resources were stretched thin even without AIDS. Moreover, there was no relief in sight. The project had no natural limits—unlike other diseases, they could not expect a decline in incidence after treatment that might ease a handover.

> We've opened the door to take care of AIDS here in Arua. Now 10 percent are com-
> ing from outside the district. We must take referrals, but originally just from Arua
> hospital. We're not refusing patients yet, but that may happen. MSF is asking why
> we're letting people in from outside. But it's the same in Kenya, same in Malawi. . . .
> Even if we get rid of them this would still be very busy. If no one comes from the
> ministry then we'll need more staff from MSF. If not, we feel we have to stop and
> become more restrictive. And that's not easy when you have someone in front of
> you crying.[27]

She expressed enthusiasm about NACWOLA and ADMACHA as well as a Muslim patient group that was just forming. Some of their goals, however, ran well beyond MSF's collective sense of expertise and its medical team's capabilities. The staff could help a little but not a lot. She also thought that the practice of providing free care to AIDS patients when other patients in the wards had to pay only contributed to stigma, and she hoped to phase it out.

Over drinks one evening a group of foreign staffers discussed their work while waiting for a lunar eclipse. As everywhere near the equator, evening fell quickly and the moon rose orange, sharply edged against the stars. One recent arrival, an Australian nurse tasked with improving standards of care in the hospital, expressed dismay at a story involving corruption. The others laughed knowingly and proceeded to pass on their accumulated store of local knowledge. An engineer responsible for maintenance spent most of his time running a private business out of a hospital building. A doctor had been notorious for not showing up to appointments. Some medical staff quietly charged for consultations, and the laboratory did the same for test results. When "out of film," the X-ray department required an additional fee to produce an image. Families and even some hospital staff were known to push a patient out of bed so that a relative might have it. The list went on and on.

Amid frustration and dark humor, however, veteran members of the team had learned to respond philosophically and to recognize the rationale behind behaviors they found abhorrent. The hospital was also a business, after all. Like the aid industry itself, it was subject to material pressures and contradictions. "You do the best you can with the materials you have," one summarized. Another took the point further. A construction expert also from Australia, he had supervised MSF's expansion of the clinic buildings, spending some three years in the area in different capacities. By now everyone knew him, and he felt at home everywhere in town. "It's all about survival," he said. "All about making ends meet. Really it's a game, but played to feed the children waiting at home. Construction here isn't that different from Australia in the forties. Nor are the little tricks." He paused for a long sip of beer. Arua was a poor district, viewed with suspicion by the central government in Kampala due to its political history. That was the key fact to understanding the context. When one of his colleagues suggested she was trying to convert lab staff to greater professionalism through persuasion, he snorted skeptically: "Convert to what? It's all about survival." Government employees could not depend on their salaries to meet all their obligations to extended kin, so of course they had to supplement things. "People are the bloody same everywhere," he concluded jovially, with an expansive wave of his hand.

Near the end of my visit I met with two nurse counselors involved in the project from the Ministry of Health side, Sister Joyce and Sister Patience. Joyce, a large and forceful woman, wore a starched headdress with her insignia on it. Her colleague Patience was more reserved but similarly imposing. Together the two of them projected an authority born of decades of hospital experience, fully inhabiting their professional honorifics. As we talked it became clear that they took the anthropologist's visit as an opportunity to express themselves in more immediate terms to MSF. They began our discussion by lamenting the shortage of personnel and space, themes they returned to repeatedly. Although the counselors functioned as the entry point to the whole system, only three or four were available at any time, working in cramped quarters. They realized that MSF had limitations on employment but complained that the Ministry of Health was not hiring, even with the increasing workload. At times patients were thus left waiting long periods, all day even, and were told to come again.

The greatest professional change in their long careers, they told me, had been the arrival of MSF. In addition to inaugurating the AIDS program, the group had created new structures and even improved the buildings. Fewer supplies were out of stock since MSF kept supplementing. They also saw colleagues working harder than usual, and in response, Joyce observed wryly, "We're trying to pull up our socks." The government had planned a PMTCT (Prevention of Mother-to-Child-Transmission) project, but nothing had actually started until the NGO came. Moreover, MSF had brought ARV drugs, free of charge. After years of talk and hand wringing, things finally started to happen, things heard of only in far-off places like Europe and the United States. From a professional standpoint these were, they intimated, exciting times.

All the same, they felt stretched and pressured by the spiraling workload and MSF's ever-expanding projects. "You may find yourself working beyond capacity," Joyce said, "People are still there, so you don't leave at five. If I work beyond my capacity it's affecting the quality of the work I do." They had approached MSF to ask if they might receive supplemental pay, but they had been told that it was not the organization's policy to substitute for the government, and their salary was a Ministry of Health problem. Joyce suggested the matter merited further discussion. "Here we can't finish the work at five," she emphasized again. "There's not enough time to work elsewhere for money, so at least they could give us lunch, if not an allowance." Cracking her knuckles, she gave me a meaningful glance. The implication seemed clear; anyone expecting the standards of wealthier countries should be prepared to pay accordingly.

Following a long moment of silence, Patience introduced a conciliatory note, observing that individual interest and devotion were also involved. After all, AIDS was a new field, and the knowledge they were gaining might prove valuable. If so, that would more than compensate for the small sums they had been seeking. Besides there were other opportunities, being picked to go to training workshops, for example. That was another form of motivation, one that could prove financially rewarding. For example, at a well-funded AIDS workshop you might be given a higher allowance for lunch, because you were working on HIV. And finally seeing a patient improve would give any nurse satisfaction, "more payment than money." There were deeper reciprocities at work in the world. "Man is a social animal," she concluded firmly, "and the person you are helping could help you tomorrow."

Like others, Joyce and Patience were skeptical that their own employer, the Ministry of Health, could reliably manage such a project. "One week we would have things, another no," Joyce speculated. "But ARVs are lifelong." Her colleague took up the thread: "If we have problems of supply with other cheap drugs, then with ARVs what would it mean to be out of stock? Patients need to keep their dose daily. . . . It's not like Septrin that I am supposed to take for five days but can take for three days if I have no money." The ministry, they observed, covered what it could afford at any given moment, not what was needed. Joyce summarized their concerns, shaking her head: "If integration means phasing out MSF support, I wonder how we will manage. We're having challenges now. If MSF thinks of pulling out as in emergencies, then it will be a problem. We are partners, yes, but for how long? I hope it will not end tomorrow. . . . It's as if you invite many people to a party and then you don't serve them."

When they stood to leave, Joyce first grinned and said jokingly, "You now know us better than MSF does!" She then fixed me with another meaningful glance, adding, "I hope one day your study will help us here."

When the opportunity arose, I dutifully conveyed the gist of these concerns to MSF staff involved in administration. It was not clear to me, however, how much they could respond without altering the scope of the project. Like with the patient groups, the larger questions of continuing care extended beyond a mobile organization's reach. To meet them would require even greater transformations. MSF would likely need to select a smaller number of project sites and settle into the practice of community development in the mode of less mobile NGOs. Alternatively it could invest in local spinoffs like THETA, moving into a donor role to fund the work of others. Or it could throw itself fully into advocacy, agitating for structural changes in international health. Even if successful, however, results on that front followed a timeline measured in protocols and treaties, as well as the budgets and elections behind them. A long-term crisis had no immediate solution. "With HIV there is always a question," an administrator with MSF-Holland told me in 2006. "Should you start lifelong treatment if you're leaving?" By initially answering in the affirmative, the group had opened a Pandora's box of ethical complications. Was temporary treatment better than none at all? To what extent should it rely on partner organizations and alter fundraising, lobbying, and advocacy? What were the risks of increasing drug resistance, and how to ensure medical supplies? In short, given a chronic problem, where to find a responsible limit?

THE MORAL ECONOMY OF ACCESS

MSF's conversion to AIDS treatment went hand in glove with a more general reorientation to issues of pharmaceutical access. In this respect the sleeping sickness program again proved emblematic. By approaching its work epidemiologically and treating key diseases over time, the group began to recognize recurring patterns of failure associated with drug resistance in its mission sites, and the importance of affecting official protocols. At the same time its essential drug supply proved increasingly uncertain. Within some quarters of the organization, concern was rising over the perennial problem of unequal access to medicines, as well as a general lack of drugs to combat unprofitable conditions.

Another pivotal step toward MSF's pharmaceutical epiphany also occurred in the early 1990s. Combating meningitis in Sudan, MSF found that its usual treatment, oily chloramphenicol, did not translate to the former British Empire, where protocols inherited from the colonial era favored ampicillin instead. To justify the French preference, Epicentre conducted a study demonstrating the French treatment's effectiveness, while its parent organization lobbied the World Health Organization to include oily chloramphenicol's inclusion on its list of essential medicines. At the very moment of triumph in 1995, however, the manufacturer of the drug abruptly ceased production after finding its profit margin too minimal. The scramble to find an alternative supply confirmed the significance of drug issues, while bringing the group in closer contact with generic manufacturers and the assistance of the International Dispensary Association.[28]

Over the ensuing years MSF sponsored a conference and subsequently formed a working group to address the issue. In 1999—on the eve of receiving the Nobel Peace Prize—the group launched what it called the Campaign for Access to Essential Medicines (quickly abbreviated to the "Access Campaign" in daily reference). Denouncing global inequities in biomedical supplies, this campaign demanded new measures to address the problem. The subsequent award of the Nobel prize, together with the publicity and funds it generated, helped to fuel the rapid growth of MSF's advocacy work over subsequent years. The group threw itself into analysis of legal documents and industry trends, issuing briefings on topics such as "What to Watch for in Free Trade Agreements with the United States."[29] It made alliances with other organizations working toward a common goal. It sought to raise public awareness with press releases, public petitions, and even traveling exhibits.

From its inception the Access Campaign included an even more significant departure for MSF: a collaborative effort to directly fund and coordinate the research and development of drugs for "neglected" diseases. Surveying the greater terrain of human afflictions from a global perspective, MSF distinguished four categories of conditions relative to the pharmaceutical market. The first was that of "global diseases," maladies such as cancer or cardiovascular disorders, which affect all populations, including wealthy ones from which profits could be made. Unsurprisingly, the focus of pharmaceutical corporations rested here. MSF's second category was that of "neglected diseases," maladies such as malaria and tuberculosis, which might occasionally strike people who live in wealthy countries but largely affect poorer ones. Such conditions remained marginal to pharmaceutical profits and hence research. The third category was that of "most neglected diseases," vector-driven maladies such as sleeping sickness and leishmaniasis, which exclusively afflict the marginal poor. Offering little opportunity for profit, these conditions received almost no corporate attention. The fourth and final category was that of conditions "other than purely medical," defects such as wrinkles, cellulite, or baldness, which obsess wealthy populations and thus have constituted a growing area of commercial drug research.[30]

Facing this constellation of diseases only partially addressed by commercial drug development, MSF eventually decided to join with several partner organizations and launch an effort known as the Drugs for Neglected Diseases Initiative (DNDi).[31] Incorporated as a legal entity in Geneva in July 2003, DNDi began the task of identifying both shorter- and longer-term projects that would modify or enlarge the arsenal of medications available to combat neglected diseases, especially the most neglected. Rather than plunging directly into comprehensive research and development itself, the initiative sought to operate as a virtual drug development organization, eliciting, supporting, and coordinating a portfolio of projects within existing infrastructures. The goal was to circumvent the marketplace by focusing on medical need and treating drugs as "public goods."

Throughout the development of the Access Campaign and DNDi, MSF's project on sleeping sickness played something of a prototypical role. By the group's own criteria, this was clearly a neglected disease. Furthermore, the drug eflor-nithine had become a topic of public controversy. Originally developed as a can-cer treatment, eflornithine had emerged as a key alternative to melarsoprol in treating the second stage of sleeping sickness. However, its manufacturer, Aven-tis, discontinued manufacture in 1995 after finding the drug unprofitable. Fol-lowing lobbying by MSF and WHO (as well as a fortuitous discovery that the compound could also treat unwanted facial hair in postmenopausal women), production resumed in 2001. The terms of the agreement guaranteed availability of a supply designated for the treatment of sleeping sickness, at least for the short term.[32] This minor victory—like the larger struggle over AIDS drugs around the same time—suggested the potential for a pharmaceutically focused humanitari-anism. Beyond suffering individuals and endangered collectives, MSF could defend life in the form of "neglected diseases" and the resources needed to com-bat them.

"The biggest killers aren't Taylor or Mobutu but rather malaria and HIV," a member of MSF's Epicentre team told me in Kampala in 2003, referring to infa-mous dictators and repeating the view that life was valuable, no matter how lost. "I find the MSF campaign for access to essential drugs only logical. Then the next step is to say why not do our own research, so we can say, 'That drug is not working.' " Of course, he quickly went on to note, "Even if you identify one drug that works better than another, it's meaningless if there's no money to pay for it." Rich coun-tries, focused on epidemics and security threats, might not care if their own popu-lations were not suffering. Nevertheless, this potential disinterest only confirmed the issue as a legitimate matter of humanitarian concern. As my man from Epi-centre himself immediately asked, "Don't we have responsibility as humans?"

The moral logic behind MSF's new foray derived from a simple principle: lives should not depend on the price or availability of medication. Certain things, in other words, lay beyond market rationality and its determination of production and value. In this sense the group's assertions echoed the riotous sentiment of eighteenth-century English crowds upset by grain prices, described by the histo-rian E. P. Thompson as "moral economy."[33] Exchange should not forget other things held dear; economy was a matter of principle as well as profit. MSF's ven-tures into pharmaceutical advocacy and research resulted in something like a rights claim. It emerged in practice, however, rather than adherence to doctrine, and remained articulated in terms of the material state of populations. The re-sponsibility might be a broadly human one, but fulfilling it required attention to an expanding universe of detail.

With AIDS and the Access Campaign, MSF confronted the enormity of need stretching beyond medical conditions. The focus on diseases extended the group's sense of crisis beyond emergency. There it found plenty of activity, but again, no simple solution. One could count lives saved in a satisfying fashion, but how to measure the fluid value of their living?[34] An American volunteer in Arua puzzled over this problem. Trained as an engineer, he had grown tired of the corporate treadmill. His pursuit of a meaningful alternative led him to MSF, which sent him to help with the AIDS program. Now, he told me, he was unsure "what kind of metric to use" to evaluate success. He did not perceive his work to be all that technical, but "just what anyone who does things in an ordered way would do." And yet he found himself regularly frustrated by what he saw as apathetic government bureaucracy and his inability to solve problems amid the inefficiencies of poverty. Why had the organization attempted to take on AIDS, where the scale was so daunting? Fresh out of industry, he spoke in its idiom when expressing his doubts about this grand experiment: he could not think of another market where a company (MSF) would get flack for sticking to its market niche (emergency). In fact, he personally wished he were on an emergency mission, where things might seem sharp and clear. Then he might feel more effective and useful.

On a group level, engagement with HIV/AIDS revitalized MSF's sense of mission. At the same time, as several people pointed out to me, it reoriented the organization "more than it realized." With such a protracted crisis, treatment extended well beyond an emergency moment and involved a vast array of actors and issues. Beyond questions of life and death, it raised questions of living. In a landscape of marginal means such questions extended broadly, diffusing into the larger problem of poverty and ordinary suffering. MSF might be able to diagnose the injustice but could only offer a limited medical remedy. To do any more it would have to transform.

When visiting the sleeping sickness program in 2003, I met a patient in the last stage of the disease at a dilapidated hospital not far from the Sudanese border. Wearing a green T-shirt with "Versace" printed across the front, she exhibited signs of dementia when awake, dancing slightly and chanting phrases only she fully understood. She had recently given birth, and her own mother now attended both her and her child, since she herself was beyond maternal duty. The nurse accompanying me explained loudly (presumably for the benefit of others in the ward as well as the anthropologist) that no drug could reverse the neural damage now, and so this patient was beyond the reach of cure. For her, any therapy was too late. On seeing me the woman in the Versace T-shirt shouted two words with foreign significance—"America!" and "Entebbe!"—before returning to her song. Both the staff and other patients around her seemed to recognize this woman as already departed; it was only a matter of time before her body followed. Her madness and impending demise lent her a degree of fleeting visibility, soon to be erased by the continuing flow of human misery. In this corner of Uganda, sleeping sickness was far from the only health problem, and hardly anyone's priority. The very unremarkable nature of her fate, however, revealed both another horizon of humanitarian ambition and its continuing frustration.

The Verge of Crisis

*For you people coming here, you may see war, but we here, we think of this
as a peaceful time.*

UGANDAN DRIVER IN GULU, 2006

AMIN'S DEATH

In the summer of 2003 Idi Amin lay dying. The symbol of Uganda's period of
crisis, once the very embodiment of postcolonial excess, now clung to a final
thread of life in his Saudi Arabian hospital room. Uganda's media outlets blared
updates in breathless type, along the lines of "Still in a coma! . . . Doctors give up
hope!" Some also turned a suspicious eye on the dictator's old home district in the
country's northwest: "Arua Gripped by Amin Nostalgia."[1] Rumors flew about the
possible return of his body, dead or alive, to the land of his birth. In Amin's native
region, popular sentiment ran strongly in favor of this idea, presented as a moment of reconciliation with a whiff of redemption. Amid a landscape of rural
poverty and both national and international neglect, the fallen dictator retained
an aura of magnificence; while people admitted that he may have committed some
crimes, he remained a native son grown larger than life—simultaneously local
and extralocal in his sphere of recognition.

Before this public resurrection, Amin's presence had largely faded from daily
experience. Two decades had passed since the end of his rule, and younger
Ugandans—the bulk of the population—had little or no memory of that era or the
tumultuous period that followed. Beneath the surface scars certainly lingered,
both on the landscape and in divisions between regions and ethnic groups. In the
national parks, game animals were still said to be recovering from the slaughter
of the time, when hungry soldiers hunted them for food. From time to time someone would show me a bullet hole or ruin said to date from that era. And when
describing current conflicts, people might reference lingering tensions from past
tribal favoritism and the warfare of the 1980s. But times had changed. The coun-

try's current president, Yoweri Museveni, had now held office far longer than any predecessor, and word had it that some Indian business interests were back from exile by way of South Africa, reinvesting busily in the capital city of Kampala. Most people focused on more recent problems and events. Thus even northwest residents who had long taken pains to distinguish themselves from Amin's legacy might afford a minor lapse into nostalgia.[2]

The moment proved brief. In the end Amin did not return and following his death in Saudi Arabia received a quick and distinctly quiet burial. The brief flurry of international interest died down, reviving only a few years later with the release of the Hollywood film *The Last King of Scotland*. The Ugandan media reverted to its usual mix of political events, scandal, and tabloid fare. The former dictator's non-homecoming had offered a reminder of the past but no clear sign of closure. Although highly suggestive and full of potential ramifications, the threatened storm passed without breaking. It was, ultimately, something of a non-event, or better, a near-event, a moment that came and passed while suggesting much more.

At the time of this particular near-event I was in that corner of Uganda for other reasons, visiting MSF projects in the field. Doing so at a moment when the Amin era resurfaced in the news also emphasized the varying time scale of what might constitute a crisis. Which was worse, a dictatorial regime or a deadly disease? What conditions indicated a significant rupture? And how to determine when a threat was over? Uganda, I began to realize, posed something of a puzzle for describing humanitarian action. The country's uncertain landscape offered groups like MSF an array of potential problems and a regular stream of near-events. Such a setting made it more difficult to avoid structural problems such as endemic poverty, or to draw firm lines between exceptional and everyday suffering, physical and mental anguish, or humanitarianism and development. Longer-term needs lurked among the near-term ones, inviting regular and continuing judgment calls. Humanitarian action became a matter of question marks as well as exclamation points.

Situations like this, balancing on the verge of future disaster—or possible recovery—only infrequently surface in the media. Yet as a quick glance through MSF's annual report shows, even many emergency projects occur in such settings. Humanitarian organizations regularly respond to less spectacular forms of suffering in more ambiguous contexts, ones that might or might not represent states of emergency. Although MSF might narrate its history in terms of watershed tragedies, the larger record of its missions includes many more near-events than spectacular catastrophes. In this sense Uganda represents something of a revealing norm. The actual landscape of suffering appears both more common and less certain than its dramatization might indicate. As a consequence, decisions grow diffuse, drifting away from clear imperative to a wider complex of possibilities.

THE RELATIVE POVERTY OF "AFRICA LITE"

Of the many shorthand ways to divide and map the world in social science writing, the humble terms *rich* and *poor* appear the simplest. Yet even these pose a problem. "Although suffering is absolute, it is also relative," an MSF administrator once told me about the quandary of decision-making. The same holds true when describing the circumstances of a country or its people. Lives are inherently unique to those living them. But terms like *poverty* or even *the state* require some comparison to render them meaningful for discussion or analysis. Statistics can sharpen vague impressions and ease comparison, but when the information they contain is fragmentary or flawed, they suggest false certainty. Conversely the ethnographic tenor of anthropology offers a more reliable tie to experience but often leaves the material aspects of life hazy. So to portray the Uganda I encountered between 2002 and 2006, I provide a brief sketch of the country's infrastructure and the practical contrasts it suggests between places where things generally "work" and those where they frequently do not.

The condition of money and transport can serve as two raw indicators of the shape of government services. At that time in Uganda, most bills people exchanged were creased and weathered from circulation, their texture slightly greasy and their colors darkened by their passage through many fingers. On the scale of international finance most transactions seemed distressingly small, with the largest commonly available denomination converting to around US$10. At either end of the economy other forms of exchange displaced the national currency, with large sums for travel frequently negotiated in dollars and rural exchanges often conducted by barter. Funds rarely traveled electronically in local commerce, even for foreigners equipped with the proper means. In terms of everyday economic encounters, then, the state had a national presence, but it appeared worn and thin.

Roads were largely dirt, many deeply rutted and slippery after rain. Vehicles negotiated them with some abandon, largely ignoring the ever-present crowds of pedestrians and lesser transport like bicycles, which scattered to the side as best they could. It remained the responsibility of the weak to make way for the strong, although drivers also feared crowd retribution should they actually hit someone. In packed Kampala, traffic impatiently pushed and wedged forward at every intersection, exploiting small advantages to inch along. A motley of two-wheeled vehicles offered relatively fast and cheap if risky transport. Known generically as *boda-boda* (in honor of their origin along the Kenyan border), their drivers fearlessly maneuvered through stalled traffic and carried all manner of cargo. In cities such conveyances usually boasted motors. The other main option for urban public transport came in the form of collective taxis known as *matatu,* colorful vans packed with as many customers as could fit. The wealthy few who could afford

their own cars not infrequently employed professional drivers, as did most organizations. Still, traffic was a daily urban challenge, even for those with the most
expensive and reliable transport. In the countryside the relative shape of the roads
posed a different impediment. Some smooth pavement stretched between the
major cities, but elsewhere the road system revealed a downside of tarmac: years
of neglect and destruction had reduced it to irregular chunks of asphalt, producing a surface at times more treacherous than dirt alone.

Electricity can serve as another useful barometer of political and economic
capacity. Immediate and tangible to much of contemporary life, its availability
sharply demarcates settings where infrastructure remains invisible from those
where it constitutes a focal point. At the time, even the areas of Uganda with power
lines only enjoyed service for part of the day, due either to outages or planned
rationing. Wealthier individuals and institutions commonly deployed generators
to cover the down time, and the less wealthy simply waited. Nonetheless, power
did exist in urban settings. Consequently machines could function, if not all the
time. The key question was thus less one of presence or absence than of access at
any given moment. Few had the luxury of assuming there would be constant
power. At the same time, cell phone reception had rapidly grown quite good in
many areas, bypassing the meager landline system, and even people of modest
means could expect to communicate with each other without meeting face to face.
Given the difficulty of transportation this had proved a boon for professionals as
well those less well equipped, allowing business to continue even when travel
proved difficult.

The availability of health services—the infrastructure of most immediate
concern for a medical organization like MSF—largely mirrored the electrical
supply. A few gleaming exceptions aside, the country's hospitals and clinics were
short on renovation and long on dingy concrete, often crowded and thick with
the sour smell of sickness. Many of the buildings dated to the colonial period and
owed their existence to charitable and religious organizations as much or more
than to government expenditure. Uganda's laboratories and pharmacies suffered
from infrequent supply of key materials, and by and large its medical professionals felt overworked and underpaid. Transport and personal care generally
remained the responsibility of the patient's family, while official and unofficial
fees rendered treatment expensive. Nonetheless, services did exist, and a patch-
work of institutions public and private covered the country. The Ugandan Ministry of Health might appear frail and derive a hefty part of its budget from foreign
donors, but it remained clearly in charge, authorizing projects and protocols at a
national level.

The Uganda I describe also enjoyed a good deal of commerce, readily evi-
denced by roadside signs. Like many travelers I kept track of the more interesting
and poignant examples, jotting down names like Uphill Nursery School, Titanic

Barbershop, and Tick Hotel. Here a truck sporting the logo True but Why might pass Senior Breakdown Service or The Fact of Life. One could visit Gradual Enterprises, the Real Happiness Store, and the Pork Joint ("Welcome for Unique Services"), not to mention the Jesus Cares Supermarket, the God's Will Shopping Center, and God's Grace Pool Joint. Hand lettered and unregulated—a number reprising corporate trademarks famous elsewhere—the very existence of these signs indicated economic ambition, if not necessarily its fulfillment. They suggested faith that any gains would be protected from pillage on the one hand, and little fear of lawsuits on the other. All in all there was ample evidence of a flourishing vernacular market stretching beyond the official economy. It was a landscape, to quote a friend's favorite sighting, rich in "Business without Regrets."

At this material level, then, the sum impression was of a country partway between prosperity and devastation. Compared to Western Europe or even much of Latin America, Uganda appeared strikingly poor. Compared to neighbors like Sudan or the Democratic Republic of the Congo, the country appeared relatively stable and prosperous. Depending on which direction one turned, the state looked weak, strong, or fragmented. Life prospects could seem alternately opulent, desperate, or routinely meager. It was possible to envision outcomes of bright ascent, shattering decline, or, of course, continuing uncertainty.

Major problems stood ready for any who might seek them, and many who did not. Uganda featured a full slate of infectious diseases beyond AIDS and sleeping sickness, including malaria, kala azar, and the occasional outbreak of Ebola. It also had a long-running insurgency in the north that produced significant population displacement, if relatively few casualties, due to a potent mix of fear and government policy. Dramatic abductions and mutilations left haunting images but did not appear to threaten the regime. To quote a message I received from a well-traveled aid worker bemused by the flow of adventurers and agencies in the country's north, "It's one of the few places I've ever seen that qualifies as an armed conflict with victims in the hundreds of thousands and yet curious, well-meaning Westerners can get a ringside seat."[3]

At the turn of the millennium, then, Uganda lay amid several significant humanitarian concerns without being the center of any. Compared with much of the tumultuous Great Lakes region of Africa, the country had its period of greatest upheaval relatively early. The government's prescient policies on HIV/AIDS appeared to have reduced infection rates, rendering the country a potential model for other African governments in the eyes of aid donors. Moreover its relatively mild physical and social climate, together with the institutional prominence of the English language at a national level, made it an attractive site for NGOs and medical research. Although the public health infrastructure—large bits of which derived from the colonial era—might be strained and creaky, at least it existed. Uganda was not only an easy place to work, but also well positioned from a humanitarian perspective. South of Sudan, east of the Democratic Republic of the Congo, and north of Rwanda, the country could also serve as a base for missions in volatile areas nearby, or for administering to refugees who spilled over its borders. All in all, this appeared a place with considerable activity but little damaging drama. From an organizational perspective like MSF's, Uganda offered a good training ground, an engaging but safe setting for international personnel on their first assignment. In the memorable, dismissive phrase of a weathered American expatriate I encountered at a party in Kampala, this was "Africa Lite."

FINDING HISTORY IN PLACE

Uganda, of course, was not always a gentle training ground for aid groups or the infamous site of Amin's repression. But humanitarian organizations rarely delve deep into the past of any setting before they arrive. The rationale of emergency response dictates against devoting time to anything without obvious and immediate utility. The different sections of MSF largely perceive the world through what they call "situation reports"—a genre shared by military and business—which feature a brief synopsis of current issues, the political equivalent of taking a pulse. As field teams come and go they add and subtract details and offer bits of practical advice about local customs, along the lines of a travel guide. The longer teams stay, however, the more apparent elements of what historians and anthropologists like to call "context" come to be. History, then, appears for humanitarians in place, slowly, sporadically, and usually when it forces itself into view.

Nonetheless, elements of the past do register on the surface, even for the most casual visitor. As tourist brochures never fail to recall, Winston Churchill once christened Uganda the Pearl of Africa, perceiving in it a shining example of British colonial governance by proxy, or indirect rule.[4] The country certainly offers grounds for effusive appreciation; in geographic terms much of it proves an attractive place to be, combining a lush landscape with a temperate climate. If small compared to some of its African neighbors, its population is relatively dense and diverse. Ugandans practice Catholicism, Protestantism, and Islam while speaking an impressively diverse range of languages—over forty by some counts. As such quick profile facts indicate, the area has long been a meeting ground for different streams of people and beliefs.[5] When the British arrived they forged an alliance with the largest kingdom in the south, Buganda, perceiving it as the proper proxy for civilized rule, and cast some northern peoples as natural warriors. Subsequent political events have periodically reinforced such stereotypes, and tribal affiliation remains a significant social marker in much of everyday life

For international organizations like MSF this diversity registers in the practical matter of hiring local staff or shifting personnel from one region to another. The local here trumps the national, as the vernacular language of one mission site does not necessarily translate to another. Although many people may know Swahili as a trade language, it claims no national role like in neighboring Kenya or Tanzania. Rather, English serves as a common lingua franca for much interaction and education, which in turn places a premium on schooling. The hope of many families rests on sending at least some of their many children through all primary grades, or, with greater fortune, a full secondary sequence.

A number of aid veterans also noted that they found racial tensions more muted in Uganda than in other parts of Africa. British rule in the country had remained indirect. Colonial officials and Indian business interests may have inspired resentment, but unlike Kenya or Zimbabwe, no significant settler population arrived to contest the emergence of African rule in bitter warfare or to establish a repressive state as in South Africa. Violence in Uganda may have had roots in long inequalities, amplified by colonial pressures and policies, but its most visible episodes occurred after independence. The colonial legacy thus appeared less overpowering than elsewhere, particularly in its aftermath. At times allusions to British rule even approached nostalgia—a matter of the fading façade of Makerere University in Kampala or a visceral attachment to tea—as much as enduring antipathy.

When Uganda gained independence in 1962 it was hardly the focus of international apprehension: for a former colony it appeared rich and stable. Nonetheless, regional tensions lay heavily in the air. The status of the kingdom of Buganda within the new country remained unresolved, and its hereditary ruler, the Kabaka, became the country's first president, even as a northern politician named Apollo Milton Obote emerged as its first prime minister. Following a period of factional contest and maneuvering, Obote suspended the constitution and took control of the army in 1966, forcibly evicting the Kabaka and seizing the presidency. His subsequent regime increasingly aligned leftist political ideology with a practice of military rule. At Obote's side stood a military officer known as Idi Amin Dada. Originally from the northwest borderlands, Amin had been a heavyweight boxing champion as well as a career soldier in the colonial army. After serving as Obote's henchman, he subsequently replaced him, engineering a coup while the civilian leader was out of the country in 1971.[6]

Amin enjoyed an initial wave of support from Bugandan and British leaders alike, all relieved to be done with Obote. However, his subsequent actions gradually unnerved domestic and foreign allies, even as his personality loomed ever larger in the press. A massive and flamboyant man, Amin was given to theatrical gestures and fit easily into the stereotype of a depraved native leader, alternately charming and terrifying. In 1972 he expelled Uganda's significant Indian population, seizing their assets in the name of "Africanization." This sudden, populist reversal of colonial policy, which had explicitly fostered the growth of an Indian merchant class, had the effect of upsetting foreign governments and destabilizing the country's economy. Responding to real and perceived threats from Obote, now exiled in neighboring Tanzania, Amin began to arrest and eliminate potential opponents. He also ruthlessly purged the army of northern elements loyal to the former president, replacing them with people from his own northwestern region. The bodies multiplied—some floating ominously in Lake Victoria—and the dictator's security forces and secret prisons only continued to expand. Figures vary, but sources commonly credit the regime with several hundred thousand casualties.[7]

In 1979 Amin invaded Tanzania. The move ultimately backfired as Tanzanian troops and Ugandan exiles quickly routed his forces. In the counter-invasion the regime collapsed; Amin fled into exile, and a period of political instability ensued. Following two short-lived governments, Obote returned to the presidency. In the northwest a sizeable portion of the population fled across the border to Zaire. In the south another former exile named Yoweri Museveni led a rebellion known as the National Resistance Movement (NRM) against the new government. The conflict grew increasingly bloody, particularly in a region of Buganda known as the Luwero Triangle. Obote's support slowly crumbled, and in 1985 two northern generals deposed him in a coup. Their attempts to salvage the regime failed, however, and Museveni's guerilla forces took Kampala at the beginning of the following year. Although a series of insurgencies continued in the north, the NRM government proved far more durable than its predecessors. Restricting political parties, encouraging investment, and accepting foreign aid, Museveni's movement gradually shifted its political rhetoric from left to right, trading combat fatigues for business suits. Relative calm gradually settled over most of the country. From an international perspective—particularly an Anglophone one—Uganda appeared, if not quite a pearl, at least something of a modest success.

Relative to the landmark chronology of professional humanitarianism, Uganda's time of political crisis transpired relatively early in the cycle of optimism and despair. Occurring during the later stages of the cold war, the country's problems also appeared comparatively straightforward. Here was a large, suddenly needy population, fully accessible to humanitarian intervention in geopolitical terms. The agencies of the day responded by sending a small army of eager volunteers. Thus a generation of foreign aid workers passed through Uganda in the late 1980s and early 1990s, involved in projects assisting refugees of the era and seeking to foster economic development.[8] Many developed a lasting affection for the country, turning it into a point of connection and reference. This included adherents of MSF; some veterans of early Ugandan missions later rose to positions of influence, particularly within the French and Dutch sections of the organization. Others remained in the country or returned to it by working for other agencies. Their attachment then did not derive from the ease of the posting; indeed, conditions in the early years following the regime change remained distinctly chaotic.[9]

Nonetheless, Uganda was a place where foreigners returned, both by vocation and choice. Aid workers ebbed and flowed with the tides of crisis, like the refugees who filled camps on both sides of the country's borders. As the regime stabilized, new waves of development professionals arrived, followed by specialists in international health. Church groups and schools sponsored service projects. Even as the country receded from the news spotlight, it remained a veritable bazaar of international aid.

Such was the immediate background to the period in which I encountered MSF there. One could go much further, to be sure. Traces of older movements also lie beneath Uganda's surface: a thread of Amin's family history, for example, leads to a migration of Sudanese and Egyptian troops led by Emin Pasha, a German doctor who achieved his own brief moment of international fame. Some of the current population distribution derives from British colonial policy, including relocations made in the name of public health at the start of the twentieth century.[10] So, of course, do the boundaries of the contemporary nation-state itself.

These sorts of connections, however, require research and speak only indirectly to present concerns. Thus they do not appear in NGO situation reports, which share the terse style and immediate horizon favored by diplomats and business journalists. Indeed, the authors of this genre rarely bother even with the details of past aid projects, including those sponsored by their own organization. Instead they focus on a series of current facts and events thought to be related to the problem at hand. For example a report from MSF-France's mission in 1999 opens by delineating perceived challenges to Uganda over the first part of that year, including corruption and the economic policies of the International Monetary Fund, as well as by providing assessments of the domestic and international security situation. It then immediately launches into a detailed discussion and prognosis of the group's current projects in the country. The framing remains emphatically instrumental and resolutely focused on the present, in keeping with the greater logic of emergency. It defers all deeper history to a reader's background knowledge. With a few exceptions that knowledge is likely to be slender, even about the organization's own history in the country. In settings where people come and go, working under time pressure, even the thinnest sense of continuity remains far from assured.

MSF IN UGANDA

MSF first arrived in Uganda in July of 1980, during the turmoil following the collapse of Amin's regime. This was the initial famine response by the organization, still a minor actor in the aid world, and as described earlier, the effort hardly proved a resounding success. The crisis did feature on the cover of MSF's newsletter bulletin of the day, however, along with an image of an emaciated child

shown from the rear, clutching a bowl.[11] The same bulletin also provided a summary list of mission activity and a quick reference page regarding the history of
the Karamoja region and its relatively exotic pastoralist population, clarifying
that this famine had political as well as ecological roots. During the fall of that
same year the situation deteriorated on the other side of the country, amid renewed fighting in the West Nile. The town of Arua suffered considerable destruction, and MSF moved to take over its hospital in January of 1981. Working alongside hospital staff (who stayed on without pay), and in cooperation with Oxfam,
MSF managed to reestablish service by May. However, according to another bulletin story, the mission subsequently grew "impossible" and became a matter for
témoignage. Soldiers increasingly acted with impunity, and fearing military in-
timidation, much of the civilian population stayed away from the hospital. In June
fighting again erupted between the remnants of Amin's forces and the new Ugandan army. The hospital lay in the crossfire, and the team found itself treating
combatants from both sides. Under continuing threat it welcomed the assistance
of a German medical group and worked to evacuate patients with the help of the
Red Cross. Soldiers looted the hospital, shot indiscriminately at civilians, and
conducted summary executions. The drama continued through an evacuation
convoy to a neighboring town and a standoff at a military camp, where a stolen
MSF vehicle sat, loaded with booty. Upon reaching their destination, the team
decided to terminate the mission, noting bitterly that the situation was now back
to where it had been when they started six months earlier.[12]

Meanwhile the organization continued to assist Ugandan refugees in northern Zaire and responded to a new wave entering southern Sudan at the end of
1982.[13] When some of these displaced people began to return home, MSF, working with sponsorship from UNHCR, sent a team to respond to a meningitis outbreak around the town of Arua. The group then extended its work in the West
Nile around the town of Moyo, reopening clinics and the hospital. It also launched
a third project in the southwest of the country for Rwandans resident in Uganda
who had been forced out of their homes and into camps. Thus by 1985, MSF found
itself involved in a variety of activities in Uganda, ranging from preventative
medicine and vaccination to surgery, and sent a medical coordinator to Kampala
to help "harmonize" the three missions.[14] In the meantime other national sections
of the organization had emerged, and during the later 1980s they began to open
their own missions alongside those of the French. The country became a significant site for MSF-Holland, which likewise concentrated on refugee assistance,
expanding its attention to engage structural health issues. The Dutch also grappled with security questions, first refusing a request by field staff for bulletproof
vests in 1987 and then having two members of its team shot the following year.[15]
Meanwhile the small Swiss section sent its own first emergency mission, assisting
Sudanese refugees who had crossed into the country.[16]

Like the initial French foray, these later refugee projects continued to meet with mixed success. An American epidemiologist who had volunteered for a nutritional assessment run by MSF-Holland early in her career described the experience to me in terms of its "amateurish feel." In retrospect she was struck by the high turnover, exemplified by the fact that she reported to four different superiors in one year. Moreover, she felt the organization had displayed little ability to navigate local culture or collaborate with local professionals and struggled to express a long-term vision. Anthropologist Tim Allen published a similar assessment in 1996, suggesting that projects sponsored by the French and Swiss sections in the north had a limited impact. Although recognizing their altruism and the fact that they "certainly saved lives," he felt that the groups remained restricted by their artificial compound existence. Combined with larger institutional failings of the UNHCR and the Ugandan Ministry of Health, the mission's emergency orientation stood in the way of establishing sustainable programs.[17]

Whether or not MSF's projects became more effective, they gradually accumulated a more varied timeline. Rather than withdrawing, MSF stayed on after Museveni solidified power and the situation finally began to stabilize. To do so the group altered the parameters of its approach, gradually addressing a wider range of concerns beyond camp settings. Indeed, some later reports by the organization would give this year as the beginning of their "continuous presence" in the country, a fitting choice in that it coincided with the acceptance of engaging longer-term problems. For the French section this engagement took the form of combatting diseases beyond immediate epidemics, starting with the sleeping sickness venture detailed earlier.

The 1990s saw a mix of emergency missions and disease-specific work. As the decade got under way, the French section opened a small mission in the south to assist Rwandan refugees following the start of the neighboring civil war, offering medical care and vaccinating against measles. That project soon closed, only to be followed by a similar one on the western border to respond to an influx of people fleeing Zaire. Activity continued on both borders through the middle years of the decade and the Rwandan genocide, as well as on the northern border with Sudan. Indeed, in its annual reports the organization noted the regular presence of refugees as a justification for staying in Uganda.[18] The Dutch likewise continued to respond to classic refugee issues, conducting assessments and combating outbreak diseases. The Swiss section followed suit, sometimes in dramatic fashion (during renewed fighting in 1990 two Swiss vehicles were reportedly strafed with gunfire), while also beginning its pioneering forays into AIDS work.

Throughout, the French continued their project on sleeping sickness in the north, shifting between neighboring districts (Moyo, Adjumani, and Arua) as incidence rates fell. They also added a research component and in 1995 stationed an epidemiologist from Epicentre in Kampala. An upsurge of violence the following year caused them to relocate the program temporarily to the Arua hospital. The French and Dutch opened another refugee program along the border with Zaire in 1997; in addition, because of the civil war in Zaire, they ran some of their programs in that country from the Ugandan side of the border. They also responded to internal population displacement in northern Uganda, treating cholera, vaccinating against measles, and providing supplemental nutrition in addition to briefly staffing clinics. Following a significant outbreak of cholera across much of the country in 1998, an intersectional emergency team from MSF-International offered treatment across most districts in cooperation with the Ugandan Ministry of Health. At the end of the decade MSF-France conducted an exploratory mission to determine a suitable site to begin an AIDS program, debating the merits of various locations before settling on the familiar ground of Arua. Together with MSF-Holland and MSF-Switzerland, the French monitored refugee health for outbreaks of cholera and meningitis. The Swiss also opened a project on the Kenyan border, treating pastoralists suffering from kala azar, and MSF's international office contributed a team in response to an Ebola outbreak in Gulu. The last sleeping sickness site closed in late 2002, just as the Arua AIDS program began offering antiretroviral therapy.

Thus at the time of my initial arrival, MSF had been running one project or another in Uganda for over two decades. This extended presence was not the result of conscious planning or long-term policy. Rather, it represented a fitful string of initiatives implemented at different moments by an ever-changing set of personnel. Not all of MSF's constituent sections played an equal role or agreed what constituted the greatest need. In 2001 the Dutch even pulled out and closed their projects, transferring their resources elsewhere (though their departure would soon prove temporary). Over time, however, MSF's presence in the country became something of a tradition, particularly for the French. Some members of earlier missions returned years later in a new capacity, others rose to positions of influence within the wider organization. Increasing numbers of international staff arrived from beyond Europe, while others brought their families. Meanwhile some Ugandan personnel ended up working for years with the group in one setting or another. Even without creating "sustainable" projects or developing long-term commitments, MSF grew into something of an institution at a local level.

For an organization ideologically committed to mobility in response to need, extended presence in one setting raised the troubling prospect of stasis and the burdens of development. The head of the French mission noted this for me during my first visit, while outlining the current roster of projects in his office in Kampala with the aid of a large map. Speaking about one potential new program, he cautioned, "We don't want to put a foot in the hospital, or we will be there ten years later. We only want to maintain two to three programs per country in order to stay flexible. Five or more is a heavy investment, and then you can't move or be flexible. We always want to be ready for emergency." Subsequent meetings with his counterparts in later years echoed this sentiment. MSF always needed to be alert that it did not grow complacent or get caught off guard. Over time I came to recognize this as a common theme, particularly among people with some decision-making capacity. On the one hand it made perfect sense for a humanitarian organization like MSF to be in a setting like Uganda. On the other hand the need was neither singular nor indisputable, given that there appeared to be no obvious, overwhelming crisis but rather a range of partial and potential ones. The horizon in this context thus extended beyond immediate concerns and into a cloudy future. The very uncertainty that troubled the group's presence, however, also cautioned against its departure, providing an alternative justification for staying. After all, Uganda had no shortage of imaginable disasters. Should one strike it would pay to be present on the ground.

It is this edge of ambiguity and anticipation that I wish to explore in some ethnographic detail. Unlike moments of dramatic action it does not lend itself to repeated narration. Nonetheless, I suggest, uncertainty weaves through the very fabric of everyday humanitarian experience. It also complicates the temporal sense of emergency, along with its aura of moral action. If the problem itself grows unclear, so might the virtue of responding to it. For MSF, then, Uganda exposes a seam of doubt.

A BELATED EMERGENCY

In 2002 the Ugandan government launched a military offensive named Iron Fist, seeking to eradicate the main northern insurgency. Although relatively insignificant as a fighting force and unlikely to seize power, the Lord's Resistance Army (LRA) had waged a highly effective campaign of regional destabilization. The successors of earlier insurgent movements, and part of a conflict with deeper colonial roots, the LRA had acquired a lurid reputation.[19] Numbering at most a few thousand and spending considerable time over the Sudanese border, the group's sporadic raids included episodes of brutal mutilation and abduction of children. Such practices, combined with elements of spirit possession and references to the biblical commandments in place of an elaborated political agenda, propelled the LRA beyond the pale of conventional journalistic storylines. The LRA spread fear among northern rural populations, including the very Acholi people who theoretically provided the rebels with their primary base. At the same time, the government pursued a policy of concentrating people into resettlement camps for defense. Many northerners speculated that elements of the central regime and national army had a stake in keeping their region weak; from this perspective the government and rebels effectively conspired to keep the conflict alive. Nonetheless, Museveni was also under pressure to take action, and Iron Fist was the latest attempt at a military solution. The result was a dramatic escalation in violence. Although the army chased the rebels and destroyed bases in Sudan, the LRA also pulled off attacks in new areas in 2003 and 2004. The population of displaced people surged, by some estimates tripling to 1.5 million. Uganda had the makings of another real crisis on its hands.

Humanitarian groups took notice of the deteriorating situation. The different sections of MSF monitored all available information while sending exploratory teams northward to evaluate whether to open a mission, and if so, where to locate it. At a party in Kampala during the summer of 2003, the local heads of the French and Swiss missions discussed the need to start operations in the region. Although hardly a decision-making forum, their animated exchange reflected the mood of moment. Something, it seemed, was bound to happen.

I left the country shortly afterward. By the time I returned the following year, both MSF sections had new programs in the north, gearing up into full emergency mode. In addition, MSF-Holland had come roaring back to Uganda and established the largest program of all in the northern town of Lira. I went to see their new head of mission at their reopened office in Kampala, now a hive of activity. A dynamic woman originally from Spain, she spoke passionately about the new project, part of a Dutch effort to get back to the basics of emergency response while incorporating lessons from the group's nonemergency work on AIDS and malaria. The latest upsurge of violence in Uganda had coincided with this effort and provided a good context for implementing the latest model of intervention. Uganda, after all, had many medical problems beyond human conflict. At the same time there were people in the Amsterdam headquarters who felt strongly that the group never should have left the country. Indeed, in retrospect that decision now looked potentially short sighted. The head of mission suspected the aid community in Uganda had grown too complacent, lulled by the relative calm in the south and the existence of a semifunctioning state. Whereas the Congo might suffer from rich resources, this country, she suggested, was "cursed by a good image." In the north things were different, with the real brutality of force on display. NGOs were all too often overly cautious, she felt, and became the easy targets of cynical manipulation. The time had come to take more risks.

The original Dutch plan had been to focus on the area around Gulu, the long-standing epicenter of the conflict. However, the Swiss section of MSF had arrived there first, while the French were exploring areas to the east around Soroti. The Dutch thus settled on Lira, a town located between the two, where the violence had unexpectedly shifted. A commercial center usually outside the conflict zone, Lira had been quite unprepared for a sudden influx of displaced people, many suffering from malnutrition. The local hospital found itself quickly overwhelmed. In full emergency mode, the Dutch team concentrated on moving at high speed, sending as many people as possible and working out the details afterward. They also launched twin efforts at research and advocacy, to better establish the scope of the problem and to publicize it in the national and international media.

Due to a series of contingent circumstances, I visited the French and Swiss missions that year rather than the Dutch. By the time I arrived, the French were already winding down their operation in the town of Soroti and shifting focus to the smaller community of Amuria further north. Although Soroti had experienced an unexpected influx of rural people fleeing the fighting and suffering from hunger, conditions had stabilized and the problem seemed to be dissipating. The therapeutic feeding center MSF had established in the local hospital was largely empty, with only a few painfully thin children still receiving treatment. There, the emergency appeared to be over. Amuria, however, still had plenty of needs. The French team struggled to expand the water system to cope with the thousands of new arrivals, while running a health clinic and assessing conditions in the neighboring areas. I participated in a couple of these rapid assessments, the results of which proved ambiguous: the crisis could have been moving in either direction.

Meanwhile, in Gulu the Swiss faced both a cholera outbreak in a nearby camp and a sudden influx of children sent by their parents to sleep in the relative safety of town. Known as "night commuters," they flooded local institutions, including the hospital where MSF was working. The Swiss team helped set up a center for them and established a counseling program to respond to the potential psychological effects of violence and displacement. The cholera response went smoothly and the disease was quickly contained. The night commuter program, on the other hand, offered less clear possibilities for closure. Numbers had declined since the peak but now held steady. The phenomenon derived from a complex mix of social causes, and unlike cholera, mental health was hard to treat quickly. The center also attracted considerable media attention, to the exasperation of some of the staff. Although pleased with the overall publicity, they feared its effects on the program, which they suspected might be acquiring an unintended role as a quasi youth center. Here the sense of crisis was varied, particular, and unresolved.

In November 2004, MSF Holland released a research survey assessing baseline health among camp residents in two northern districts. Preliminary findings indicated that crude mortality and under-five mortality rates were above emergency thresholds. Morbidity and insecurity measures were also high, and water supplies appeared deficient. Nonetheless, most respondents indicated they would stay in the camps until the situation eased.[20] A second study focused on mental health. It found evidence of trauma and domestic violence as well as depression and thoughts of suicide, particularly among women. Action was needed in order to "achieve normalization and improved quality of life."[21] Even as the conflict in Uganda began to attract greater attention from the international media, MSF included it in its annual list of "underreported humanitarian stories" for 2005. The different arms of the United Nations swung into action; these included the newly established International Criminal Court, which began its first official investigation in response to a request from President Museveni. From a distance, at least, a state of crisis had clearly arrived: once again, Uganda's time was now.

On the ground, however, things remained far less uniform or sharply defined. While I was in Gulu in late 2004, yet another MSF section arrived to town. A small team from MSF-Spain conducted an exploratory mission around the area, evaluating the situation and looking to see where humanitarian conditions might warrant a project. For several days they roared off in one direction or another, traveling from camp to camp following news of misery. In the evenings they discussed their findings and talked to the Swiss group already in place. Both the severity and the trajectory of the situation were uncertain. Conditions were clearly not good, with many people in undesirable circumstances. But to the team's eyes, the level of misery hovered on a borderline between exceptional disaster and endemic poverty. It was also unclear whether things were disintegrating, improving, or merely holding steady. The decision whether or not to open a mission would not be a simple one, the team leader told me. "We want to act, but don't want to force it. What we see is lots of work around, but no one obvious center." Given the presence of other organizations in the area, including other sections of MSF, they leaned toward a negative recommendation.

When I returned to Uganda in 2006, I was therefore surprised to find that MSF-Spain had indeed launched a mission in Gulu. After debate, it turned out, the central office had decided to override the initial exploratory team and open a project. Part of the rationale for doing so was that establishing a presence would allow the group to monitor the situation. Should conditions deteriorate, the Spanish would be prepared. The resulting project itself, however, had been slow to take off. The team experienced personnel issues and chafed at restrictions placed on its movement in the name of security. Several team members lobbied to stay in the camps overnight, as originally planned, in order to expand their activities. All thought the situation far calmer than it might appear from Barcelona. Thus far their work had been limited to providing basic health care and working on health infrastructure, and it was going more slowly than anticipated. "I'm not always sure what we're doing," a Spanish nurse told me, expressing frustration over the slow pace of a government clinic with which she was collaborating. "Nothing has changed in a year. You come, do something, and then pfft!—there's nothing left. OK, we save some lives, but . . . " Her voice trailed off. Nearing the end of her posting, she was annoyed at the lack of progress and the continuing sense of limbo.

Alex, the Québécois engineer who served as the new project coordinator, took a longer-term view. "It really irritates me when MSF is worried that they'll get stuck in one place for ten years," he told me. "Like an old washing machine, get sucked in and that's that. There are lots of places where we know we'll be in ten, twenty years' time. Cambodia, after the genocide, for example." Northern

Uganda, he implied, might be just such a setting—less dramatic perhaps, but requiring similar measures of patience. Beyond their evaluations of this particular program, these two divergent views suggest the deeper problem of humanitarian time frames and assumptions about crisis. How long could an emergency last? Or, in terms more appropriate for this setting, how long should a group like MSF wait for one to appear or disappear?

The problem was hardly an absence of good works to do. Most health indicators in northern Uganda were (and remain) far from ideal. The question, rather, was whether they were the right good works for MSF to undertake. Would the group find itself contributing to an aid economy, offering health services that it felt the government should provide? Would it become an effective accomplice of those seeking to prolong the status quo? Would it succumb to the alluring mirage of development and engage in projects beyond its expertise or capacity to deliver? As an entity committed to worldwide engagement MSF feared investing too heavily in one place and thereby missing a worse problem elsewhere. But conversely, pulling away too soon risked missing a sudden deterioration. Leaving altogether would abandon local populations to the continuing misery of camp life.

A member of MSF-Holland's office staff in Amsterdam gave me a cogent summary of the challenge the situation presented for her organization:

> In a sense Uganda is at the edge of crisis. The situation isn't as dramatic as many other contexts. But the population is almost completely dependent on foreign assistance. For whatever reason, the government hasn't been able to protect many people from five hundred LRA soldiers. Uganda managed to convince the international community and has been a model of "good development." But everyone has ignored the north up until now. It's a difficult situation to assess. The conflict doesn't translate into high mortality but has been enough to keep 1.2 to 1.5 million people hostage for twenty years. So it's difficult to pinpoint just what's going on and to get a handle on this crisis. It's not always visible; it's not like there have been bombing of buildings or anything like that. Rather it's small scale, a few killings, or one car attack at a time. Everyone has a story to tell, but it's not comprehensive, only piecemeal. And there are lots of tensions with the government military. For MSF it's a destroyed society, and we're struggling to try and deal with that. Ultimately, most of it's a social and domestic issue. Put a lot of people together with no space to move for several years and you'll have your own crisis. In such a chronic sort of crisis, though, what is our role?[22]

The different sections of MSF responded to this question in somewhat different ways. MSF-Holland and MSF-Switzerland opened major projects, supplementing more classic refugee relief with programs to treat social problems like night commuting, attempts to provide counseling for trauma, including sexual violence, and (in the Dutch case) offering some treatment for nonemergency conditions like HIV/AIDS. MSF-France, which had a large AIDS program elsewhere in the coun-

try, offered basic health care, therapeutic feeding, and water and sanitation programs, while continuing to make exploratory forays and shifting location when
it deemed conditions to have suitably improved. MSF-Belgium, which had never
had a significant presence in the country, simply stayed away. And MSF-Spain,
late on the scene, tried to find a place to fit in.

All these efforts encountered moments of uncertainty, even the relatively brisk
French forays ("Are we fishing for an emergency?" one project coordinator wondered in 2004, when a nutritional screening in one camp again yielded borderline
results). But the Spanish team had the greatest difficulties of all. It had arrived
uncertainly, following an inconclusive initial survey, and was subsequently delayed for months by security concerns. Working in the shadow of the nearby Swiss
team, it struggled to get its project fully off the ground and to come to an agreement with local officials about the extent of its operations. In a moment of
reflection, the coordinator compared the problems he faced in this setting to those
of his previous one in the Democratic Republic of the Congo:

> Up until now I don't think we had a precise idea what we're doing in the field here.
> Things are fuzzy. I don't feel our project is here yet. It's unlike in the DRC; there it
> only took a week to be clear. There they were lost and needed a leader. But there was
> no crisis or dissension, like this team has had. In DRC it was a similar project, pri-
> mary health care. But there we had a setting where there was no service at all. Here
> we have to establish a partnership with the Ministry of Health. They could always
> just continue what they are doing, however inefficiently, so we're not in a powerful
> position. In the Congo it was the reverse: they could do nothing without us.

Beyond personality conflicts between team members, he faced a more fundamental problem of finding a role in a semifunctional state. Health services in
Uganda might be poorly funded, erratically staffed and supplied, and generally
inefficient, but they did exist. MSF might build a better clinic or latrine, but providing primary health care quickly led to a morass of questions about the organization's role. The Spanish anticipated expanding operations to address other aspects of suffering in the camps, including mental health and sexual violence, as
other sections had done. But as yet the team had not found the right venue. In the
interim it offered emergency care in uncertain conditions, warily cooperating
with a semifunctional (but hardly "failed") state.

Even in classic emergency settings, the end of any crisis is often less clear than
the moment of its identification and the initial response to it. According to MSF's
authoritative volume, *Refugee Health Care: An Approach to Emergency Situations,*
one common criterion suggests that a postemergency phase begins when the
crude mortality rate of a population falls below one death per 10,000 per day,
which is taken to be a norm. "However," this guidebook hastens to add, "the border between these two phases is not that clearly defined and the evolution from

emergency to post-emergency is not unidirectional." Moreover, "The post-emergency phase ends when a permanent solution is found for the refugee problem (repatriation, integration into the host country or re-settlement in a third country). The duration cannot therefore be defined."[23] As the work goes on to note, some refugee crises persist for years if not decades. A humanitarian health response therefore must shift from a concentrated focus on infectious diseases to a wider range of chronic concerns, including such things as reproductive health, tuberculosis, and psychosocial and mental health. At some point the problems facing the population no longer appear exceptional, however significant they may be. At that juncture, humanitarian action grows indistinguishable from more general concerns about development and public health.

THE PSYCHOSOCIAL HORIZON

Here I focus on one such project with an uncertain limit, the one launched by MSF-Switzerland in Gulu at the height of that town's emergency. As well as offering a classic menu of health services to people living in neighboring camps, the MSF mission confronted a more novel problem: the regular influx of children seeking temporary shelter, known as "night commuters." In an effort to respond to this problem the organization found itself helping to administer a center on the grounds of a major hospital (the very site of an Ebola outbreak several years before). Here several thousand children crowded into the gates every evening, fleeing the fear of abduction. During the day they would disperse and return home. While at first they huddled in the open, MSF soon built a hygienic environment for them within the hospital compound, with tents and latrines. It also offered basic clinical care and psychological counseling, particularly aimed at those among the children who might have experienced violence firsthand, including escaped abductees and former members of the LRA. Although many of the elements of the center were features of any refugee camp, the total assemblage represented a newer variant, with the additional psychosocial services serving as a hallmark of the expanded humanitarian project.

The night commuter phenomenon quickly achieved a relatively high degree of publicity, helping to place the Ugandan crisis on the international map. Child "commuters" fearing for their safety provided a vivid, tangible symbol of continuing security problems and instability. Beyond being photogenic, some of the children had wrenching personal stories of violence, which made for excellent copy. One shelter in town, I was told, would host five or more journalists a night. By the time I visited in late 2004 MSF refused many media requests for access, fearing the children were becoming over-photographed and over-interviewed. The organization readily deployed them, however, for its own advocacy and fundraising purposes.

At that point the MSF center operated far below peak levels and under capacity. Where once some six thousand had massed inside, regular numbers now ran a third of that. Still, as darkness fell children ran about the orderly row of tents that had been shifted from a cholera project just down the road. Some were young, perhaps six or seven years old, but many were older, if all officially under sixteen. The MSF project coordinator outlined the basic features of the center while leading an impromptu tour and inspecting the latest work. Although officially in charge of MSF's side of the enterprise, he voiced skepticism about its long-term effects, noting that the organization had a weakness for "committing to things we can't or don't want to do." MSF might improvise something like the commuter shelter in response to a specific need, but it exceeded the group's core mission. Consequently the team was already searching for another entity, perhaps local authorities or an international organization like War Child, to step in and take over operations.

Beyond the tents, the water system, the latrines, and the health clinic, MSF helped sponsor a counseling center, where the tour inevitably led. The therapy tent emitted a glow of neon light against the evening sky. Inside the décor was sparse, limited to a poster outlining the Convention of the Rights of the Child that hung on one wall. Four Ugandan counselors sought to meet the varying needs of the young population. As well as group sessions, they offered talks to both the center residents and members of neighboring communities to discuss topics such as sexual violence and its aftermath. The community visits presented a special challenge, one of them noted, not only due to the sensitivity of the topic, but also because community leaders expected tangible returns for attendance. In this poor setting, if a meeting did not offer food, then attendance was guaranteed to be low. The counselors focused more on girls than boys, especially those fourteen and over. As well as the threat of rape (incidents of which had occurred just outside the hospital walls), they navigated a wider field of potential problems, including harassment, pregnancy, risky abortions, and suicide attempts. When it seemed warranted, the counselors would try to follow up with home visits. But beyond the center itself the children had few resources available to them. The focus of their kin groups lay in immediate subsistence, not long-term therapy, and unless they could achieve official classification in a category of current international donor interest—former child soldiers or AIDS orphans—few organizations would help. As an MSF doctor noted with dark irony, in the short run they might have been materially better off by having HIV.

By now the war had returned to a lull, with the rate of abductions slowing. The project director in Gulu, less enamored with the night commuter project than his Genevan headquarters was, thought the experiment would not last long. If demand kept shrinking, then MSF would surely shift its resources to projects with a clearer medical focus and a more definable outcome. On my return visit in mid-

2006, I was therefore surprised to find that the center not only continued to operate, but also remained the responsibility of the Swiss. By this point the overall security situation indeed appeared to be improving, although local optimism remained guarded. MSF had a new team in place, and they puzzled over why, now that the war seemed to be winding down again, a large group of children in the night commuter shelter had yet to return home. Why were they not reintegrating?

Over drinks at a bar, members of the project team discussed the issue. On the one hand, a small number of children clearly had nowhere else to go or had been deeply scarred by violence. Many more, however, defied such a straightforward diagnosis. Although poor and needy, they were not former child soldiers and appeared to have numerous living kin. Some staff speculated that members of their households may have grown accustomed to their absence and rather enjoyed the regular baby-sitting service. Or perhaps the children themselves preferred the experience of staying with a lively, fluid group of their peers to facing more restrictive roles at home. Had the program effectively grown into a de facto community center? At the same time, there was the larger question of the change in the social landscape. If communities had altered as a result of conflict and displacement—kin groups scattered and under economic stress—then where *was* their home? One team member argued forcefully against reintegration, suggesting it was an illusion. Although aware that the local residence patterns did not conform to European norms, the MSF team possessed only a limited sense of the ethnographic terrain and was uncertain of the degree to which it might have altered. Had norms changed? Was the "general atmosphere of violence" that a staff psychologist noted earlier that year now dissipating?[24] Just as the surrounding crisis faded but did not end, this specific project resisted any easy resolution. MSF would clearly move on to another front line, even within the same country. It was unclear, however, what it would leave behind.

The category of psychosocial care in aid work is fluid and expansive, addressing a much broader category of potential need than that usually tackled by emergency medicine. For an organization like MSF it has proved simultaneously seductive and threatening, offering both the expansive possibility of innovative engagement and the risk of lost focus. Even as the group increasingly embraced the practice mental health, it remained deeply ambivalent about it. The possibility of attending to psychological as well as physical conditions began with a famous response to the Armenian earthquake of 1988. A decade and a half later such intervention had become something of a normative expectation, and the category of trauma had established a firm foothold in the diagnostic vocabulary. As Didier Fassin and Richard Rechtman note, by the time of the Iranian earthquake of 2003, psychological intervention had gone from being an afterthought to the primary medical justification of a mission.[25] Nonetheless, the practice of humanitarian mental health work encountered considerable resistance within the organization itself. As with AIDS work, many members initially saw the endeavor as exceeding the bounds of their proper function and as promising more than they could deliver. One of the very first MSF volunteers I ever interviewed had been involved in a mental health effort in Kosovo. She complained bitterly that the medical team repeatedly made its skepticism about her role apparent. Well after humanitarian psychiatry had grown routine, a 2006 roundtable discussion about MSF's mental health activities still produced considerable sparks. Rony Brauman, by then MSF-France's senior resident philosopher, compared cheerful assessments of such projects to the all-encompassing illusions of magic. The integration of such work into MSF's larger endeavor and identity remained a point of tension even for mental health advocates in the debate. Despite the fact that that group might routinely engage with counseling, therapy, and trauma, it had, in the words of its mental health officer, "failed to take ownership" of this choice.[26]

Like chronic disease, psychological and social phenomena confronted MSF with an expansive timeline. The effects of a catastrophic event can ripple through an extended family, affecting not only individual psyches but also the very tissue of their sociality. A rape or a disappearance might alter lives for a generation. The habits and suspicions of a given social order do not simply vanish with the fall of a political regime, and the world remade often remains fragile. In this sense the shared commonality of species biology still carries the scars of history.[27] From such a perspective the aftermath of violence remains a distinctly public problem, a deep question of extended relationships. Confronting northern Uganda's turmoil in the form of its night commuters, MSF not only explored the horizon of its therapeutic expertise, it also returned to the unsettled heart of its own certainty.

UNCERTAINTY IN UGANDA

It's not doubt that drives men mad, it's certainty.

FRIEDRICH NIETZSCHE, AS QUOTED BY MILTON TECTONIDIS
IN *MESSAGES*, 2005

Following my departure from Uganda, things both changed and remained the same. The war in the north hovered on the edge of a peace deal without achieving one. Under the threat of warrants issued by the International Criminal Court, the LRA moved across international borders to pillage neighboring countries. In Uganda people began to leave the displacement camps, and as the crisis subsided, humanitarian attention ebbed into a postconflict phase.[28] After brief visibility, the country again submerged beneath the level of media headlines. MSF continued to support a range of endeavors but again rearranged its focus. In 2007 the organization handed over several projects in northern health centers to the Ugandan Ministry of Health, while expanding others to include support for HIV/AIDS and

TB as well as emergency obstetric care. MSF also joined the government and WHO in vaccinating against a meningitis outbreak, and it shifted nutritional resources back east to Karamoja, the site of its first famine project, subsequently transferring one malnutrition project to Action Against Hunger (ACF) and opening another. The French section continued its main AIDS project in Arua, decentralizing service delivery and placing some patients on second-line drugs. The following year saw the group combating hepatitis E in the north as well as an Ebola outbreak in the west. It briefly opened a cholera treatment center in Arua and cared for refugees from the Democratic Republic of the Congo. In 2009 MSF continued to toil against hepatitis and malaria in the north, while also providing for Congolese refugees. That year it proudly reported having treated more than 16,000 in its Arua AIDS program since 2002, as well as providing over 20,000 consultations, including to 2,500 pregnant women, in Karamoja. At the end of 2010 the group estimated that 95 percent of the formerly displaced population had returned home, but it cautioned that the health care system remained fragile. The 572 staff active in the country devoted themselves to HIV/AIDS, tuberculosis, malaria, and sleeping sickness as well as maternal and child health.[29] It was, so to speak, business as usual.

By recounting the trajectory of a particular NGO in one country at some level of detail, I seek to illustrate the complexity involved in defining crisis. Part of MSF's continuing challenge in Uganda has been simply determining whether or not it should act, and if so, on what and where. The result, to quote a summation in MSF-France's internal newsletter, is "questions, but no answers."[30] Such an expression of uncertainty, while quite familiar in discussions of humanitarian ethics, rarely appears in discussions of humanitarian action or analysis of states of exception.

The seductive appeal of crisis is that it offers moral clarity.[31] Even if that clarity only fully emerges retroactively, the framing of contemporary humanitarianism divides action from inaction in anticipation of it. A failure to respond can become a potential sign of moral collapse, a source of future anguish and recrimination. In this sense the reluctance of the Red Cross to speak out during the Second World War has weighed heavily on its humanitarian successors. Once the Holocaust acquired retroactive coherence as a defined narrative, it cast a long shadow on presents future and past, even in vastly different contexts. Most crucially, one's response to a given, defining moment determines one's relative virtue. In this sense the present grows vital—an essential point of reference for both action and evaluation.

For MSF the operational category of emergency constitutes the most specific form of a vital present. Within the parameters of a sharply defined emergency, humanitarian morality narrows reassuringly: lives are at risk and should be saved. At a wider aperture, however, the view grows clouded. A need for evaluation and decision expands, and with it critical doubts. Rather than one drowning victim, an indistinct crowd struggles in the surf. It is not obvious who needs assistance and one might wonder why are they there at all. At the verge of crisis, it grows harder to maintain an "ethic of refusal" (in the terms of MSF's Nobel acceptance speech) or to ignore questions of accountability. For if crisis is no longer a given—defined through a clear state of emergency—then its determination becomes an active problem. Faced by an array of near-events in Uganda, MSF has confronted the ongoing quandary of recognizing exceptional outrage, not simply responding to it.

Action beyond Optimism

"What's optimism?" said Cacambo. "Alas," said Candide, "it is a mania for saying things are well when one is in hell."
VOLTAIRE, *CANDIDE*, 1759

There aren't any happy endings. You need to learn that first thing in college and get on with it.
MSF PROJECT COORDINATOR, NEW YORK, 2006

THE RHETORIC OF ACTION

It has become difficult to discuss a problem without offering a solution. Our era prizes the idiom of problem solvers, no matter how often or how spectacularly they might fail. Nowhere, perhaps, is this truer than in the contemporary United States, where goodwill and earnest effort remain deeply held articles of faith, and the suggestion that they might not ultimately prevail nears heresy. When faced with unpleasant questions or facts related to values they hold dear, people often react with predictable dismay. Sometimes they simply dismiss those questions or facts. At other times they resort to a more sweeping form of defense: how dare one reject optimism, the faith in success against all odds? Without hope of success, after all, what is the use of even trying? In historical terms this reaction exhibits a strikingly narrow sense of ethical possibility, one devoid of noble defeats or unrewarded virtue. Nonetheless it remains insistent, heartfelt, and not simply a norm of legendary American naiveté. Surely action demands hope and hope demands optimism, if not a fully articulated utopia. A solution *must* lie in the future and so be implied even as one raises a question.

Given its topic this book can only run against the grain of such expectation. I began the project to follow a particular ethical stance—concern for human life and suffering—as embodied in a medically oriented organization and put into global practice. The trajectory of Médecins Sans Frontières suggests anything but a straight line or an obvious conclusion. However seductively simple the group's message may be, it has yielded no clear solutions. Indeed, the record offers few examples of "success" in any longer-term sense.[1] MSF's classic form of humanitarianism responds to immediate needs, after all, and makes few claims on anything beyond survival. When venturing beyond emergency, the group encounters the broader wasteland of human need. There its machinery—often impressive at an individual level—appears suddenly frail and diminished. Even its best projects rarely yield lasting results; when handed over to states or less well-funded organizations they frequently dissipate. Sustainability, so easy to desire, remains hard to achieve. Moreover, the group's commitment to mobility dictates against permanent partnerships. Having defined itself as "without borders," MSF remains nomadic and hence a creature of transitory relations. Sympathies aside, it does not claim to promote social justice beyond medical issues, let alone to save the world.

Nonetheless, MSF undeniably saves lives. A survey of relevant details evokes more than such a stock phrase can indicate. The organization's balance sheet of activities for 2005, for example, includes a full 10 million outpatient consultations and close to 400,000 clinical admissions worldwide. These figures encompass a range of medical activities, both exceptional and routine. The group conducted 75,000 major surgeries, 8,000 for trauma suffered in conflict. It delivered 91,000 babies. It oversaw 161,000 people with HIV/AIDS and supplied 60,000 of these with antiretroviral drugs. It also cared for 22,000 cases of tuberculosis and well over 2 million of malaria. It provided 806,000 vaccinations for measles and 361,000 for yellow fever. Some 130,000 children received therapeutic feeding and 12,000 women treatment for sexual violence. Nearly 150,000 patients benefited from mental health services of some kind.[2] Such statistics aggregate specific stories, some happier than others. Even the few individual narratives selected for the organization's reports suggest different outcomes that stretch beyond the moment—dramatic recovery, mundane survival, continuing despair. But the raw force of the combined result remains: among the many facing likely death, a few more lived. What might appear modest for a horizon of world history can measure the very limits of a personal one.

Thus while MSF may offer no grand solution, it certainly addresses an impressive array of smaller problems. Indeed, the group defines itself explicitly in terms of action and the language of engagement. It runs projects and prides itself on being operational. Its version of humanitarianism demands activity to bolster its claim to moral worth. Indeed, it views abstract advocacy with suspicion, feeling that authority derives from presence in the field. Resolutely secular, its rhetorical practice nonetheless positions field missions as something like sacred sites. Truth derives from action, not contemplation.[3] At the same time the group's tradition favors argument, dispute, and a measure of self-reflection. Its self-presentation includes not only the arrogance of moral claims, but also restlessness and discontent. One finds few traces of optimism.

The work of MSF, then, provides an example of acting in the absence of expected solutions, and indeed of acting while questioning the action itself.[4] However much specific conduct may vary, the very ethos remains interesting. What might happen to the status of a category like "hope" in such circumstances? To approach this question I first detour through one small moment in the history of optimism, both to decouple that term from hope and to recall the tradition of the bildungsroman as a cautionary tale, not simply a heroic project of formation.

A CONTEMPORARY CANDIDE

During the period Europeans consider their Enlightenment, the contrarian French writer Voltaire penned his most celebrated work, a scathing indictment of rosy outlooks. Entitled *Candide* and subtitled *Optimism,* it featured a sublimely naive protagonist stumbling through a cascade of mishaps large and small. Voltaire gave this hapless youth an even more resilient mentor: Dr. Pangloss, the notoriously monotone philosopher who persistently interpreted every event in light of his favored maxim—that we indeed inhabit "the best of all possible worlds." The book's satire indicted the views of Gottfried Leibniz and Alexander Pope, and more broadly, any form of theological optimism that would soothingly suggest that all events, no matter how unfortunate they may appear, reflect a divine master plan. Partly inspired by the Lisbon earthquake of 1755, *Candide* grapples with what would later become the lodestone of humanitarian ethics: How to respond to tragedy? How to live with a shortage of happy endings?

Voltaire's famously ambiguous answer undercuts philosophical reflection with a note of pragmatism. The survivors of his epic tour of suffering finally reunite in Turkey, where, fortunes won and lost, they work a small farm together. There, each learns to exercise a particular talent, and all prove useful. Pangloss offers one final, grand summation, demonstrating how they have reached this happy state only by enduring their many misadventures. Candide affably acknowledges his teacher's conclusion as "very well put" but then reiterates his new, prosaic maxim: "We must cultivate our garden."[5] Voltaire's work appears a bildungsroman of sorts, recounting a journey of enlightenment. How precisely to read its protagonist's formation, however, remains unclear. Should one indeed "work without speculating," an approach that Martin, the tutor's main foil, suggests as "the only way to make life bearable"? If so, would such work imply a final acceptance of things as they are? Or conversely, would it signal continued skepticism and a rejection of any philosophical justification of the status quo? Satire resists simple summation.

Candide appeared in 1759, the same year as Adam Smith's *Theory of Moral Sentiments.* As noted earlier, Smith's work likewise displayed an embryonic humanitarian sensibility, if in a more systematic and ponderous vein. Over the course of four sections of fastidious speculation, this earnest author lays forth his vision of human morality. Unlike Candide's chaotic adventure, Smith's is an orderly world revolving around the twin suns of human nature and the judgment of an inner "impartial observer" who stands at an appropriate remove from the actions and fates of others. Smith is no Pangloss; he recognizes misfortune and does not explain it away. Nonetheless, the celebrated hero of classical economics does display something akin to optimism. Reason may not save us, but our emotions, particularly our natural moral sentiments, offer a guide for collective conduct. If not dwelling in the best of worlds, our nature is still for the best. We are caring as well as selfish creatures.

In terms of sensibility MSF's ethical stance echoes Voltaire's jaundiced satire more than Smith's tidy moralism. Whether or not Smith ultimately intended his two famous figures of speech to unite—the judicious "impartial observer" of moral sentiment balancing the rapacious "invisible hand" of market exchange—his worldview consistently sought a natural system amid human affairs. Things are as they are for a reason; any effort to improve them should divine and perfect their underlying principles. By contrast, Voltaire depicts a corrupt and capricious universe full of undeserved harms and fatuous justifications. A faith that simply excuses it grows obscene, and a philosophy that explains it appears farcical. Candide perseveres through a world beyond his control, finding his place through experience rather than philosophy. His closing words affirm an ongoing project rather than offering an explanation. Although far less serene than this fictional protagonist, MSF shares something of his final, world-weary ambiguity. Its collective metaphorical garden may appear far larger, with less certain boundaries, but the focus on working remains. Speculation, however well put, cannot substitute for action. And even action offers no guarantees, reveals no redeeming qualities of human nature.

Alluding to this now-distant juncture of European thought serves as a reminder that current predicaments are rarely entirely new. It also helps distinguish between varieties of optimism and hope. Voltaire's Panglossian caricature offers one optimistic extreme. Within it, hope becomes essentially superfluous since the world is already ideal. Past, present, and future flow together in a seamless web of justification; while we may not understand why things are the way they are, time will reveal them all to be for the best. Smith's moral philosophy provides another, more secular form of optimistic possibility. At once more systematic and open ended, it does not attempt to justify every moment of experience, but rather suggests the possibility of discerning a deeper order within those moments. Hope thus emerges as a personal affair, a glimmer of better prospects amid varied fates. Optimism lingers in the possibility of recognizing human nature and better adapting human affairs to accommodate it. Just as fostering market exchange might channel human selfishness into economic efficiency, cultivating the human propensity for sympathy might produce a harvest of fellow feeling. In broad terms, this Smithian perspective marks the boundaries of common sense for much contemporary aid. Capitalism remains an economic given and moral sentiment the primary basis for promoting a common cause. Such a vision has proved enduringly popular in donor settings, however belied by much actual human experience.

Humanitarians of MSF's variety tend to peer through a darker lens, perceiving what Fiona Terry calls—contra Pangloss—a "second-best world."[6] Humanitarian rhetoric, after all, specializes in issuing calls to arms rather than reassurance. Only a quick response promises to save lives amid needless suffering. What lies beyond the moment of rescue grows less clear. The life saved is simply a continuing future, one that may prove as dark as the past that precedes it. There are no sure grounds for optimism in life itself. Likewise I encountered few practitioners who professed much faith in either capitalism or human nature. Confronting repeated panoramas of human agony, they rejected the economic theodicy that the market remained an absolute good no matter what casualties it might produce. They also recognized that civilian suffering inspires political manipulation as well as human sympathy. Morality is never pure or certain; sometimes it flows in contradictory and even damaging ways. By the time of my research, a chorus of observers had warned of the "dilemmas" and "hard choices" of international aid for many years, some of the most withering analyses coming from former adherents.[7]

Nonetheless, humanitarianism remains a favored screen for projections of something like a happy ending, particularly in settings otherwise devoid of them. MSF's oppositional legacy hardly serves to immunize it from this affliction. Indeed, if anything it would appear to add a patina of rebellious flair and heroic affirmation to the humanitarian value of life. Profiles of the group regularly play on this redemptive theme, well summarized by the evocative title of a lucid Canadian study of MSF, *Hope in Hell*.[8] Along with the slogans of countless humanitarian fundraising brochures, this title implies the possibility of redemption through sufficient generosity coupled with energetic action. But what sort of hope could exist in hell? Or more accurately, what might follow optimism in a second-best world?

LIFE BEYOND PLANNING

In the centuries after Voltaire mocked theological complacency, secular versions of a happy ending generally took political form. For classic liberalism, faith resided in individual liberty and the wonders of market innovation. Leftist alternatives endorsed a harder line of revolutionary upheaval, seeking to reshape the social order. Utopian visions could endow suffering with worldly meaning; one

died for the greater good. Even where revolutionary fires burned low, the modern-
ist political idiom remained that of progressive change and the redemption of
remaking. It had little patience for traditions of charity or any activity that implied an acceptance of given conditions and existing inequalities.

The generation that brought MSF into being inherited this wider political
sensibility. Key figures had activist biographies, after all, and the organization
itself emerged at a time of social and political turmoil. Being "without borders"
was a claim to conceptual as well as geographic liberation; its members would
refuse complacency and remain rebellious. When I first encountered the group I
was surprised by the degree to which it avoided terms like *charity* and *relief*
(memorably, the then-director of the Amsterdam office excised such offending
language from my proposal with a red pen). I subsequently realized that the aid
world had its own shifting sense of vocabulary, within which MSF saw itself as an
oppositional conscience. However much it might act like a charity in delivering
aid, it had no desire to be one.

Nonetheless, veterans of the organization rarely sounded sanguine about
either the state of the world or the greater benefits of their work. When I asked the
head of communications of the Paris office about his views on hope in 2005, he
responded in the following way:

> Hope? Hope for whom? The beneficiaries? Those in contact with MSF for sure, it
> helps them with living conditions, health, and the like. Hope for global society or
> something like that? Well, that's putting a lot of hope in something that doesn't
> really have this pretense. We deliver the means of life survival, tents, water, medi-
> cine. That's our objective, being rescue workers. For some, medical action is just a
> means to obtain changes of some sort in society, through God knows what, *té-
> moignage* and so on. Yes, there are some spin-offs we can point to, say medical ac-
> cess proving that ARV treatments work, but these spin-offs are hard to account for
> or measure. We can account for the number of patients we have saved over a year,
> but a medical article and the like, that's harder. So, hope for those patients or some-
> thing more global?

Warming to the topic, he then enlarged the reflection to a more general analysis of the limits of any nongovernmental organization:

> There have been surveys that show people putting MSF on a pedestal, "a factor for
> peace" and things like that. But it's absurd to pretend that NGOs can be a factor of
> peace. NGOs can be a safety net of sorts, but to replace states? No, not in any sys-
> tematic way. Privatization and all that, it's just not very realistic. If you look at the
> beneficiaries of specific programs, [people] suffering from a specific problem, like
> AIDS, malaria, and so on, then we can talk about hope. But that's specific to this
> NGO, not anything grand like solidarity or a global village. Fighting poverty, or
> something like that, that's way beyond our reach. We're like rescue workers on a
> highway after a car crash. Should they stop just because tomorrow there will be

another crash? MSF tried to narrow what we mean by humanitarianism. Not health for everyone, that's political, that has to be dealt with at a political level. Humanitarianism should be the third party in the battlefield. It can extend beyond war to other crises, pandemics like AIDS, et cetera. But change the world? That's something else.[9]

As befit this individual's professional role as a spokesman, the comments struck common themes. Although the group might be a frequent recipient of laudatory approval, its members generally resisted any heroic mantle. Instead, when commenting at this level they emphasized their limitations and the inherent modesty of the enterprise. Aware of the charge that humanitarianism served as either a handmaiden for the status quo or a mask for imperial designs, they deliberately deflated its role, repeatedly insisting on realism.

In addition to avoiding abstract language and utopian claims, MSF's variant of realism stressed action, less in the sense of any grand gesture than in that of daily practice. A former member of the group later answered my query by email:

> I don't really know how to respond to "hope" in a humanitarian context. My instinctive reaction is allergic, I confess. In fact I don't associate hope with any humanitarian motivations at all, but this I guess is a personal matter. Sacrifice is similar; I've heard senior MSF-ers talk nonsense (to my ears) about how humanitarian work is a "sacrifice of one's ego"—Buddhist self-effacement kind of stuff. . . . The ones who've managed to retain my respect on those matters just never talk about it at all. What can you say?—The most sound approach is humility, of course . . . in the big scheme of things, humanitarians are "a sparrow fart in the winds of history," as a friend says.[10]

Like the communications officer quoted above, he too made a comparison to less glamorous forms of care giving: "I prefer the view that humanitarians are really no different than any other kind of social work, or even menial labor, like janitorial work. It's just cleaning up other people's messes. Maybe there's some remotely ethical dimension to that kind of work, and if so it's no different than the remotely ethical dimension of humanitarianism."

Such a comment may go to extreme lengths in its rhetorical refusal of heroic rescue and in its portrayal of humanitarianism as routine maintenance work. The sort of mess confronting humanitarianism would appear far more morally charged than that usually facing a janitor. Yet its author had considerable experience with several other humanitarian organizations and was obviously quite committed to this activity at the level of practice. Moreover, he was well read in philosophy. One wall of his Amsterdam office even featured a quotation from Theodor Adorno's *Minima Moralia:* "The only philosophy which can be responsibly practiced in the face of despair is the attempt to contemplate all things as they would represent themselves from the point of redemption."[11]

What then to make of such statements? Do they express contradictions, false modesty, or sincere turmoil? Even taken at a literal level they signal an abiding ambivalence about the expectations placed on humanitarian work, expectations that the urgent language of fundraising only helped promote. Whatever else, humanitarianism constitutes a sensibility, like environmentalism, one that similarly lends itself to moral feeling and public campaigns. People readily contribute to save lives, whereas they rarely do so to perform routine maintenance. And yet emergency response only addresses problems that remain narrowly defined. By itself it offers little in the way of an agenda, and it hardly substitutes for political platforms or social policies. Reflective individuals who have spent considerable time doing such aid work fully recognize this limitation.

Simply put, MSF has no plan. That is not to suggest that it lacks specific goals, strategies, projections, and expectations, nor that it avoids "planning" at the level of ordinary bureaucratic procedures. The complex, plural federation of national sections produces an endless supply of documents both short and long to track the present, evaluate the past, and anticipate the future. But unlike most governmental agencies—and even philanthropic donors like the Gates Foundation—it does not attempt to steer a certain predetermined course.[12] Rather, the group responds to specific situations while maintaining a looser version of Red Cross principles. Its action thus remains reactionary in the technical sense, defined against given preexisting conditions rather than imagining hypothetical alternatives.

The group's emergence, furthermore, coincided with a period of political disillusionment and an erosion of intellectual faith—in the prospect of Marxist revolution, in the romance of decolonization, even in politics itself. The original French branch took form against the human wreckage of conflicts in Nigeria and Bangladesh, followed by the excesses of revolution in settings like Cambodia and Ethiopia. Amid the debris of political regimes its members found refuge in medical work and asserting the value of human life. In concert with an expanding consortium of quarreling cousins, they gradually defined an uneasy ethical stance around this minimalist moral principle, which would eventually be designated in the Nobel acceptance speech as "an ethic of refusal." The group would focus on political failure and reject justifications for human suffering. In making pronouncements, however, it would resist straying far from actually existing problems or health affairs.

Nonetheless, MSF's adherents are radically egalitarian in at least one respect: they wish for a world where all humans receive equal care, no matter their location or the nature of their suffering. No one should die a needless death. Many also believe in an active welfare state, at least in the sense of expressing dismay at its absence and a resulting failure to provide populations with adequate medical services. In this sense they may participate in the "neoliberal" moment—even embodying certain aspects of its forms—but they do so with reluctance and suspicion.[13] Moreover, the group's inherited ethos remains that of rebellion. Like the range of its actions, the field of political desire running through MSF quite exceeds its self-representation. Its members alternately embrace and rebel against moral minimalism.[14] Thus an organization established to defy borders finds itself perpetually proclaiming and debating limits.

THE PATHOS OF MINIMALISM AND RESIDUAL HOPE

I thought after doing something like this I'd have a more realistic view about changing the world. But I still feel like I want to go over there, to fix it all, even if I know I can't.

MSF NURSE, CHAPEL HILL, NORTH CAROLINA, 2009

An administrator in MSF's New York office remarked to me brusquely in 2006, "There aren't any happy endings. You need to learn that first thing in college and get on with it." She was speaking about the organization's continuing struggle to retain good people, despite having a reliable oversupply of eager volunteers. "Younger people do one mission and then are off," she observed. "How to disabuse them of the notion that this might be glamorous and attractive, but at the same time instill real spirit? As opposed to the Angelina Jolie image . . . I wonder if it's about astrological characteristics, or maybe children of people born in the sixties? But it's an issue with Europeans as well as Americans." Her comments echoed those of other experienced members contemplating inheritance and the future of the organization. At first glance, MSF hardly suffered from a recruitment problem. It regularly received far more inquiries than it could ever accept, turning away the vast majority of applicants. Most of these eager souls, however, were people without experience. They would require training and orientation, not only with technical skills but also with organizational culture. In addition they began as unknown elements whose personal qualities remained to be tested and who might unbalance a team. Some regularly proved to have unrealistic expectations, of both the world and themselves. The divide between first-mission volunteers and veterans could thus at times loom almost as large as that between expatriate and national staff. Within the structure and logic of the organization, only experienced members—with tested international perspective—possessed the requisite knowledge and judgment to fill leadership roles.

MSF's problem was that not enough of those who survived their initiation continued in other missions. Those who did struggled not only with career concerns but questions of burnout. The life proved demanding and the work all-consuming. One could always do more, and yet results remained elusive. At the same time, the thought that this would become just a job haunted the organization and unsettled many within it. MSF feared complacency, to the extent that it institutionalized turnover. Just as it fretted about naive children of privilege, it also worried about national staff from poor countries and anyone else suspected of joining for a paycheck. Neither group was certain to display the proper spirit or tireless commitment.

For their part experienced members of the organization vacillate between expressions of abiding loyalty and deep frustration. The pages of its internal newsletters include exhortations and denunciations, tributes and dark humor. After-hours discussions, particularly at mission sites, regularly involve banter and often self-interrogations or confessions of doubt. I was warned early on not to take these moments too seriously, since the same individuals would rise the next day and return to work. Nonetheless the pattern remains. So does a record of fiercer dispute, sometimes leading to angry rupture. An impressive number of MSF's pioneers stormed away from the organization, some more than once. Although life might now be calmer than in the era of the "dinosaurs" (as aging veterans are known), the well of emotional tensions remains. Most of the group's missions raise as many questions as they resolve. Indeed, recognizing that might at times appear something like a rite of passage.

Sample scene: an MSF compound in northern Uganda, 2004, with a Canadian doctor on her first mission, a visiting Canadian journalist, a Ugandan driver, and this anthropologist. We have recently returned from a visit to a clinic in a distant refugee camp, and the others turn contemplative after asking about my research.

> *Doctor:* Should we all just leave? The project is great when we're there, but it's clear it will collapse when we leave. (She looks at the driver, who merely smiles and shakes his head.)
>
> *Journalist:* The problem is a nonfunctioning government. That's the issue.
>
> *Doctor:* But people at home are thinking it's all such great work. That we're making a real difference.
>
> *Anthropologist* (trying out a new question): Do you need to feel optimistic to act?
>
> *Doctor:* I think it's easier as a doctor, being on the medical side of MSF. People are going to die no matter what, you know that, but you can still work for health.
>
> *Journalist:* I won't agree that development is a failure. The problem is the government.
>
> *Doctor:* Then maybe we should just stay on and on.
>
> *Journalist:* The new missionaries?
>
> *Doctor:* It took me five years to find someone to fill in for six months![15]

The moment passes, as such moments do, and we return to other topics and our respective roles. Nothing has been resolved. Nonetheless, the exchange touches the undercurrent of uncertainty running through MSF's larger enterprise.

I should add that this particular project seemed more promising than many; the population had clear needs, and no one else stood ready to meet them. Unlike the mission's other project site, a camp nearer to the regional town and swarming with jockeying organizations, it was not yet "aid-fucked," to use the pungent description of the group's field coordinator. The doctor liked to work there, feeling useful. It was precisely because the project seemed promising that it raised anxieties about its future. We all knew that MSF would pull back when the crisis eased. It was not a development organization. It did not wish to substitute for a state. Its project remained a small one with limited goals. None of this, however, felt particularly satisfying. Of the individuals present, only the driver had a direct stake in Uganda's government. While judiciously silent during this discussion, his earlier remarks suggested he personally had little faith in the political future. Indeed, as several other Ugandans reminded me at various junctures, "change" could always mean things getting worse as well as getting better.

"Africans must solve African problems," an Argentinean doctor proclaimed a few years later, sitting at a bar in the same town. "That's why I want to return to Argentina. The medical staff I worked with today were good—as good as I am or better." He seemed to be speaking to himself as much as the others around the table, affirming a strongly held belief shared by many within MSF. A newcomer who had just started in a larger clinic, Ernesto was acutely aware that his medical degree gave him little real advantage among less credentialed but more experienced Ugandan colleagues. Brought up with leftist political sympathies and facing a tight job market for young doctors in his home country, he had decided to volunteer for international work. MSF was a famous and professional organization, even paying for the plane ticket that allowed him to interview. So far he was glad he had joined; he wanted to practice real medicine among people who needed it. However, solidarity should only be taken so far. Ultimately he was not a Ugandan, and it was not his place to dictate a lasting solution. Local professionals should take the lead.

"We have to accept that we're not fixing anything, just working on something and moving all the time," a more weathered coordinator had told me emphatically at MSF's Brussels office in 2003. "To think that we're fixing anything is wrong." His point nicely summarized the organization's moral minimalism. One should act for the best, but without undue expectations. Together with Ernesto's anticolonial sensibility, it outlined a limit of what MSF should attempt as a mobile entity driven by emergency. What about hope, however? Might it hold any residual place within a recipe of acting with minimal expectations? Beyond pointing to small triumphs of individual lives saved, MSF members sometimes indicated another potential benefit of action: one never quite knew where it would lead. Refugee camps were hardly sterile spaces, after all, as another old hand reminded me in

Brussels. Amid all the problems they generated they also could, from time to time, "accelerate history." Once people had enjoyed better health care, they might expect more, and so demand more of their political leaders. A space of normality amid crisis might help restore a sense of dignity, and with it the possibility of greater self-determination.

I stress that such claims as emerged were made in a qualified way—as a possibility, not a given certainty. Often the speaker would point to a specific case known to collective experience, but whether as an exception or a rule was not always clear. Rather than any sure chain of causality, these claims indicated a more fundamental dynamic of uncertainty in practice, what Bruno Latour refers to in another context as the "slight surprise of action."[16] Without elaborating a philosophy of being, in these moments members of MSF recognize the gap between intention and deed, and through it, a glimmer of hope. The fact that the group is there has effects that are never fully predictable beforehand. This unpredictability leaves room for small countercurrents, exceptions amid a larger pattern of setbacks. Should its engagements fail to affect public health at a population level, they might still achieve disruptive significance through their clinical outcomes, defending human life and dignity "one patient at a time," in keeping with one of MSF's favored lines. Thus something like hope becomes embodied and realized in specific individuals and actual lives. The results may not establish good public policy, but they potentially disrupt the bad while benefiting a tangible few in the process.

What I am describing as moral minimalism and residual hope resides at the intersection of a concern for values and effects. As Craig Calhoun notes, humanitarianism labors beneath Max Weber's distinction between value rationality and instrumental rationality, phrased as a question of whether to favor good deeds for themselves or to concentrate on their outcomes.[17] Within the contemporary aid world, the categorical concern for life and suffering that motivates humanitarian organizations encounters expectations of accounting and results. From a humanitarian perspective, to let people suffer would be wrong. But what if trying to help only makes things worse? In embracing action and an ethic of refusal, MSF seeks to limit abstraction and emphasize practice. To accept justifications for suffering, even in the name of other goods, would risk leaving true humanitarianism behind.

Such austere minimalism, however, is not easy to maintain. Members of MSF frequently chafe at the restrictions of their own organization. Field teams are often loathe to leave mission settings after the official crisis is over and look for other reasons to stay. Moreover, individuals regularly denounce aspects of the group's positions that they find wanting. MSF's tradition of internal discussion and debate absorbs much of this turmoil, sometimes redirecting it to new projects that can extend well beyond emergency care. But other concerns raise more fundamental questions for those with a progressive conscience. Why does MSF keep insisting it is not a pacifist organization when it constantly finds itself in war zones? Why is it so tentative about issues related to poverty and so allergic to development? Why not claim human rights or social justice? Why not embrace movements to counter existing forms of globalization? Even experienced members wonder aloud from time to time within their continuing commitment. Humanitarianism, it seems, always leaves one wanting more.

MSF's chosen path leads to a resolutely bleak horizon. Once there, many eventually leave for other endeavors, a few taking the haunting exit of suicide. Some soldier on, however, even in the face of repeated failure. "The hopelessness of human beings is not a reason to abandon them," a Spanish doctor proclaimed at a public forum in Amsterdam. "Should we only get involved in beautiful, sexy emergencies or also in hopeless places? Our work is to keep trying amid pessimism." His words echo famous formulations of others who saw the world darkly while actively engaging it, for example, Antonio Gramsci's motto "Pessimism of the intellect, optimism of the will" or Michel Foucault's description of himself as a "hyperactive pessimist."[18] Similarly, MSF keeps acting amid dissatisfaction. It thus reluctantly participates in the greater humanitarian illusion that "something is being done." One saving grace might rest in the slight uncertainty between action and outcome. Another could reside in dissatisfaction itself, and in a continuing attitude of restless refusal.

ACTION, CARE, AND DISCONTENT

Casting the story of Médecins Sans Frontières as a bildungsroman, the narrative arc might go something like this: A young organization sets out boldly into the world, following a simple principle. Through the weight of experience it discovers the shortcomings of its original project and pushes in new directions. Realizing its limits it then pulls back, reaffirming its priorities. If older and wiser, it remains restless, suggesting a cycle that repeats.

People should not die for want of health care. A vision of volunteer doctors on the front lines of international emergencies grows into a professional organization. This collective develops expertise in refugee camps, perfecting a form of humanitarian health. It acquires a tradition of speaking out when confronting moral outrage. It learns to finance itself in order to grow more independent. It worries about becoming less medical, about losing its soul. Faced with genocide it calls for war. Later, faced with military humanitarianism it denounces such intervention. Recognizing the problems with emergency programs, the collective intervenes with social problems and specific diseases. When wary of development it pulls back. It invests heavily in AIDS treatment, launches a drug access campaign, and sets up a project for pharmaceutical development. It discovers mental health and, later, gender-based violence and nutritional foods. Over time the group realizes its personnel are aging and changing, and it seeks to become more egalitarian. Throughout it makes difficult decisions and quarrels about them. It tries to stay young.

Life remains hard for many people on the planet. This simple fact underlies discussions of human suffering, a grim qualification to any hopeful claim. That life is hard does not render it devoid of pleasure or the small dramas of relative success and failure. It simply means that few people enjoy the luxury of forgetting about the elementary aspects of daily existence. For those at the cruel edge of survival, the margin for error becomes razor sharp. This is MSF's chosen terrain for action, its garden, if you will. Here it wrestles loudly and unhappily with the politics of life, offering minimalist welfare and standing witness to violation.

MSF's medical sensibility fits loosely into a larger rubric of "care." It assumes a relation of concern about the well-being of others and a value of life. Unlike some recent efforts to explore an ethics of care, however, it remains committed to expertise.[19] While fundamental, human feeling is no substitute for medical treatment. The spiritual labors of a figure like Mother Teresa, providing comfort to the dying, or the even the patient work of lay nurses, remain of another order. Here the body comes first, the body as understood in moments of rupture and rendered universal through the clarity of emergency. In caring for it MSF holds true to a biomedical vision of shared humanity. It recognizes populations beneath the mosaic of kin and ethnic relations and seeks to treat them in common, whatever differences they may have. Its political imagination runs liberal in the larger historical sense, placing emphasis on self-determination alongside normative expectations of a welfare state. Nonetheless its course remains restless with conventional forms and ever unhappy with the status quo.

Two moments may help outline this ethos of continuing discontent. On one of my initial visits to MSF, in this case to an office in Amsterdam, I interviewed a veteran staff member, then readying to work for another organization. After a lengthy discussion of the politics of intervention, he paused, lit a cigarette, and noted with a wry smile: "The beauty of MSF is the anarchy as well. We're not always consistent." The comment stayed with me throughout my subsequent research. Beyond reflecting the essential style of the group, it also summed up and celebrated its de facto embrace of contradiction. Keeping things unsettled was a moral ethos as well as a way of life.

Several years later I found myself at a party in Kampala. Near its end, amid empty bottles of wine and eddies of conversation, the local heads of MSF-France and MSF-Switzerland discussed the state of affairs of their larger organization. They agreed that people were now being pushed too quickly into leadership roles. To really take up the charge one needed self-confidence and a full grasp of the habits of a complex, far-flung entity, something hard to develop without four or five years of experience. Most crucially of all, one needed a visceral understanding of MSF's calling. Both were native French speakers, and they used a term I hadn't heard before: *hargne,* or irascibility. For them the MSF spirit went beyond passionate commitment. It required an ever-cantankerous edge, not for its own sake but as an aversion to accepting things as they were. The fact that these two individuals were known for their calm and cheerful personalities only underscored the point. Here again the official, circumscribed ethical stance did not translate simply into practice. Nor did it satisfy the larger hunger to appear rebellious and questioning, to convert crisis back into critique. One might not know what to say or do, but one should stay irascible.

Who can argue with water, hygiene, and basic health care? A clean tap, a latrine, a simple clinic. These are all essentially good things in their way, especially when surrounded by glaring absence. Of course meager, temporary presence only highlights the continuing inequality of circumstances. Charity offers only minor ameliorations, not justice. Too, the delivery of any good has multiple effects and mingles care with control. All generate new possibilities for regulation: a tap can be turned on and off, a latrine requires maintenance, and a clinic preaches the gospel of healthy behavior. Such control extends to the basic functions and conditions of life—life in its most elemental and animal form. It is precisely this aspect of life that MSF often confronts, both literally and rhetorically. At our present moment it produces a compelling vision, matters of life and death, the raw stuff of personal concern filtered through mass media. But it remains important to recall that humans have prized other values, sometimes deeming them a worthy trade for existence. Love, honor, belief, utopian futures—the list runs through the moral range of causes for which people have both killed and died, sacrificing being for something else. Humanitarians have good reason to remain discontent, not only with others but with themselves. Surely there is more to life than saving it.

An aging 1991 French documentary about MSF, *À coeur, à corps, à cris,* contains a particularly telling scene.[20] It features Xavier Emmanuelli, one of the organization's famously large early personalities, sitting on a windswept hillside in Kurdistan, wearing a bright yellow raincoat and giving an interview to an attentive reporter. An older woman, dressed in a head scarf and carrying a long stick, moves into the background of the frame. She gestures toward the camera and begins speaking rhythmically, her words indistinct and untranslated on the soundtrack. Emmanuelli carries on unperturbed, authoritatively describing the situation and MSF's unfolding response. The interviewer looks more uncomfortable, glancing toward the woman and adjusting the dial on his recorder. She then pokes his leg with her stick. A hand appears on the side of the screen and gives her money. She accepts it, carefully refolding her dress. She then recommences her chant, poking the reporter again. He ignores her now, trying to focus on the ever-voluble Emmanuelli. For a moment the two men look almost vulnerable, in a way as exposed as those who have lost their homes. Their earnest narrative of emergency has met a chaotic welter of refugees in cold mud. Some will not stay silent no matter what is said, perceiving a smaller personal crisis or a wider world one. The scene thus deflates the very center of MSF's certainty, casting it back into doubt. But here doubt is hardly the end of action. Rather, like a burr in the shoe, it can be a seed of renewal. When contemplating the organization and the larger value of discontent, then, I recall this old woman and her insistent long stick.

EPILOGUE

Over the years I spent slowly writing this book, MSF continued to evolve. The period after the La Mancha meeting saw some retrenchment, with sections both reorganizing their operational structure and renewing their fundamental commitment to emergency response.[1] On that front there was always plenty to do. The group's updates chronicled a steady stream of human suffering due to disaster and war. Although the crisis in Uganda may have eased, many of the same countries continued to occupy the annual top ten list of crises, with the Democratic Republic of the Congo, Sudan, and Somalia all seemingly assured a permanent place in the upper tier. Following the devastating 2010 earthquake in Haiti, the group embarked on its largest emergency project ever. Even with the aid of an inflatable hospital, surgeons quickly found themselves overwhelmed, performing amputations as if in wartime. Given the subsequent appearance of cholera and continuing problems of displacement, that particular mission seemed unlikely to close quickly. Amid lively debate, the organization laid plans to establish and staff a general hospital, accepting a longer-term commitment of at least a decade. In Haiti at least, emergency reopened the door to development.[2]

MSF did undertake new initiatives, for example loudly advocating ready-to-use therapeutic food (RUTF) as a response to malnutrition. However, much of its work remained familiar if not routine. The rise of humanitarian rhetoric around war and expansion of rights discourse by other NGOs altered the context for *témoignage*. The group increasingly adopted an orthodox humanitarian line, to the extent that some feared the witnessing tradition might atrophy altogether. Meanwhile, the Access Campaign forged ahead with pharmaceutical advocacy and DNDi developed three products, two for malaria and one for sleeping sickness.

The antiretroviral programs likewise continued to expand in both size and scope, extending their timeline and taking on associated conditions like TB. The encounter with AIDS had clearly changed MSF, perhaps even more than it realized. At times the organization resembled a set of conjoined twins, sharing a body but pulling in different directions.

By serendipity, I found myself in South Africa while finishing this text. In the township of Khayelitsha near Cape Town, MSF had sponsored what was likely its most famous and influential HIV/AIDS treatment program. The project quickly cast the organization in an unexpectedly prominent role in the struggle for antiretroviral treatment. Allied with a South African group known as the Treatment Action Campaign (TAC), MSF helped challenge both the Mbeki government's reluctance to accept medications formulated around theories of HIV and their exorbitant pricing by pharmaceutical companies protected by patents. In 2011 the Khayelitsha program celebrated its tenth anniversary in style, sponsoring a day-long event at the township's community center. An impressively large crowd turned out. The ample building reverberated with speeches, dancing, award presentations, and the general excitement of a milestone event: by now the project could claim to have treated 20,000 patients. Although not every individual responded to treatment, the overall effect had clearly proven transformative, both for the patients and the surrounding community. This was the closest, perhaps, MSF had come to a success story.[3]

The Khayelitsha program had also been an epiphany of sorts for the instigating organization. When MSF embraced AIDS work, it acquired a rejuvenated sense of activism and engagement beyond its specific project sites. Nowhere was this truer than in South Africa, where a confluence of political and medical histories turned a small effort to deliver antiretroviral medications into a cause célèbre. The resistance of the postapartheid regime to the HIV explanation for AIDS created a complex political field quite different from that found elsewhere, including in Uganda. Consequently the antiretroviral project proved not just controversial but openly confrontational, and at times it proceeded in a clandestine fashion. To act, MSF relied on local partners, particularly TAC. South Africa was different terrain from the group's classic field context, featuring a relatively rich endowment of infrastructure alongside extreme social inequity. Moreover, the country's charged colonial history made it difficult for an outside organization—particularly a European one contesting the health policy of an anticolonial minister—to claim moral legitimacy or operate independently. Such government opposition set South Africa apart from other countries with AIDS projects. As a consequence MSF learned to operate in a coalition; humanitarian action there moved through demonstrations and up courthouse steps.

A few weeks before the anniversary celebration I had attended the annual assembly of MSF-South Africa. Established in 2007, the new outpost still relied on the Brussels office for much of its funding. Nonetheless it appeared determined to pursue its own path, fulfilling its charge to bring an African perspective to the table. In a high-rise building in Johannesburg, delegates addressed a range of issues, from the wording of a T-shirt protesting xenophobic violence to the question of whether or not to endorse a right to health. This latter topic, framed as a debate of sorts involving several invited speakers, largely replicated similar discussions I had witnessed in other sections. Its purpose appeared to be to demonstrate the importance of serious reflection as much as to reach any conclusion. MSF was unlikely to join in proclaiming any such right even if it actively sought to fulfill it. In this setting, however, the discussion seemed oddly superfluous. Most people in the room came from Africa. The vast majority of them lived where they worked, many being national staff involved with AIDS projects in South Africa or neighboring countries. The evening opened with a rousing revolutionary cry of "Viva!" and both the antiretroviral and antiapartheid struggles served as intimate points of reference. Itself turning forty, MSF had tentatively opened one door on its Land Cruiser. The route forward remained unclear. But at least for this moment, another politics traveled alongside medical humanitarianism, another politics for its ethic of life.

NOTES

INTRODUCTION

1. To emphasize the internationalization of the group's acronym, I deviate from French convention and capitalize all components of its name throughout the text.

2. See Marc Redfield 1996 on the limits and instability of the genre. Joseph Slaughter (2007: 328) provocatively connects the bildungsroman with human rights law, suggesting that they work in concert to project a conservative vision of "the international human rights person." As should become apparent, I am applying the term more loosely here to a nongovernmental organization, although a number of Slaughter's observations remain of relevance.

3. For an enthusiastic assessment of Cuba's version of medical internationalism see Brouwer 2011. The Cuban program, which began in 1961, combines medical care with a revolutionary social platform that also seeks "to save lives" (Kirk and Erisman 2009: 188). Similarly, Kidder (2003) examines the trajectory of Paul Farmer and Partners in Health in search of social justice, while Adams (1998) explores quandaries of politics and medicine for doctors in Nepal.

4. Paul Rabinow and George Marcus suggest that "untimeliness" can prove anthropologically fruitful (Rabinow et al. 2008: 55–71).

5. For MSF's own belated efforts to understand its host communities see Abu-Sada 2012.

CHAPTER 1. A TIME OF CRISIS

1. "The Nobel Peace Prize 1999," press release, available at http://nobelprize.org/nobel_prizes/peace/laureates/1999/press.html (last accessed July 14, 2012).

2. The phrase holds more nuance in French and can also be translated as the "duty to

interfere," a moral formulation preferred by Koucher and other humanitarian proponants, if often ignored by the press. See Allen and Styan 2000 for background, as well as Ticktin 2011a: 76.

3. Vallaeys 2004: 745–750.

4. MSF press release, December 9, 1999.

5. See Corine Lesnes, Franck Nouchi, and Claire Tréan, "MSF: Les defies d'une genera-tion; tout commence au Biafra. Le besoin de soigner, de témoigner," *Le Monde,* October 18, 1999. Kirsten Sellars, "Medical Hippies Go Mainstream: Doctors' Organization Spawned Era of Humanitarian Occupation of Third World Countries," *Gazette,* October 25, 1999, p. B5. *Canard enchaîné,* October 20, 1999, cartoon titled "Le Nobel de la paix à Médecins sans frontières."

6. Acceptance speech elivered by James Orbinski, president of the MSF International Council, Oslo, December 10, 1999, http://nobelprize.org/nobel_prizes/peace/laureates/1999/msf-lecture.html (last accessed July 14, 2012). The Nobel speech was the product of fevered last-minute negotiation among the movement's constituent sections and individual mem-bers. Here I treat it as a unitary public statement through which to locate the contested vision of the organization. For more on the context of its final production and the moment of the prize reception, see MSF's "Nobel Peace Prize Journal" published in December, 1999 , as well as Vallaeys 2004: 744–751.

7. The *Oxford English Dictionary* traces *crisis* from a turning point in disease, a critical conjuncture of planets, and a point of imminent change to "times of difficulty, insecurity and suspense," the sense closest to MSF's usage. *Emergency* drifts from a rising above water into "a state of things unexpectedly arising, and urgently demanding immediate action." Amid the homogenization of the aid world (now dominated by the English language) I have discerned little difference between the French and English cognates in recent usage. Some analysts, such as Craig Calhoun, prefer *emergency* to *crisis,* given the latter's vague-ness and hint of potential resolution. As this work suggests, however, the very elasticity of *crisis* itself can prove revealing. For more on the intellectual history of *crisis* see Koselleck 2006 and Starn 1971. With regard to *emergency* see Calhoun 2010 and Nurok 2003.

8. Unless otherwise indicated, all quotations derive from field notes I took primarily between 2000 and 2006 in Uganda, France, Holland, Belgium, Switzerland, and the United States. In keeping with anthropological convention I name only those who are public fig-ures, presenting others with pseudonyms or in terms of their group identity.

9. The camp exhibit was originally a project of MSF-France, and it toured Europe before reaching the United States. A virtual, updated version of it can be found at www.refugeecamp.org/ (last accessed July 14, 2012).

10. There are debates about the adequacy of middle upper arm circumference (MUAC) measures to evaluate nutritional status within a population. The cut-off norm of 12.5–13 centimeters was defined by well-nourished Polish children of the early 1960s, and refer-ence to additional factors such as height would be more sensitive to age and sex differences (see Mei et al. 1997). However, by virtue of its speed and simplicity, the MUAC bracelet remains in wide use as a rapid assessment tool. It has also appeared in a MOMA exhibit on risk and design (www.moma.org/explore/multimedia/audios/20/510, last accessed July 14, 2012).

11. Arendt 1998: 97.

12. Redfield 2005: 328.

13. See the World Health Organization World Health Observatory, www.who.int/gho/
mortality_burden_disease/regions/dalys_text/en/index.html (last accessed July 14, 2012),
as well as Kleinman and Kleinman 1997 for analysis.

14. Foucault 1990: 138; 2003: 240–241. Both Foucault's version of *biopower* and multiple
iterations of *biopolitics* have grown into familiar concepts for many anthropologists. For
discussions of the concept see Rabinow and Rose 2006. I also thank Carol Caduff and
Tobias Rees for preparing and sharing a discussion paper on this topic (Rees and Caduff
n.d.). For a provocation highly relevant to MSF see Fassin 2009.

15. MSF acceptance speech, Oslo, December 10, 1999, http://nobelprize.org/nobel_
prizes/peace/laureates/1999/msf-lecture.html (last accessed July 14, 2012).

16. See, e.g., Dunant 1986 and Kouchner 1991. Not all humanitarianism focuses on
emergency or is practiced by nonstate actors. For a broader history of the term and alternative uses, including relations to human rights claims and efforts at human improvement, see Barnett 2011; Bornstein and Redfield 2011; Calhoun 2008; Fassin and Pandolfi
2010; Feldman and Ticktin 2010; and Wilson and Brown 2009. For a more complete analysis of humanitarian reason, including its appeal within domestic state policies, see Fassin
2011.

17. The quoted phrase is from MSF's Nobel acceptance speech. There are, of course,
other possible reactions to suffering; a politics of revenge, for instance, might manipulate
the same images in an effort to define retribution. By contrast, humanitarianism can
neither overlook present suffering nor embrace its potential utility. In this sense its moral
reasoning remains implacably categorical as well as sentimental (Festa 2010).

18. Agamben 2005: 1. See also Agamben 1998 and Schmitt 1985.

19. Benjamin 1969: 257.

20. Agamben 1998: 133–134. If ultimately skeptical of aspects of Agamben's sweeping
analysis, anthropologists addressing humanitarianism have found it generative. For a
broader, provocative portrayal of humanitarian "mobile sovereignty" see Pandolfi 2003,
and for states of emergency see Fassin and Pandolfi 2010.

21. See again the entry under crisis in the *Oxford English Dictionary*. Milton Friedman
echoes Marx on this score: "Now, you never have real changes unless you have a time of
crisis," www.pbs.org/fmc/interviews/friedman.htm (last accessed July 14, 2012). I thank
Janet Roitman for sharing her unpublished work related to crisis.

22. This phrase became a touchstone for the organization in the early 1990s; see MSF
1992.

23. Fox 1995: 1609. See also Taithe 2004 and Fassin 2010.

24. A repeated phrase; see, e.g., MSF *Activity Report, 2002–2003*. Brussels: MSF International Office.

25. See Feldman 2007 on the politics of population claims.

26. Calhoun 2004.

27. Rieff 2002.

28. See the phrase "stupid deaths" in Farmer 2003: 205; 2010.

29. Field notes, Paris, France, June 2003.

30. Here I borrow a phrase from Achille Mbembe and Janet Roitman (Mbembe and Roitman 1995: 323). "'The crisis,' according to the Hippocratic treatise *On Affections*, 'occurs in diseases whenever the diseases increase in intensity or go away or change into another disease or end altogether'" (Starn 1971: 4). Although present in a range of other decisive domains of ancient life—politics, war, theology—it was through the dominant medical lineage that it spread into the vernacular languages of modern Europe as a temporal concept. See Koselleck 1988; 2002: 237–238; 2006.

31. Luc Boltanski nicely captures this dual nature of immediacy and its importance to organizations like MSF: "Ultimately what justifies the humanitarian movement is that its members are on the spot. Presence on the ground is the only guarantee of effectiveness and even of truth" (Boltanski 1999: 183).

32. See Malkki 1995, Hyndman 2000, Agier 2002, Feldman 2007. On the wider use of *emergency* see Fassin and Pandolfi 2010; also Barnett 2011 and Calhoun 2004.

33. See Cooter and Luckin 1997; Fassin and Rechtman 2009; Guly 2005; Haller 1992; Hutchinson 1997; and Zink 2006. Nurok (2003) provides an incisive analysis of the "epistemological alignment" of emergency in medicine.

34. See Moyn 2010 on the recent chronology of human rights and its uncomfortable status as the "last utopia." In unpublished work Tobias Rees makes a similar point about the emergence of the phrase "humanitarian crisis," which he dates through bibliometric study to the 1970s era of the boat people.

35. See Kidder 2003: 101.

36. Fassin 2012: 253–55. See also Brown 2001: 22 on moralism.

37. See Barnett 2011; Bass 2008; Fassin and Pandolfi 2010; Fassin 2012.

38. Koselleck 2006: 359. Koselleck further identifies the "moral totalism" of humanistic appeals to a sovereign recast in human rather than absolute terms: "As a man, the prince was defined; he could only be one thing, namely the humane executant of humanitarianism" (Koselleck 1988: 150).

39. Foucault 2000a: 448. See also Faubion 2001; Fassin 2008; and Caduff 2011.

40. Bourg 2007; Eribon 1991: 296–308; Kouchner 1985.

41. Foucault 2000a: 444. See Fassin 2011 on the limits of humanitarian self-interrogation.

42. MSF 1992: 7.

43. The cartoon appeared in MSF-France's internal newsletter *Dazibao*, June 2002: 1.

CHAPTER 2. A SECULAR VALUE OF LIFE

1. I take this list of events largely from the assemblage presented by Wikipedia, which can stand as a situated archive of popular memory: http://en.wikipedia.org/wiki/1971 (last accessed July 14, 2012); see also http://fr.wikipedia.org/wiki/1971.

2. See Festa 2010; Haskell 1985a, 1985b; Hunt 2007; Laqueur 2009; also Moyn 2006: 399.

3. Smith 1976. See also Laqueur 2009.

4. Several commentators have astutely noted the vital role of visual media in the dynamics of contemporary aid (e.g., Benthall 1993; Boltanski 1999; Bornstein 2009; Ignatieff 1984).

5. Rawson (1969) observes that the story circulated in the Roman Empire, via Plutarch's *Apophthegmata Laconica*.

6. See Darnton 1985 and Pfeifer 2004. Animal cruelty, inhumane punishment, and infanticide have all served as targets for humanitarian reform movements; see, e.g., Foucault 1979.

7. Hubert and Mauss 1964: 101.

8. It bears emphasizing that many human traditions include ideals of generosity, kindness, and giving, to guests as well as kin, and acts of mercy may also represent something of a pan-human heritage (see Isaac 1993 and Bornstein and Redfield 2011). Religious examples of charitable action include Buddhist doctrines of compassion, Christian alms, Islamic *zakat*, and Hindu *dān*. Although differing widely in form, they accept suffering as part of the general human condition and do not present living as an end in itself.

9. Brauman 1996: 7. See also Rieff 2002: 93.

10. MSF's background involves additional inspirations, such as Eugène Jamot, a doctor with the French colonial service who pioneered an impatient frontier style at odds with both bureaucracy and missionaries (Lachenal and Taithe 2009).

11. For more about the context of Voltaire's poem see Aldridge 1975. Ray (2004) suggests the Lisbon earthquake played a significant role in the modern sense of the sublime. For a comparative sense of human responses to disaster see Hoffman and Oliver-Smith 2002 and Lakoff 2010.

12. Rousseau 2000: 109–111.

13. See Dynes 2000.

14. Asad 2003: 68.

15. In making this claim Arendt (1990: 78–79) drew a distinction between compassion for particular individuals and pity for a mass condition. See also Boltanski 1999: 3–19.

16. Pupavac (2010) underscores the conservative cast of humanitarianism in the British context, while Taithe (2004) emphasizes how the recent French version bridged both Revolutionary and Catholic legacies.

17. Hochschild (2005) makes the analogy to contemporary human rights most explicit. See also Bender 1992; Haskell 1985a, 1985 b; Drescher 2009; and Dubois 2004 on Haiti's revolution.

18. The focus here is on the International Committee of the Red Cross, based in Geneva, rather than national Red Cross and Red Crescent societies or the International Federation of Red Cross and Red Crescent Societies. For more background see Moorehead 1998; Hutchinson 1996; and Forsythe 2005.

19. Sontag 2003. See also Slaughter 2009.

20. Hutchinson 1996; Moorehead 1998; Dunant 1986 (1862).

21. John Hutchinson notes that the documentary record fails to clarify the precise rationale for the emblem, only later suggesting a reversal of the Swiss flag (Hutchinson 1996: 35). See also Benthall 1993 and Taithe 1998.

22. This Christian legacy proved a problem once the movement reached religious frontiers, and the Ottoman Empire's substitution of a red crescent prompted a struggle (Benthall 1997). Tensions over the appropriate symbol for aid have continued, particularly in the case of Israel, leading to the inclusion of a Red Crystal in 2006.

23. See Hutchinson 1996: 14–18 on the class assumptions structuring Dunant's account. Slaughter (2009) provides a more extended reading.

24. Dunant 1986: 61–62, 66–67.

25. Dunant 1986: 66.

26. Dunant 1986: 73–74.

27. Dunant was ultimately a visionary rather than an organizational founder; the scandal of his business failure forced him to resign from the fledgling Red Cross in 1867. Only late in his life did he enjoy rehabilitation and regain renown.

28. The exceptions to this rule involved settings at the threshold of European recognition, e.g., the Ottoman Empire. Conversely, see Sven Lindqvist's unconventional *A History of Bombing* (2001) for an account of colonial experiments in violence.

29. Headrick 1981; Hardiman 2006. See also Lyons 1992; Vaughn 1991.

30. Vaughn 1991; Headrick 1994.

31. Vaughn 1991: 56–57.

32. Vaughn 1991: 62–63.

33. Nobel Peace Prize Presentation Speech, 1952, at http://www.nobelprize.org/nobel_prizes/peace/laureates/1952/press.html (last accessed July 14, 2012).

34. "I wanted to be a doctor that I might be able to work without having to talk. . . . Medical knowledge made it possible for me to carry out my intention in the best and most complete way, wherever the path of service might lead me" (Schweitzer 2009: 92).

35. As he wrote in a 1905 sermon, "For me, missionary work in itself is not primarily a religious matter. Far from it. It is first and foremost a duty of humanity never realized or acted upon by our states and nations" (Schweitzer 2005: 75–76).

36. Mazrui 1991: 98–101.

37. Fernandez 1964: 537. The quotation is from Joseph Conrad's *Heart of Darkness*.

38. Quoted in Headrick 1994: 258–270. Headrick underscores that Schweitzer's work resonated more strongly in English- and German-speaking countries than in France. See also Lachenal and Taithe 2009.

39. Schweitzer 2009: 88–89.

40. Calhoun 2008; Barnett (2011) stabilizes the term but adds modifiers.

41. Moorehead 1998.

42. Forsythe 2005: 52–53.

43. Universal Declaration of Human Rights (http://www.un.org/en/documents/udhr/ , last accessed July 14, 2012). As Paul Rabinow (1999: 102–103) notes, this appearance of the term in official discourse marked a significant philosophical claim: now dignity adhered not to reason but the very fact of being—by implication, inalienable, and shared by all.

44. Lemkin 2002.

45. Westad 2007: 5, 39.

46. The United Nations High Commission for Refugees (UNHCR) appeared in 1950 to replace earlier problem-specific entities. The United Nations Children's Fund (UNICEF), begun to assist European children after the Second World War, became a permanent part of the UN in 1953. The World Food Program (WFP), established in 1961 as an experiment, quickly transformed into an enduring fixture of international relief.

47. Waters 2004.

48. Benthall 1993: 92–108; de Waal 1997: 72–77; Moorehead 1998: 622–3; Black 1992.

49. Guillemoles 2002; Vallaeys 2004: 39–51. Although consistently popular with the

French public, Kouchner has long been a controversial figure. For a caustic assessment of his trajectory as a generational icon see Ross 2002: 147–169. See also Taithe 2004: 147–158, as well as Caldwell 2009 for an account of recent controversy. Allen and Styan (2000) describe his role in advancing a "right to interfere." Within MSF his public legacy has proved a source of continued frustration.

50. One provocative article implied a generational current of innovative ambition, suggesting that in 1963 Rastignac, Balzac's social climber in *La comédie humaine*, would be "communist, bourgeois and creative" like himself (Guillemoles 2002: 55).

51. Vallaeys 2004: 61, 75. Kouchner 1991: 113.

52. Vallaeys 2004: 22

53. Emmanuelli 2005.

54. Vallaeys 2004: 107–126. Philippe Bernier, "Sommes-nous des mercenaires?" *Tonus* 442 (November 23, 1970): 1, 6.

55. Philippe Bernier, "Inde: Aidez-les à survivre!" *Tonus* 486 (November 15, 1971): 1, 7.

56. Quoted in Vallaeys 2004: 116.

57. Philippe Bernier, "La reponse à tous ceux qui doutaient de vous," *Tonus* 493 (January 3, 1972): 1, 3.

58. Here I have largely followed the detailed rendering of Anne Vallaeys (2004) in addition to the few available contemporaneous documents (e.g., the *Tonus* articles). In Olivier Weber's (1995) account Kouchner plays a more decisive role in the genesis of the group and its name, as he does in his own (e.g., Kouchner 1991).

59. Jeunes sans frontières and "Jeux sans frontières." Interview with Rony Brauman in 2003; Benthall 1993.

60. Jean-Paul Ryst, "L'oiseau blanc et rouge," *Bulletin Médecins sans frontières* 3 (April–July 1975): 14–15. This design resembles the later blue and white symbol of Kouchner's breakaway group, Médecins du monde.

61. The Association Law of 1901 emerged from the struggle between church and state in the French Third Republic. It extended state sanction over free associations and limited the autonomy of religious congregations (Archambault 1997). MSF's secularism, however, was far from anti-Catholic. Brauman and Kouchner both cite the inspiration of Abbé Pierre, who turned away from politics to address poverty, and Emmanuelli would eventually announce his own religiosity (Taithe 2004; Emmanuelli 1991: 249–250).

62. Vallaeys 2004: 125, 121–122.

63. Report on the first congress of MSF. Philippe Bernier, "La médecine d'urgence peut-elle être efficace sans 'professionels'?" *Tonus* 536 (December 18, 1972): 1, 3.

64. Vallaeys 2004: 139.

65. *Bulletin Médecins sans frontières* 3 (April–July 1975): back cover.

66. *Bulletin Médecins sans frontières* 5 (January–August 1976): 47. This would have converted to about US$67,000 at the time (see http://research.stlouisfed.org/fred2/data/EXFRUS.txt, last accessed July 14, 2012).

67. See Vallaeys 2004: 189. By 1977 MSF's rising star Claude Malhuret was denouncing the Khmer Rouge on French television, and the following year the group determined that staff would report human rights abuses and inform the public "in cases where MSF was the sole witness." Weissman 2011: 178.

68. "Dans leur salle d'attente 2 milliards d'hommes," *Bulletin Médecins sans frontières* 6 (April 1977): cover. See also Vallaeys 2004: 190–191.

69. Vallaeys 2004: 233.

70. Brauman 2006: 51. Vallaeys 2004: 260–271.

71. Field notes, Paris, France, June 2003.

72. For a less abbreviated cast of characters and greater social analysis of their context see Dauvin and Siméant 2002.

73. Ross 2002: 156–157.

74. Quoted in Vallaeys 2004: 254–255.

75. Vallaeys 2004: 248.

76. Xavier Emmanuelli, "Un bateau pour Saint-Germain-des-Prés," *Quotidien du médecin*, December 4, 1978. See also Emmanuelli 1991: 129–135; Brauman 2006: 71–79; Vallaeys 2004: 295–297; Bortolotti 2004: 52–54; and Benthall 1993: 128–131.

77. Vallaeys 2004: 299.

78. Brauman, in Groenewold and Porter 1997: xxii. See also Bortolotti 2004: 55.

79. Raymond Borel, "Choisir une 'Verité,'" *Bulletin d'informations de Médecins sans frontières* 3 (September 1979): 7.

80. Xavier Emmanuelli, "L'âge de raison," *Bulletin d'informations de Médecins sans frontières* 2 (April 1979): 1, 8.

81. Vallaeys 2004: 372.

82. Bernard Kouchner, "Relations avec les organisations humanitaires," *Bulletin d'informations de Médecins sans frontières* 3 (1975): 32–34.

83. Vallaeys 2004: 491–492.

84. MSF Holland 1995; Bortolotti 2004: 56–57.

85. Stany Grelet and Mathieu Potte-Bonneville, "Qu'est-ce qu'on fait là?" interview with Rony Brauman, *Vacarme* 04/05 (Summer 1997), www.vacarme.eu.org/article1174.html (last accessed July 14, 2012). For a more comprehensive historical overview of the political context around MSF see Westad 2007.

86. See Weissman 2011: 180–182, who notes that LSF received funding from the National Endowment for Democracy in the United States. Its trajectory also followed the emergence of human rights discourse among dissidents of socialist regimes (Moyn 2010). As with the schism, bitterness surrounding the episode lingered. Decades later in Uganda I met a doctor still upset about LSF, and the moment re-emerged briefly in discussion about globalization in MSF-France's newsletter *Messages* (132 [October–November 2004]). By the time I interviewed him in 2003, Brauman described the feud as a youthful mistake. The French operation believed in centralization and felt deeply imbued with the rebellious "Jacobin spirit of France." The Belgians, he now saw, had a different understanding of the state and resented the imperious attitude of their colleagues. See also Bortolotti 2004: 58 and Vallaeys 2004: 461–509.

87. Vallaeys 2004: 511–550. MSF's internal history offers rich elaboration, particularly the MSF Speaking Out series devoted to Ethiopia (Laurence Binet, 2005. *Famine and Forced Relocations in Ethiopia, 1984–1986*. MSF Speaking Out. Paris: MSF-France and CRASH).

88. "Médecins Sans Frontières, 1971–1991: Who Are You?" twentieth anniversary brochure.

89. Siméant 2005. MSF-Luxembourg was largely a satellite of MSF-Belgium, while MSF-Greece would be temporarily disowned by the family in 1999 following disagreements about its actions in Kosovo. After its reinstatement it began running operations in cooperation with MSF-Spain. See "The Odyssey of MSF-Greece," a 1997 memorandum of MSF-Greece, and "MSF victime du conflit du Kossovo," a 2000 memorandum of MSF Greece.

90. "Les chartes de Médecins sans frontières / The Charters of Médecins Sans Frontières," *Dazibao* 116 (July–August 2001): 1–2.

91. Philippe Bernier, "La reponse à tous ceux qui doutaient de vous," *Tonus* 493 (January 3, 1972): 1. See Givoni 2011 on MSF's trajectory through witnessing.

92. Blumenberg 1983: 65. See also Arendt 1998: 314–321 and Benjamin 1978: 299. For discussions of secularism from the perspective of anthropology see Scott and Hirschkind 2006 and Cannell 2010.

CHAPTER 3. VITAL MOBILITY

1. On cold war technopolitics see Hecht 2011, and on proxy wars and their significance during the post-Vietnam period see Westad 2007.

2. First aid instruction manuals date to at least the seventeenth century. As Roy Porter notes, "The medical chest awaits its historian" (Porter 1997: 102). For more on the late-nineteenth-century European fascination with accidents, aids, and ambulances see Cooter and Luckin 1997 and Hutchinson 1997.

3. See, e.g., Druett 2000, Lynn 1993, and Lindqvist 2001.

4. JRCIRC 1944: i.

5. JRCIRC 1944: i.

6. JRCIRC 1944: i.

7. JRCIRC 1948: 245.

8. The 2004 edition of the *Red Cross Logistics Field Manual* does not mention the *MMM*, though it does note the dispatching of family parcels during the war and the evolution of purchasing and transport between the late 1970s and early 1980s (ICRC 2004: 24). For other discussions of humanitarian logistics see Cock 2005, Kaatrud et al. 2003, and Payet 1996. For an account of the packages that gave rise to CARE see Feldman 2011, and for the history of "essential pharmaceuticals" see Greene 2011.

9. Zink 2006: 5–15.

10. Nurok 2003: 569–575.

11. See Guly 2005 and Zink 2006 for respective histories of emergency medicine in Britain and the United States; Nurok (2003) provides a conceptual overview.

12. For more on the ambulance see Haller 1992. For more on SAMU see Drouet 1982 as well as the SAMU website, www.samu-de-france.fr/en/System_of_Emergency_in_France_MG_0607#1 (accessed July 14, 2012). Rony Brauman and Xavier Emmanuelli underscore the significance of SAMU for MSF's history; see Brauman 2006: 58; Emmanuelli 1991: 21–25; as well as Taithe 2004: 150–151 and Tanguy 1999: 226–244.

13. For a portrayal of the ethos and images of the time see Guibert et al. 2009.

14. Kurt Jansson, the head of UN operations in Ethiopia at the time, gives a caustic

assessment of MSF's actions. Describing them as "very young" and having "little previous experience of Africa and of Ethiopia," he allowed they may have done some good with health but also proved "excitable" and prone to assisting the press in its generation of sensational material "highly exaggerated and unreliable in facts" (Jansson et al. 1990: 24–25). Alex de Waal (1997: 124) dismisses Jansson's reports as fiction and suggests that MSF was mainly guilty of the political naiveté of "reporting on what they had seen." For more on MSF's Ethiopian experience see Vallaeys 2004: 511–550.

15. See Harrell-Bond 1986 and Leopold 2005 for historical background.

16. See the collected papers in Dodge and Wiebe 1985. Karl-Eric Knutsson (1985) uses the evocative phrases "at best chaotic" and "disaster within a disaster" in his contribution. Several contributors note that the Karamoja famine stemmed not only from drought, but also colonial land management policies in the region and increased availability of automatic weapons that altered the balance of cattle raids. Harrell-Bond (1986) provides an extensive review of this Ugandan moment and Lakoff (2007) an incisive analysis of preparedness in the American context.

17. Well 1985: 177–182. The model for Well's strike force was a Swedish government team known as the Swedish Special Unit, whose efficient work in the West Nile region received accolades. On the other side of the cold war divide, Cuba also developed a disaster relief form of its medical brigades (Brouwer 2011: 45–47).

18. Knutsson 1985: 187–188.

19. Rony Brauman, "Karamoja: Les difficultés d'un sauvetage," *Bulletin d'information de Médecins sans frontierès* 7 (August/September/October 1980): 9–12. Unlike Oxfam or Action Contre la Faim (Action Against Hunger), MSF primarily focuses on therapeutic aspects of nutrition. Nonetheless, famine relief has played a significant role in its history.

20. This and all subsequent descriptions refer to the 2003 English edition of the *MSF Catalogue.*

21. Known as *intendant* in French. See Irène Nzakou's twentieth-anniversary interview with Jacques Pinel in MSF-France's house journal, *Messages:* "Log Story," *Messages* 142 (September 2006): 30–31; also Vallaeys 2004: 374–384 and Payet 1996: 12–14.

22. This account of the origins of MSF's kit system draws from an interview with Jacques Pinel conducted in French by Johanna Rankin, December 21, 2004. The translation is mine from the transcript of the exchange (included as an appendix in her undergraduate honors thesis, Rankin 2005: 152–170). In this interview Pinel—like every MSF logistician I have ever queried—presents the kit system as an inspired but ultimately commonsense response to an inherent technical problem. Akrich (1992) outlines a more complex reading of technical transplantation beyond emergency.

23. Vidal and Pinel 2011: 27.

24. Vidal and Pinel 2011: 29.

25. Rankin 2005: 166–167.

26. I take this description from the *MSF Catalogue,* 2003 edition. Corty (2011a) gives additional historical background on the development of this kit. The designation 001 derives from a WHO designation for cholera, a famous and influential disease. See Hamlin 2009 for general background and Briggs and Briggs 2003 for a situated account.

27. Vidal and Pinel 2011: 30.

28. Jacques Pinel and Irène Nzakou, "Log Story," *Messages* 142 (September 2006): 30–31.

29. Payet 1996: 14.

30. MSF 1997.

31. Quoted in Oliver Falhun, "Probing Surgery," *Messages* 144 (March 2007): 2.

32. Vidal and Pinel 2011: 31.

33. MSF Field Library List, as recorded by the author in Brussels, July 2003.

34. Vidal and Pinel 2011: 30.

35. An account of the ICRC reaction to the kit appears in Oliver Falhun, "Probing Surgery," *Messages* 144 (March 2007): 1–3; several informants noted the logistics migration to Geneva. However, the ICRC also began its own logistics developments in the late 1970s and established a unit to centralize vehicle purchase and management in 1984. See ICRC 2004: 24. Following the 1996 crisis in eastern Zaire the UN established the United Nations Joint Logistics Center to better coordinate between agencies (see Kaatrud et al. 2003).

36. Corty 2011a: 94–95.

37. Lévi-Strauss 1966.

38. Field notes, Kampala, Uganda, May 2004.

39. Field notes, Paris, France, August 2001.

40. The following observations and quotations are drawn from the author's field notes, Kampala, Uganda, July 2003 and May 2004.

41. Caroline Livio, "Medicines, an Indicator of Our Activity?" *Messages* 138 (November 2005): 11.

42. See Lakoff and Collier 2008.

43. MSF press releases issued April 30, 2003; March 24, 2005; May 23, 2005; as well as *MSF Activity Report 2001–2002,* 35.

44. De Laet and Mol 2000.

45. See Latour 1987: 226–227 and 1999.

46. Field notes, Amsterdam, Netherlands, July 2006.

47. See "Kit Culture" by Jean-Hervé Jézéquel, www.msf-crash.org/crash/sur-le-vif/2009/06/04/281/kit-culture/ (last accessed July 14, 2012). If MSF was also guilty of lapsing into kit culture, the organization found itself trumped when the United States Air Force dropped both aid packets and bombs over Afghanistan following the attacks of September 2001.

48. Foucault's use of the French term Brauman cited—*dispositif*—is notoriously slippery. In a 1977 interview he described it not only as a "heterogeneous ensemble" involving a range of discursive and nondiscursive elements, but also as a formation that "has as its major function at a given historical moment that of responding to an *urgent need*" (emphasis in original). Foucault 1980: 194–195; see also Rabinow 2003: 49–55 and Cock 2005. Here I take Brauman's observation seriously in order to situate MSF's moral reasoning about emergency—its "regime of living" (Collier and Lakoff 2005)—within the larger humanitarian enterprise it both enacts and criticizes.

49. For example, the French training institute Bioforce offers programs in management and logistics: www.bioforce.asso.fr/ (last accessed July 14, 2012).

50. For similar health initiatives see the WHO's guidelines for "health actions in cri-

ses," www.who.int/hac/techguidance/en/ (last accessed July 14, 2012), and Laurie Garrett's "Doc-in-a-Box" project at the Council on Foreign Relations, www.cfr.org/project/1247/docinabox_project.html (last accessed July 14, 2012).

51. See the special issue of *Messages* focusing on MSF's international scope, "The International Movement: How Many Divisions Does MSF Have?" *Messages* 136 (May 2005): 1–21.

52. As noted by a number of speakers at the American section's annual meeting in 2003 and reflected in annual reports. By 2008 donors from the United States contributed some 13 percent of MSF's combined worldwide income of $979 million: www.doctorswithoutborders.org/donate/donorcommitment.cfm (last accessed July 14, 2012).

53. An unpublished report of a small survey by MSF/Factanova suggests that the group's positive image with supporters rests on its perceived authenticity. See MSF-France/Factanova, "Résultats étude qualitative phase entretiens donateurs," 2004. A larger survey conducted for MSF-France in 2010 indicates that most donors care deeply about transparency and efficacy beyond a given cause ("Résultats enquête à l'écoute des donateurs de Médecins Sans Frontières," June 1–7, 2010).

54. See Bornstein 2009 on the Hindu tradition of *dān*, which implies no continuing interest and expects no direct return.

55. MSF-USA's website further outlines its commitment to donors as to how funds will be spent: www.doctorswithoutborders.org/donate/donorcommitment.cfm (last accessed July 14, 2012).

56. There is, of course, a vast literature on the gift and its moral standing, well beyond Mauss 1990, e.g., Schrift 1997. Here I am treating the transaction as literally as possible.

57. On the discourse of corruption see Nordstrom 2004.

58. This particular solicitation dates from 2008.

59. See the donor surveys sponsored by MSF-France cited in note 53 ; see also Slovic 2007.

60. December 19, 2006, news release from the Center for Philanthropy at Indiana University, www.philanthropy.iupui.edu/News/2006/pr-Tsunami.aspx (last accessed July 14, 2012). According to this study small donations made up the vast majority of contributions (the median amount being $50), with a quarter of American households participating.

61. "Following the Wave," *Messages* 134 (March 2005): 25–27. See also Stirrat 2006 for context.

62. In the United States watchdog evaluators such as Charity Navigator (www.charitynavigator.org/) and the American Institute of Philanthropy (www.charitywatch.org/) actively monitor and grade nonprofit organizations on a number of standardized criteria.

63. Reviewing a set of campaigns conducted between 2001 and 2004, an article in MSF-France's journal *Messages* confirms that natural disasters outperformed other crises, advertising notwithstanding, and that conventional campaigns proved more successful than experimental ones. Ann Avril, "Donors Particularly Reactive to Natural Catastrophes," *Messages* 134 (March 2005): 15.

64. On the issue of inflation see Collier et al. 2004: 7; also Michel Foucault 2000b: 373.

CHAPTER 4. MORAL WITNESS

1. See the Nobel Peace Prize acceptance speech delivered by James Orbinski on behalf of MSF, http://nobelprize.org/nobel_prizes/peace/laureates/1999/msf-lecture.html (last accessed July 14, 2012).

2. See for comparison the lay expertise developed in the AIDS activist movement (Epstein 1996).

3. Camus 1991: 163; 1947: 132. Adopting a translation that renders *honnêteté* more literally as *honesty*, Alex de Waal (1997: 221) positions this quotation at the end of his extended critique of humanitarian efforts to intervene in situations of famine.

4. James Orbinski, "Taking a Stand: The Ethics of Intervention," 2001, www.peace.ca/orbinski.htm (last accessed July 14, 2012). Also see the Nobel speech cited above.

5. Kouchner 1991.

6. Miles (2004: xiv, 149–151) gives this rendition and suggests that the proscription is against the physician using "privileged information to dishonor persons." For additional context for the oath and its historical reception see Nutton 1993.

7. The initial charter appeared on the front page of the January 3, 1972, issue of the medical journal *Tonus*. The current charter can be found at www.doctorswithoutborders.org/aboutus/charter.cfm (last accessed July 14, 2012).

8. Kouchner 1991: 112.

9. *Bulletin Médecins sans frontières* 2 (January–March 1975): 3.

10. Heyster 2000: 1.

11. *Bulletin Médecins sans frontières* 6 (1977): 4–5.

12. Soussan 2008: 14. See also Givoni 2011 and Weissman 2011 for insightful analysis.

13. Advocacy action by these two sections was not entirely unprecedented; the Dutch section had been evicted from Suriname in 1987, accused by the regime of aiding Maroon rebels, and provided information for journalists about atrocities in Sudan the following year. See de Haan et al. 1995: 27–30.

14. Quoted in Soussan 2008: 15.

15. For a close analysis of several controversial cases of humanitarian action by an MSF insider see Terry 2002. Dauvin (2004) gives a discussion of sectional differences in Kosovo.

16. Heyster 2000: 4.

17. Soussan 2008: 31.

18. Soussan 2008: 34–35.

19. Bouchet-Saulnier and Dubuet 2007, esp. 14, 19, 32–36. Also the discussion with Françoise Bouchet-Saulnier, "Grounds for Divorce? MSF and the International Criminal Court," www.msf-crash.org/en/rencontre-debats/ (last accessed July 14, 2012).

20. See the dossier "Freud in the Field," *Messages* 142 (September 2006): 1–15.

21. Fassin 2004, 2012; Fassin and Rechtman 2009.

22. Soussan 2008: 32, 42. Ticktin 2011b provides more detailed description and analysis.

23. Hannerz 2004: 135.

24. Rackley 2001: 3.

25. Rackley 2001: 9.

26. Rackley 2001: 13.

27. Rackley 2001: 20–21.

28. This point is reemphasized in a final footnote: "It is a sad misunderstanding that humanitarianism can 'save the world,' as is apparently believed by many of our first mission volunteers, donors, and general public as well. When we succeed at what we do, at best it can be called 'keeping people alive,' but this is hardly 'to save the world' or even to affect the root causes responsible for the suffering of a given population. That *témoignage* aspires to a kind of justice is in part an extension of this recognition of the limits of medical relief alone" (Rackley 2001: 27).

29. See the series "MSF Speaking Out," www.msf-crash.org/en/publications/ (last accessed July 14, 2012).

30. Field notes, Paris, France, June 2003.

31. Field notes, Paris, France, June 2003.

32. Van Herp et al. 2003.

33. Van Herp et al. 2003: 151.

34. Alison Marschner, "A Scientific Approach to 'Témoignage,'" *MSF Annual Activity Report, 1998–9*. Brussels: MSF International, 1999: 18–19.

35. To quote Annelise Riles (2000: 18) in another context: "The achievement, then, lies not in the discovery of new knowledge, but in an effort to make what we know analytically accessible."

36. Organizations like MSF are acutely aware of the need to enumerate casualties before, during, and after any disaster in order to attract media attention. At the same time some recognize the dangers of doing so, particularly in a context as fluid and vast as the Congo. Retroactive mortality studies, including the one sponsored by the International Rescue Committee between 1999 and 2001 that suggested a figure of 2.5 to 3.5 million deaths in the region, have encountered methodological criticism (www.theirc.org/health/mortality_2001.cfm).

37. MSF 2002.

38. A similar collection, entitled "The War Was Following Me" and issued by MSF-Holland, likewise matched selected testimonials with stark black-and-white photographs of suffering to chronicle the preceding decade of violence in the Congo (MSF-H 2002). For a discussion of tensions of voice in global projects see Butt 2002 and responses by Irwin et al. 2002, as well as Malkki 1996 on refugees. Spivak (1988), of course, would suggest inherent difficulties for any project seeking transparent expression on behalf of the oppressed.

39. Soussan (2008: 39) suggests an increasing emphasis on medical action beyond simple presence. For religious parallels to MSF's secular practice, see Bornstein 2005: 39 on World Vision's sense of the field as a sacred site of "real work" and Giri 2002: 45 on Habitat for Humanity's emergence from "love in action."

40. His point finds echoes in many other accounts I have received. Arriving in the former Yugoslavia near the beginning of that state's disintegration, an emergency team from MSF-France was embarrassed to find that its medical expertise was both less crucial and less well-adapted than expected; a hospital in Split had plenty of trained personnel

and requested a list of drugs similar to one "you would find in Marseilles." The team remained in place, however, realizing that the delivery of minor services would allow it to remain and monitor the situation.

41. Ticktin (2011b) insightfully expands on this point with respect to sexual violence.

42. See Butt 2002 and Irwin et al. 2002.

43. For an etymological discussion of differing implications of testimony see Agamben 2000, especially 148–150. Fassin (2011: 200–222) further extends and complicates etymological distinctions between forms of witnessing. For Agamben as well as many others (e.g., Douglass and Vogler 2003), the Holocaust established the defining paradigm for moral witnessing.

44. Although legally independent, in practical terms Epicentre represents a subsidiary enterprise; MSF members sit on its board and most of its employees have considerable experience on MSF missions. Not all sections of MSF avail themselves equally of Epicentre's services, but they share a common commitment to epidemiological study.

45. Rademacher and Patel 2002: 176.

46. MSF-France president's "Rapport Moral 1987." MSF's move to equip itself with a better arsenal of statistical facts fits a more widespread pattern within nonprofit and advocacy organizations at the time. Even Greenpeace supplemented its tradition of guerrilla theater with a greater focus on research (Steven Durland, "Witness: The Guerilla Theater of Greenpeace," *High Performance* 40 (10 [1987]): 4, listed at www.apionline.org/hpbackiss .html (last accessed July 14, 2012); Keck and Sikkink 1998: 21).

47. Alison Marschner, "A Scientific Approach to 'Témoignage,'" *MSF Annual Activity Report, 1998–9.* Brussels: MSF International, 1999: 18–19.

48. Field notes, Paris, France, April 2004.

49. Robertson et al. 2002.

50. Soussan 2008: 49.

51. Nordstrom 2004: 5.

52. Neff 2000: 7.

53. Neff 2000: 103.

54. For a parallel argument about war and states see Nordstorm 2004. The larger point is that assumptions about linear, progressive time may sometimes generate analytic confusion.

55. Weiss 1999; Tanguy and Terry 1999.

56. Fiona Terry, "The Principle of Neutrality: Is it Relevant to MSF?" *Les Cahiers de Messages* 113 (March 2001): 5.

57. Jean-Hervé Bradol, "Motions Debated at the Thirtieth General Assembly of Médecins Sans Frontières," *Messages* 116 (July–August 2001): 2.

58. Tanguy and Terry 1999.

59. Fiona Terry, "The Principle of Neutrality: Is it Relevant to MSF?" *Les Cahiers de Messages* 113 (March 2001): 4.

60. Cited in Soussan 2008: 49.

61. Most people I talked to in Uganda recognized MSF's medical focus but little else. A multicountry study undertaken by the organization itself found that most beneficiaries were not aware of the group's independence, let alone its multiple sections, and often ascribed a

religious or political purpose to its action. See Abu-Sada 2012 ; also the Feinstein International Studies report "Humanitarian Agenda 2015: Principles, Power, and Perceptions," http://sites.tufts.edu/feinstein/2006/humanitarian-agenda-2015-principles-power-and-perceptions-2.

62. Foucault 2000c : 111–133.

63. Foucault 2000c: 129.

64. Like Gramsci (1971), Foucault historicizes the timeless figure of "the intellectual" if focusing on forms of knowledge and regimes of truth rather than class or labor per se. For general background on the sociology of intellectuals and their politics see Kurzman and Owens 2002. Krause (1996: 123–172) outlines the social history of French doctors.

65. Rabinow and Rose 2006; see also Collier and Lakoff 2005.

66. As Mario Biagioli and Peter Galison (2003: 2) note, physicists are unclear about what the Nobel Prize means "in an era when two thousand scientists sign a single paper." See Galison 2003 for an expanded discussion of the "collective author" in the context of science.

67. Boli and Thomas 1999; Fisher 1997; Keck and Sikkink 1998.

68. See Robbins 1999: 11–37 for a discussion of internationalism, cosmopolitanism, and nationalism related to Susan Sontag's denunciation of depoliticized intellectuals absent from Sarajevo.

69. Shapin 1994: 42.

70. Haraway 1997: 24. See also Slaughter 2007 on the parameters of the bildungsroman tradition of forming an autonomous subject to speak the truth.

71. Quoted in Proctor 1992: 17.

72. Brauman 1996: 76; see also Rieff 2002: 75.

CHAPTER 5. HUMAN FRONTIERS

1. See Magone et al. 2011 on the broad problem of humanitarian negotiation.

2. MSF's initial debates over longer-term missions did recognize the "personal interests and family obligations" of those leaving for extended periods. See Philippe Bernier, "La medicine d'urgence peut-elle être efficace sans 'professionnels'?" *Tonus* 536 (December 18, 1972): 1, 3.

3. To quote an internal summation: "Statistically MSF looks like this: a malaria patient receiving a consultation from a Congolese doctor who is supervised by a 34 year old nurse, recruited through a partner section and in the field for about 7 months." MSF, *La Mancha Gazette* (May 2006): 7. The line clearly intends to disrupt stereotypes and should be read in that light.

4. Shevchenko and Fox (2008: 110–111) suggest the limits of the colonial frame by examining expatriate/national tensions in MSF's Russian missions.

5. Field notes, Yumbe District, Uganda, July 2003.

6. See Geissler 2010 on the general tensions surrounding transport allowances in a research setting, and Kelly 2010 for an extreme example of bodies in place.

7. Hudson Apunyo, "NGO Sacks Staff over Low Pay Strike," *Monitor* (May 23, 2006).

8. Field notes, Kampala, Uganda, July 2006.

9. MSF-France, "Carnet de Route" (2003): 19.

10. MSF-France, "Carnet de Route" (2003): 18–23.

11. Field notes, Kampala, Uganda, December 2004.

12. In many settings where MSF works, particularly the sub-Saharan African heartland of humanitarianism, biomedical personnel remain in short supply due to limited training opportunities or out-migration (for a study of medical education in Malawi see Wendland 2010, and for history in East Africa Iliffe 2002). This is particularly true in remote rural regions. One of the clinics associated with MSF's sleeping sickness program had been waiting over a year for a doctor. At another project I visited along the country's northeastern border, most government health staff came from elsewhere in the country and lived within their own walled compound.

13. See Rémi Vallet, "Pain Management: Ongoing Pain," *Messages* 138 (November 2005): 4–5; also Françoise Duroch, "Medical Responsibility and Sexual Violence: Overcoming the Resistance," *Messages* 138 (November 2005): 6–7.

14. Anne-Sophie Coutin and Chloé Gelin, "Abortion and Medical Responsibility: Abortion, in Theory and in Practice," *Messages* 138 (November 2005): 7.

15. See *Contact* 71 (June–July 2001): 76.

16. Dauvin and Siméant (2002) provide a more comprehensive study of motivations and trajectories of volunteers in French humanitarian NGOs. For ethnographic discussion of circulating aid professionals in other domains see Mosse 2011, Rottenburg 2009, and Stirrat 2008.

17. A cartoon in MSF-France's open newsletter *Dazibao* expanded on this anxiety in 2005, showing an aid worker sporting an "MSF patch" to counteract his addiction and assuring the viewer that "you too can get out" (*Dazibao* 136 [May 2005]).

18. This corresponded with a concern about the growth of office staff and partner sections in general. Morten Rostrup, "La Croissance sans vertu?" *Dazibao* 123 (November 2002–February 2003): 2–3.

19. MSF, *La Mancha Gazette* (May 2006): 1. See also the volume *My Sweet La Mancha*, MSF 2005.

20. As the director elaborated: "Norway is different (it has no colonial past, for example, and the sentence in Norwegian has an obvious double meaning)." This snippet appeared in MSF Belgium's house journal *Contact* 56 (September 1998): 44.

21. Field notes, Kampala, Uganda, August 2003.

22. Field notes, Kampala, Uganda, August 2003.

23. Marine Buissonnière, "La Mancha, Here We Come!" *La Mancha Gazette* (May 2006): 3.

24. MSF, "The La Mancha Agreement," *La Mancha Gazette* (May 2006): 6.

25. The case of MSF's South African section, rooted in the well-known AIDS program there and stablished in 2006 to provide a regional voice, has proved notably different.

26. See Geoff Prescott, "Simply Focus on the Staff," *Ins and Outs*, MSF-Holland (June 2006): 6–7.

27. Bateson 1972; see Gibney 2006 for retrospective. For recent deployments in anthropology see Cattelino 2010, Fortun 2001, James 2010, and Mertz and Timmer 2010.

CHAPTER 6. THE PROBLEM OF TRIAGE

1. See, for example, the provocative discussion of intervention in McFalls 2010: 319.

2. For more on pastoral power see Foucault 2007, especially 125–130.

3. Maskalyk 2009: 142.

4. MSF-Holland. "Justice and MSF Operational Choices," report of a discussion held in Soesterberg, Netherlands (June 2001): 26.

5. MSF *Messages* 138 (November 2005): 14.

6. Rony Brauman, "Controversies within Health and Human Rights," February 14, 2001, www.cceia.org/resources/transcripts/93.html. See also Brauman 2000.

7. See Hammond 2008: 175–176 on relative security risk. The statistical record appears inconclusive, suggesting that any increase was likely borne primarily by national staff and that the real change has occurred in perceptions. Attacks on aid providers in battlefield settings are far from new.

8. Soussan 2008: 8–9.

9. Soussan 2008: 38.

10. Fassin 2012: 238. On the question of what makes a life "grievable" see Butler 2004.

11. www.doctorswithoutborders.org/news/article.cfm?id=895&cat=field-news (last accessed July 14, 2012).

12. Brauman 1996.

13. Cox 1911; Lippert 2004.

14. A field coordinator for MSF told me an anecdote about how the U.S. Army once purchased 300 white Toyota Land Cruisers of the sort that NGOs commonly use in such settings. Stunned by the sheer scale for potential misrecognition suddenly confronting it, MSF could only plead with the military command to at least paint them green (field notes, Gulu District, Uganda, December 2004). See also Abu Sada 2012: 11.

15. As Didier Fassin (2004, 2012) suggests, in cases like Palestine, MSF's presence itself constitutes an act of advocacy.

16. Orbinski 2008: 193.

17. Weissman 2004.

18. Bradol 2004: 4–5. The original French version identifies the international order as "cannibal" rather than sacrificial, though the tenor and argument is the same. MSF's Nobel acceptance speech of 1999 also proclaims "the refusal of all forms of problem solving through sacrifice of the weak and vulnerable" as a fundamental distinction between humanitarian and political action (www.nobelprize.org/nobel_prizes/peace/laureates/1999/msf-lecture.html).

19. Bradol 2004: 5–6. On shifting attitudes toward violence see Elias 1978, as well as Cohen 2001 and Scheper-Hughes 1993.

20. "But if sacrifice is so complex, whence comes its unity? It is because, fundamentally, beneath the diverse forms it takes, it always consists in one same procedure, which may be used for the most widely differing purposes. *This procedure consists in establishing a means of communication between the sacred and the profane worlds through the media-*

tion of a victim, that is, of a thing that in the course of the ceremony is destroyed" (Hubert and Mauss 1964: 97, emphasis in original). For an extended reading of this passage, see Christopher Roberts, "Machining the Sacred: A Critical Exploration of *Sacrifice: Its Nature and Functions,* master's thesis, Department of Religious Studies, University of North Carolina at Chapel Hill, 2003.

21. See Goldhammer 2005 on the French tradition connecting sacrifice with political violence.

22. Bradol 2004: 21.

23. See Asad 2003 and Faubion 2003.

24. Bradol 2004: 9.

25. Bradol's essay, for example, closes with a figure of 20,000 children saved by MSF in Angola in 2002 (Bradol 2004: 22).

26. Fassin 2007; 2012.

27. Fassin 2007: 514.

28. A participant in Fassin's account of the Iraq debate expressly appeals to the phrase "ethics in action" (Fassin 2007: 505).

29. From Larrey's memoirs of Napoleon's Russia campaign, quoted in Iserson and Moskop 2007: 277. In addition to this succinct two-part review (part two being Moskop and Iserson 2007), see also Baker and Strosberg (1992), who provide a more extensive discussion of Larrey.

30. See Iserson and Moskop 2007; also Gabriel and Metz 1992: 158.

31. Baker and Strosberg 1992: 104.

32. Nguyen 2010; Biehl 2007 also alludes to the tragic tension of triage with respect to HIV/AIDS.

33. Iserson and Moskop 2007: 279; Moskop and Iserson 2007: 282.

34. "Those who are dangerously wounded must be tended first, entirely without regard to rank or distinction. Those less severely injured must wait until the gravely wounded have been operated on and dressed. The slightly wounded may go to the hospital [behind the] line; especially officers, since they have horses and therefore have transport—and regardless, most of these have but trivial wounds" (Larrey, quoted in Baker and Strosberg 1992: 110. The authors argue against those who interpret Larrey as a military utilitarian, emphasizing his revolutionary egalitarianism. Since their interpretation prefigures MSF's view I have adopted it here.

35. Moskop and Iserson 2007: 282–284.

36. Field notes, Paris, France, July 2005.

37. Orbinski 2008: 226. Tellingly, a documentary about Orbinski and his work bears the title *Triage* (*Triage: Dr. James Orbinski's Humanitarian Dilemma,* 2008).

38. Brauman, "Controversies within Health and Human Rights," February 14, 2001, www.cceia.org/resources/transcripts/93.html.

39. See Zelizer 1994 on the shifting value of children in the United States.

40. See the discussion in "Limits: Closing Down Programs," *Messages* 138 (November 2005): 15–18. Quotations are from pp. 16–17.

41. Fassin 2007a: 501.

CHAPTER 7. THE *LONGUE DURÉE* OF DISEASE

1. Philippe Bernier, "La médecine d'urgence peut-elle être efficace sans 'profession-nels'?" *Tonus* 536 (December 18, 1972): 1, 3.

2. For a discussion of projects focused on "exclusion and social violence" see Ann Guibert, "Other Projects," *Messages* 146 (May 2007): 1–3. In light of reevaluation and clo-sures, the article argues for the humanitarian importance of such missions, despite the continuing struggle to establish project limits. Not all these programs, the author suggests, have been "stuck in 'charity,' managed by nice but rather naive MSF people."

3. Rowan Gillies, "The Year in Review," *MSF Activity Report, 2003–04,* 5.

4. *MSF Activity Report, 2003–04,* 40; *MSF Activity Report, 2009,* 32.

5. Bradol 2004: 8.

6. For a sample of the insightful and influential writing about AIDS in anthropology see, e.g., Biehl 2005, 2007; Farmer 2003; Fassin 2007b; Geissler and Prince 2010; Hyde 2007; Klaits 2010; Nguyen 2010; Setel 1999. Steinberg (2008) provides a vivid portrayal of MSF's treatment program in rural South Africa.

7. Lyons 1992: 70–73.

8. Hoppe 2003; Lyons 1992, chapter 4; and Ford 1971. See also Tilley 2004 and Vaughn 1991. The form initially identified in the Ugandan epidemic, *Trypanosoma brucei gam-biense,* acquired a sibling in 1910 with the identification of *Trypanosoma brucei rhodesiense* in northern Rhodesia. Precisely which form produced the Ugandan epidemic is now less clear. See Fèvre et al. 2004. The human version of this disease divided Africa rather neatly west to east, with Uganda on the fault line between "chronic" Ghambian and "acute" Rhodesian varieties, both of which proved deadly.

9. Lyons 1992: 72–75.

10. See Gerardo Priotto and Winyi Kaboyo, "Final Evaluation of the MSF-France Trypanosomiasis Control Program in West Nile, Uganda, from 1987 to 2002." Paris: Epi-centre report, 2002.

11. See Lachenal and Taithe 2009; also Corty 2011b and Headrick 1994.

12. Corty 2011b: 135.

13. Gerardo Priotto and Winyi Kaboyo, "Final Evaluation of the MSF-France Trypano-somiasis Control Program in West Nile, Uganda, from 1987 to 2002." Paris: Epicentre report, 2002: 9.

14. Corty 2011b: 137.

15. According to an AIDS researcher with deep roots in the country, in the early days Museveni would recount how he had been counseled to act by Fidel Castro. This story later disappeared, along with an early contingent of Cuban doctors.

16. Bradol and Szumilin 2011.

17. By 1998 MSF claimed 48 field projects involving AIDS (Bradol and Szumilin 2011: 184).

18. "Uganda, Traditional Healers Fight against AIDS," MSF-Switzerland annual report (June 1996–May 1997): 30–31. See also Jacques Homsy, "Guérisseurs, médecins et SIDA: Un projet—Espoir en Ouganda," *MSF Suisse* 29 (Fall 1993): 12–15.

19. This was likewise the case with MSF's early ARV project in Thailand, which was started by a nurse caring for friends with under-the-counter medications (Bradol and Szumilin 2011: 183). Early treatment in poor settings generally proceeded in an ad hoc and clandestine manner, with individuals quietly transporting donated drugs (Nguyen 2010).

20. Field notes, Kampala, Uganda, October 2002.

21. For an example of THETA's research work see Homsy et al. 1999.

22. See www.thetaug.org/ (last accessed July 14, 2012).

23. Bradol and Szumilin 2011: 183.

24. Nguyen 2010 details the "confessional technologies" of AIDS activism. As a point of comparison see Packard 2007 on the history of efforts to combat malaria.

25. Field notes, Arua, Uganda, May 2004.

26. Biehl (2007) and Nguyen (2010) outline forms of "pharmaceutical" and "therapeutic" citizenship.

27. Field notes, Arua, Uganda, May 2004.

28. See the interview conducted with Jacques Pinel by Johanna Rankin in Rankin 2005: 93–96 and appendix A.

29. "Access to Medicines at Risk across the Globe: What to Watch Out for in Free Trade Agreements with the United States," MSF Campaign for Access to Essential Medicines briefing note, May 2004. For more on the background of essential medicines see Greene 2011, and for a sense of the current terrain around drugs see Ecks 2008 and Petryna et al. 2006.

30. "Fatal Imbalance: The Crisis in Research and Development for Drugs for Neglected Diseases," MSF special report, 2001, at www.doctorswithoutborders.org/publications/reports/2001/fatal_imbalance_short.pdf (last accessed July 14, 2012).

31. In addition to MSF, founding partners in DNDi included the Oswaldo Cruz Foundation in Brazil, the Indian Council of Medical Research, the Institut Pasteur in France, the Malaysian Ministry of Health, and the Kenyan Medical Research Institute. The new organization also worked in association with the UN–World Bank–WHO program known as TDR (Research and Training in Tropical Diseases). For further details see the DNDi website (www.dndi.org).

32. "Supply of Sleeping Sickness Drugs Confirmed," MSF press release, May 3, 2001.

33. Thompson 1971. The phrase has had an extended afterlife; see, e.g., Fassin 2011.

34. See Kleinman and Kleinman 1997 for a discussion of DALYs (Disability Adjusted Life Years) as a representation of suffering.

CHAPTER 8. THE VERGE OF CRISIS

1. Kefa Atibuni, "Amin Nostalgia Grips Arua," *Monitor* (August 3, 2003): 8.

2. See Leopold 2005: 57 and Rice 2009 for a portrait of Amin's legacy.

3. Personal communication, 2007.

4. Churchill 1909: 197.

5. See, e.g., the country profile in the CIA's World Factbook, www.cia.gov/library/publications/the-world-factbook/geos/ug.html. Linguistic shorthand distinguishes between the

agrarian Bantu speakers of the south and west and the more pastoral Nilotic and Sudanic speakers of the north and east. This north-south divide continues to feature prominently in contemporary political analyses, as do finer distinctions between other regions.

6. For more on the history of Uganda and its regional violence see Chrétien 2003; Kasozi 1999; Seftel 1994; Mamdani 1996; Finnström 2008. Leopold (2005) offers a meticulous accounting of Amin's image and ties to the northwest.

7. For vivid portrayals of the period see Rice 2009 and Seftel 1994, the latter being a compilation of contemporary reports for the African magazine *DRUM*.

8. See Harrell-Bond 1986 and de Torrenté 2001 on post-conflict reconstruction.

9. See, for example, the account of Ugandan refugees in Harrell-Bond 1986.

10. Leopold 2005; Hoppe 2003.

11. *Bulletin d'informations de Médecins sans frontières* 7 (September–October 1980).

12. H. C. Kelle, "Ouganda: L'impossible mission," *Bulletin d'informations de Médecins sans frontières* 11 (August–September 1981): 10–11.

13. See Evelyne Jacqz, "Zaïre: Terre des réfugiés," *Bulletin d'informations de Médecins sans frontières* 12 (December 1981–February 1982): 13–15; J. J. Frère, "Réfugiés ougandais au Soudan: Un nouvel exode," *Bulletin d'informations de Médecins sans frontières* 15 (November–December 1982): 1–5.

14. *Bulletin d'informations de Médecins sans frontières*, special issue, "MSF en Afrique," part 1 (January–March 1985).

15. De Haan et al. 1995: 35, 51–52. The attack killed a member of the national staff and seriously wounded a Dutch volunteer.

16. *Report of the Board, Médecins sans frontières Switzerland, 2005–2006*.

17. Allen 1996: 238–239; see also Allen 1994.

18. This summary derives from annual activity reports for 1990–2001 for MSF-France as well as respective annual activity reports for MSF International. The format of and detail in these reports fluctuates from year to year. See MSF-Paris, "Rapport d'activités, 1993–1994," 65–66, for discussion of the programs and their justifications.

19. For more background on the Lord's Resistance Army and related issues, see Allen 2006; Behrend 1999; Finnström 2008.

20. MSF-Holland, "Internally Displaced Camps in Lira and Pader, Northern Uganda: Baseline Health Survey Preliminary Report," November 2004.

21. MSF-Holland, "Pader: A Community in Crisis: A Preliminary Analysis of MSF Holland's Baseline Mental Health Assessment in Pader, Uganda," November 2004.

22. Field notes, Amsterdam, Netherlands, July 2006.

23. MSF 1997: 243.

24. The phrase made it into Uganda's profile in the 2006 edition of the organization's annual report: www.doctorswithoutborders.org/publications/ar/report.cfm?id=1759&cat=activity-report (last accessed September July 14, 2012).

25. Fassin and Rechtman 2009: 163–164. For a wider sense of the shifting global terrain of subjectivity see Good et al. 2008.

26. See "Freud in the Field," *Messages* 142 (September 2006): 1–12.

27. Das 2007; see also Fassin 2007. For other insightful work on the human aftermath of conflict see Nelson 2009 and Shaw et al. 2010.

28. Branch (2011) and Dolan (2009) provide critical analyses of the humanitarian role in Ugandan government policy.

29. See respective MSF activity reports from 2006–2007, 2008, 2009, and 2010.

30. François Delfosse, "In Uganda, MSF and the 'Decongestion' Process: What Is to Be Done?" *Messages* 141 (July 2006): 26–27.

31. Kidder (2003: 101) discusses parallel "areas of moral clarity" for Partners in Health, which, however, frames its response through community development and enduring relationships.

CHAPTER 9. ACTION BEYOND OPTIMISM

1. Rony Brauman once commented, "When one speaks of a failure, one implies that there could be success. I have a hard time imagining what a humanitarian success would be in situations where violence is itself the sign of failure. As humanitarians we inscribe ourselves in failure." Quoted in Dawes 2007: 18–19.

2. *MSF Activity Report 2005–2006*, 84.

3. See Arendt 1998 on action and contemplation.

4. See Fassin 2012: 246 on the condition of simultaneously acting and expressing "ambivalence or disappointment."

5. The work's closing passages as cited in this paragraph are from Voltaire 1991: 75.

6. Terry 2002: 216.

7. The list of warning titles runs remarkably long. For relevant examples see, e.g., Brauman 1996; Rieff 2002; Terry 2002. Hugo Slim provides an incisive discussion of "dilemmas" (Slim 1997).

8. Bortolotti 2004.

9. Field notes, Paris, France, July 2005.

10. Personal communication, March 20, 2005.

11. Adorno 1974.

12. I thank Tobias Rees for sharing an essay on the Gates Foundation, which very much does have a plan.

13. For relevant commentary on neoliberalism from the perspective of anthropology, see Ferguson 2006; Ong 2006. Functioning as politics, the moral force of humanitarianism frequently erodes into reactive moralism in the sense suggested by Wendy Brown (2001: 22), foreclosing rather than opening the political horizon (Rancière 2004). While remaining resolutely reactive, MSF participates in the "politics of survival" (Abélès 2010). However, it also engages in forms of critique and the sort of "matters of concern" that Latour (2004) identifies as post-critique.

14. See Brauman 1996: 65.

15. Field notes, Gulu, Uganda, December 2004.

16. "I never *act*; I am always slightly surprised by what I do" (Latour 1999: 281). See also Tsing 2005 on friction in connection and interaction.

17. Calhoun 2008, especially 89–94. Also see Bornstein 2009.

18. See Gramsci 1994: 299–300 for a formulation and potential debt to the French writer Romain Rolland; Foucault 1984: 343.

19. On care see Mol 2008; also Klaits 2010; Ticktin 2011a; and Tronto 1993.

20. Frédéric Laffont and Christophe de Ponfilly, *A coeur, à corps, à cris: La grande aventure des "Médecins sans frontières"* (1991), Paris: Interscoop.

EPILOGUE

1. Efforts to redefine relations between the historic core of operational sections and their partners produced a new geographic vocabulary. For example, the headquarters of MSF-France became Operational Center Paris, or OCP in everyday shorthand. This muting of its own internal borders corresponded with a stronger international structure, including plans for an international association that members could join directly and sections defined on a regional rather than national basis. For its fortieth anniversary in 2011, the group welcomed new sections in Latin America and East Africa as well as Brazil and South Africa.

2. The proposed hospital was not the only sign of longer-term thinking at MSF; as the first issue of a new internal newsletter noted, since the term *emergency* was not actually in the organization's charter, development might not always remain a taboo (*MSF Borderline* 1 [March 2011]: 1). At a meeting in Paris in 2010, the group had already extended its commitment to treating HIV/AIDS. It also finally began to investigate the perceptions of those it treated (see Abu-Sada 2012) and increase its involvement with anthropology and other social sciences.

3. MSF-South Africa, "Khayelitsha 2001–2011, Activity Report: 10 Years of HIV/TB Care at Primary Health Care Level." For more on the background of the South African AIDS story and MSF's role in it, see Comaroff 2007; Fassin 2007b; Robins 2009, 2010; Steinberg 2008. It should be noted that MSF's South African section defines itself in regional rather than national terms.

REFERENCES

Abélès, Marc. 2010. *The Politics of Survival*. Durham, NC: Duke University Press.

Abu-Sada, Caroline, ed. 2012. *In the Eyes of Others: How People in Crises Perceive Humanitarian Aid*. New York: MSF USA / Humanitarian Outcomes / NYU Center on International Cooperation.

Adams, Vincanne. 1998. *Doctors for Democracy: Health Professionals in the Nepal Revolution*. Cambridge: Cambridge University Press.

Adorno, Theodor. 1974 [1951]. *Minima Moralia: Reflections from Damaged Life*. London: NLB.

Agamben, Giorgio. 1998. *Homo Sacer: Sovereign Power and Bare Life*. Stanford, CA: Stanford University Press.

———. 2000. *Remnants of Auschwitz: The Witness and the Archive*. New York: Zone Books.

———. 2005. *State of Exception*. Chicago: University of Chicago Press.

Agier, Michel. 2002. *Aux bords du monde, les réfugiés*. Paris: Flammarion.

Akrich, Madeline. 1992. "The De-Scription of Technical Objects." In *Shaping Technology*, edited by W. Bijker and J. Law. Cambridge, MA: MIT Press, 205–224.

Aldridge, A. Owen. 1975. *Voltaire and the Century of Light*. Princeton, NJ: Princeton University Press.

Allen, Tim. 1994. "Closed Minds: Open Systems." In *A River of Blessings: Essays in Honor of Paul Baxter*, edited by D. Brokensha. Syracuse, NY: Syracuse University Press, 225–246.

———. 1996. "A Flight from Refuge: The Return of Refugees from Southern Sudan to Northwest Uganda in the Late 1980s." In *In Search of Cool Ground: War, Flight and Homecoming in Northeast Africa*, edited by T. Allen. Trenton, NJ: Africa World Press, 220–261.

————. 2006. *Trial Justice: The International Criminal Court and the Lord's Resistance Army*. London: Zed Books.

Allen, Tim, and David Styan. 2000. "A Right to Interfere? Bernard Kouchner and the New Humanitarianism." *Journal of International Development* 12: 825–842.

Archambault, Edith. 1997. *The Nonprofit Sector in France*. Manchester: Manchester University Press.

Arendt, Hannah. 1990 [1963]. *On Revolution*. New York: Penguin Books.

————. 1998 [1958]. *The Human Condition*. Second ed. Chicago: University of Chicago Press.

Asad, Talal. 2003. *Formations of the Secular: Christianity, Islam, Modernity*. Stanford, CA: Stanford University Press.

Baker, Robert, and Martin Strosberg. 1992. "Triage and Equality: An Historical Reassessment of Utilitarian Analyses of Triage." *Kennedy Institute of Ethics Journal* 2 (2 [June]): 103–123.

Barnett, Michael. 2011. *Empire of Humanity: A History of Humanitarianism*. Ithaca, NY: Cornell University Press.

Bass, Gary. 2008. *Freedom's Battle: The Origins of Humanitarian Intervention*. New York: Knopf.

Bateson, Gregory. 1972. *Steps to an Ecology of Mind*. Chicago: University of Chicago Press.

Behrend, Heidi. 1999. *Alice Lakwena and the Holy Spirits: War in Northern Uganda, 1986–97*. Oxford: James Curry.

Bender, Thomas, ed. 1992. *The Antislavery Debate*. Berkeley: University of California Press.

Benjamin, Walter. 1969. *Illuminations: Essays and Reflections*. Translated by H. Zohn. Edited by H. Arendt. New York: Schocken Books.

————. 1978. *Reflections: Essays, Aphorisms, Autobiographical Writings*. Translated by E. Jephcott. Edited by P. Demetz. New York: Schocken Books.

Benthall, Jonathan. 1993. *Disasters, Relief and the Media*. London: I. B. Tauris.

————. 1997. "The Red Cross and Red Crescent Movement and Islamic Societies, with Special Reference to Jordan." *British Journal of Middle Eastern Studies* 22 (2 [Nov.]): 157–177.

Biagioli, Mario, and Peter Galison, ed. 2003. *Scientific Authorship: Credit and Intellectual Property in Science*. New York: Routledge.

Biehl, João. 2005. *Vita: Life in a Zone of Social Abandonment*. Berkeley: University of California Press.

————. 2007. *Will to Live: AIDS Therapies and the Politics of Survival*. Princeton, NJ: Princeton University Press.

Black, Maggie. 1992. *A Cause for Our Times: Oxfam, the First Fifty Years*. Oxford: Oxfam and Oxford University Press.

Blumenberg, Hans. 1983. *The Legitimacy of the Modern Age*. Translated by R. Wallace. Cambridge, MA: MIT Press.

Boli, John, and George Thomas, eds. 1999. *Constructing World Culture: International Nongovernmental Organizations since 1875*. Stanford, CA: Stanford University Press.

Boltanski, Luc. 1999 [1993]. *Distant Suffering: Morality, Media and Politics*. Cambridge: Cambridge University Press.

Bornstein, Erica. 2005. *The Spirit of Development: Protestant NGOs, Morality, and Economics in Zimbabwe.* Stanford, CA: Stanford University Press.

———. 2009. "The Impulse of Philanthropy." *Cultural Anthropology* 24 (4).

Bornstein, Erica, and Peter Redfield, eds. 2011. *Forces of Compassion: Humanitarianism between Ethics and Politics.* Santa Fe, NM: School for Advanced Research Press.

Bortolotti, Dan. 2004. *Hope in Hell: Inside the World of Doctors Without Borders.* Buffalo, NY: Firefly Books.

Bouchet-Saulnier, Françoise, and Fabien Dubuet. 2007. "Legal or Humanitarian Testimony? History of MSF's Interactions with Investigations and Judicial Proceedings." In *Les cahiers du CRASH.* Paris: Fondation Médecins Sans Frontières.

Bourg, Julian. 2007. *From Revolution to Ethics: May 1968 and Contemporary French Thought.* Montreal: McGill-Queens University Press.

Brabazon, James. 2000. *Albert Schweitzer: A Biography.* Second ed. Syracuse, NY: Syracuse University Press.

Bradol, Jean-Hervé. 2004. "Introduction: The Sacrificial International Order and Humanitarian Action." In *In the Shadow of Just Wars: Violence, Politics and Humanitarian Action,* edited by F. Weissman. Ithaca, NY: Médecins Sans Frontières and Cornell University Press, 1–22.

Bradol, Jean-Hervé, and Elizabeth Szumilin. 2011. "AIDS: A New Pandemic Leading to New Medical and Political Practices." In *Medical Innovations in Humanitarian Situations: The Work of Médecins Sans Frontières,* edited by J.-H. Bradol and C. Vidal. New York: Médecins Sans Frontières USA / Doctors Without Borders, 178–199.

Branch, Adam. 2011. *Displacing Human Rights: War and Intervention in Northern Uganda.* Oxford: Oxford University Press.

Brauman, Rony. 1996. *Humanitaire, le dilemme.* Paris: Editions Textuel.

———, ed. 2000. *Utopies sanitaires.* Paris: Le Pommier-Fayard.

———. 2006. *Penser dans l'urgence: Parcours critique d'un humanitaire.* Paris: Éditions du Seuil.

Brient, Elizabeth. 2000. "Hans Blumenberg and Hannah Arendt on the 'Unworldly Worldliness' of the Modern Age." *Journal of the History of Ideas* 61 (3 [July]): 513–530.

Briggs, Charles L., and Clara Mantini-Briggs. 2003. *Stories in the Time of Cholera: Racial Profiling during a Medical Nightmare.* Berkeley: University of California Press.

Brouwer, Steve. 2011. *Revolutionary Doctors: How Venezuela and Cuba Are Changing the World's Conception of Health Care.* New York: Monthly Review Press.

Brown, Wendy. 2001. *Politics out of History.* Princeton, NJ: Princeton University Press.

Butler, Judith. 2004. *Precarious Life: The Powers of Mourning and Violence.* London: Verso.

Butt, Leslie. 2002. "The Suffering Stranger: Medical Anthropology and International Morality." *Medical Anthropology* 21 (1): 1–24.

Caduff, Carlo. 2011. "Anthropology's Ethics: Moral Positionalism, Cultural Relativism, and Critical Analysis." *Anthropological Theory* 11 (4): 465–480.

Caldwell, Christopher. 2009. "Communiste et Rastignac." *London Review of Books* 31 (13 [July 9]): 7–10.

Calhoun, Craig. 2004. "A World of Emergencies: Fear, Intervention and the Limits of Cosmopolitan Order." *Canadian Review of Sociology and Anthropology* 41 (4): 373–395.

———. 2008. "The Imperative to Reduce Suffering: Charity, Progress and Emergencies in the Field of Humanitarian Action." In *Humanitarianism in Question: Power, Politics, Ethics,* edited by M. Barnett and T. Weiss. Ithaca, NY: Cornell University Press: 73–97.

———. 2010. "The Idea of Emergency: Humanitarian Action and Global (Dis)Order." In *Contemporary States of Emergency: The Politics of Military and Humanitarian Interventions,* edited by D. Fassin and M. Pandolfi. New York: Zone Books, 29–58.

Camus, Albert. 1947. *La peste.* Paris: Editions Gallimard.

———. 1991 [1947]. *The Plague.* Translated by S. Gilbert. New York: Vintage Books.

Cannell, Fenella. 2010. "The Anthropology of Secularism." *Annual Review of Anthropology* 39: 85–100.

Cattelino, Jessica. 2010. "The Double Bind of American Indian Need-Based Sovereignty." *Cultural Anthropology* 25 (2): 235–263.

Chrétien, Jean-Pierre. 2003. *The Great Lakes of Africa: Two Thousand Years of History.* Translated by S. Straus. New York: Zone Books.

Churchill, Winston. 1909. *My African Journey.* Toronto: William Briggs.

Cock, Emile. 2005. *Le dispositif humanitaire: Geopolitique de la générosité.* Paris: L'Harmattan.

Cohen, Lawrence. 2001. "The Other Kidney: Biopolitics beyond Recognition." *Body & Society* 2/3: 9–21.

Collier, Stephen J. , and Andrew Lakoff. 2005. "On Regimes of Living." In *Global Assemblages: Technology, Politics and Ethics as Anthropological Problems,* edited by A. Ong and S. Collier. Malden, MA: Blackwell, 22–39.

Collier, Stephen, Andrew Lakoff, and Paul Rabinow. 2004. "Biosecurity: Towards an Anthropology of the Contemporary." *Anthropology Today* 20 (5): 3–7.

Comaroff, Jean. 2007. "Beyond Bare Life: AIDS, (Bio)Politics, and the Neoliberal Order." *Public Culture* 19 (1): 197–459.

Cooter, Roger, and Bill Luckin, eds. 1997. *Accidents in History: Injuries, Fatalities and Social Relations.* Amsterdam: Rodopi.

Corty, Jean-François. 2011a. "Cholera: Diagnosis and Treatment outside the Hospital." In *Medical Innovations in Humanitarian Situations: The Work of Médecins Sans Frontières,* edited by J.-H. Bradol and C. Vidal. New York: Médecins Sans Frontières USA / Doctors Without Borders, 88–106.

———. 2011b. "Human African Trypanosomiasis: Moving beyond Arsenic." In *Medical Innovations in Humanitarian Situations: The Work of Médecins Sans Frontières,* edited by J.-H. Bradol and C. Vidal. New York: Médecins Sans Frontières USA / Doctors Without Borders, 131–154.

Cox, J. Charles. 1911. *The Sanctuaries and Sanctuary Seekers of Medieval England.* London: George Allen and Sons.

Darnton, Robert. 1985. *The Great Cat Massacre: And Other Episodes in French Cultural History.* New York: Vintage.

Das, Veena. 2007. *Life and Words: Violence and the Descent into the Ordinary.* Berkeley: University of California Press.

Das, Veena, and Deborah Poole, eds. 2004. *Anthropology in the Margins of the State.* Santa Fe, NM: School for Advanced Research Press.

Dauvin, Pascal. 2004. "Kosovo: Histoire d'une deportation, ou la chronique d'une prise de parole publique dans une ONG internationale." In *ONG et Humanitaire*, edited by J. Siméant and P. Dauvin. Paris: L'Harmattan, 35–59.

Dauvin, Pascal, and Johanna Siméant. 2002. *Le travail humanitaire: Les acteurs des ONG, du siege au terrain*. Paris: Presses de Sciences Po.

Dawes, James. 2007. *That the World May Know: Bearing Witness to Atrocity*. Cambridge, MA: Harvard University Press.

de Haan, Anke, Edith Lute, and Roderik Bender. 1995. *Médecins Sans Frontières: Ten Years Emergency Aid Worldwide / Artsen zonder grenzen: 10 jaar noodhulp wereldwijd*. Amsterdam: MSF-Holland.

de Laet, Marianne, and Annemarie Mol. 2000. "The Zimbabwe Bush Pump: Mechanics of a Fluid Technology." *Social Studies of Science* 30 (2): 225–263.

de Torrenté, Nicolas. 2001. "Post-Conflict Reconstruction and International Community in Uganda, 1986–2000: An African Success Story?" PhD diss., London School of Economics and Political Science.

de Waal, Alex. 1997. *Famine Crimes: Politics and the Disaster Relief Industry in Africa*. Oxford: James Currey.

Dodge, Cole P. , and Paul D. Wiebe, eds. 1985. *Crisis in Uganda: The Breakdown of Health Services*. Oxford: Pergamon Press.

Dolan, Chris. 2009. *Social Torture: The Case of Northern Uganda, 1986–2006*. New York: Berghahn Books.

Douglass, Ana, and Thomas Vogler, eds. 2003. *Witness and Memory: The Discourse of Trauma*. New York: Routledge.

Drescher, Seymour. 2009. *Abolition: A History of Slavery and Anti-Slavery*. Cambridge: Cambridge University Press.

Drouet, N. 1982. "Mobile Medical Emergency Units in France—Parts 1 and 2." *British Medical Journal* 284 (June 26): 1924–1928.

Druett, Joan. 2000. *Rough Medicine: Surgeons at Sea in the Age of Sail*. New York: Routledge.

Dubois, Laurent. 2004. *Avengers of the New World: The Story of the Haitian Revolution*. Cambridge, MA: Harvard University Press.

Dunant, Henry. 1986 [1862]. *A Memory of Solferino*. Translated by the American Red Cross. 1939. Geneva: International Committee of the Red Cross.

Dynes, Russell R. 2000. "The Dialogue between Voltaire and Rousseau on the Lisbon Earthquake: The Emergence of a Social Science View." *International Journal of Mass Emergencies and Disasters* 18 (1 [March]): 97–115.

Ecks, Stefan. 2008. "Global Pharmaceutical Markets and Corporate Citizenship: The Case of Novartis' Anti-cancer Drug Glivec." *BioSocieties* 3 (2): 165–181.

Elias, Norbert. 1978 [1939]. *The Civilizing Process*. Vol. 1: *The History of Manners*. Translated by E. Jephcott. New York: Pantheon.

Emmanuelli, Xavier. 1991. *Les prédateurs de l'action humanitaire*. Paris: Albin Michel.

———. 2005. *L'homme en état d'urgence*. Paris: Hachette.

Epstein, Steven. 1996. *Impure Science: AIDS, Activism, and the Politics of Knowledge*. Berkeley: University of California Press.

Eribon, Didier. 1991. *Michel Foucault*. Cambridge, MA: Harvard University Press.

Farmer, Paul. 2003. *Pathologies of Power: Health, Human Rights, and the New War on the Poor*. Berkeley: University of California Press.

———. 2010. *Partner to the Poor: A Paul Farmer Reader*. Edited by H. Saussy. Berkeley: University of California Press.

Fassin, Didier. 2004. "La cause des victimes." *Les temps modernes* 59 (627): 73–91.

———. 2007a. "Humanitarianism as a Politics of Life." *Public Culture* 19 (3): 499–520.

———. 2007b. *When Bodies Remember: Experiences and Politics of AIDS in South Africa*. Berkeley: University of California Press.

———. 2008. "Beyond Good and Evil? Questioning the Anthropological Discomfort with Morals." *Anthropological Theory* 8 (4): 333–344.

———. 2009. "Another Politics of Life Is Possible." *Theory, Culture and Society* 26 (5): 44–60.

———. 2011. *Humanitarian Reason: A Moral History of the Present Times*. Berkeley: University of California Press.

Fassin, Didier, and Mariella Pandolfi, eds. 2010. *Contemporary States of Emergency: The Politics of Military and Humanitarian Interventions*. New York: Zone Books.

Fassin, Didier, and Richard Rechtman. 2009. *The Empire of Trauma: An Inquiry into the Condition of Victimhood*. Translated by R. Gomme. Princeton, NJ: Princeton University Press.

Fassin, Didier, and Paula Vasquez. 2005. "Humanitarian Exception as the Rule: The Political Theology of the 1999 Tragedia in Venezuela." *American Ethnologist* 32 (3): 389–405.

Faubion, James. 2001. "Toward an Anthropology of Ethics: Foucault and the Pedagogies of Autopoiesis." *Representations* (74 [Spring]): 83–104.

———. 2003. "Religion, Violence and the Vitalistic Economy." *Anthropological Quarterly* 76 (1): 71–85.

Feldman, Ilana. 2007. "Difficult Distinctions: Refugee Law, Humanitarian Practice and Political Identification in Gaza." *Cultural Anthropology* 22 (1): 129–169.

———. 2011. "The Humanitarian Circuit: Relief Work, Development Assistance, and CARE in Gaza 1955–67." In *Forces of Compassion: Humanitarianism between Ethics and Politics*, edited by E. Bornstein and P. Redfield. Santa Fe, NM: School for Advanced Research Press, 203–226.

Feldman, Ilana, and Miriam Ticktin, eds. 2010. *In the Name of Humanity: The Government of Threat and Care*. Durham, NC: Duke University Press.

Ferguson, James. 2006. *Global Shadows: Africa in the Neoliberal World Order*. Durham, NC: Duke University Press.

Fernandez, James W. 1964. "The Sound of Bells in a Christian Country—In Search of the Historical Schweitzer." *Massachusetts Review* 5 (3 [Spring]): 537–562.

Festa, Lynn. 2010. "Humanity without Feathers." *Humanity: An International Journal of Human Rights, Humanitarianism, and Development* 1 (1): 3–27.

Fèvre, E. M., P. G. Coleman, S. C. Welburn, and I. Maudlin. 2004. "Reanalyzing the 1900–1920 Sleeping Sickness Epidemic in Uganda." *Emerging Infectious Diseases* 10 (4): 567–573.

Finnström, Sverker. 2008. *Living with Bad Surroundings: War, History and Everyday Moments in Northern Uganda*. Durham, NC: Duke University Press.

Fisher, William F. 1997. "Doing Good? The Politics and Antipolitics of NGO Practices." *Annual Review of Anthropology* 26: 439–464.

Ford, John. 1971. *The Role of Trypanosomiases in African Ecology*. Oxford: Claredon Press.

Forsythe, David P. 2005. *The Humanitarians: The International Committee of the Red Cross*. Cambridge: Cambridge University Press.

Fortun, Kim. 2001. *Advocacy after Bhopal: Environmentalism, Disaster, New Global Orders*. Chicago: University of Chicago Press.

Foucault, Michel. 1979. *Discipline and Punish: The Birth of the Prison*. Translated by A. Sheridan. New York: Vintage Books.

———. 1980. "The Confession of the Flesh." In *Power/Knowledge: Selected Interviews and Other Writings, 1972–1977*, edited by C. Gordon. New York: Pantheon, 194–228.

———. 1984. "On the Genealogy of Ethics: An Overview of Work in Progress." In *The Foucault Reader*, edited by P. Rabinow. New York: Pantheon, 340–372.

———. 1990 [1976]. *The History of Sexuality*. Vol. 1. Translated by R. Hurley. New York: Vintage.

———. 1998 [1969]. "What Is an Author?" In *Essential Works of Michel Foucault, 1954–1984*. Vol. 2: *Aesthetics, Method and Epistemology*, edited by J. Faubion. New York: New Press, 205–222.

———. 2000a [1979]. "For an Ethic of Discomfort." In *Essential Works of Michel Foucault, 1954–1984*. Vol. 3: *Power*, edited by J. Faubion. New York: New Press, 443–448.

———. 2000b [1983]. "The Risks of Security." In *Essential Works of Michel Foucault, 1954–1984*. Vol. 3: *Power*, edited by J. Faubion. New York: New Press, 365–382.

———. 2000c [1976]. "Truth and Power." In *Essential Works of Michel Foucault, 1954–1984*. Vol. 3: *Power*, edited by J. Faubion. New York: New Press, 111–133.

———. 2003. *"Society Must Be Defended": Lectures at the Collège de France, 1975–1976*. Translated by D. Macey. Edited by F. E. Michel Senellart, A. Fontana, and A. Davidson. New York: Picador.

———. 2007. *Security, Territory, Population: Lectures at the Collège de France, 1977–1978*. Translated by G. Burchell. Edited by F. E. Michel Senellart, A. Fontana, and A. Davidson. New York: Picador.

Fox, Renée C. 1995. "Medical Humanitarianism and Human Rights: Reflections on Doctors without Borders and Doctors of the World." *Social Science and Medicine* 41 (12): 1607–1626.

Gabriel, Richard, and Karen Metz. 1992. *A History of Military Medicine*. Vol. 2: *From the Renaissance through Modern Times*. New York: Greenwood Press.

Galison, Peter. 2003. "The Collective Author." In *Scientific Authorship: Credit and Intellectual Property in Science*, edited by M. Biagioli and P. Galison. New York: Routledge, 325–355.

Geissler, Paul Wenzel. 2010. "'Transport to Where?' Reflections on the Problem of Value and Time à propos an Awkward Practice in Medical Research." *Journal of Cultural Economy* 4 (1): 45–64.

Geissler, Paul Wenzel, and Ruth J. Prince. 2010. *The Land Is Dying: Contingency, Creativity and Conflict in Western Kenya.* Oxford: Berghahn Books.

Gibney, Paul. 2006. "The Double Bind Theory: Still Crazy-Making after All These Years." *Psychotherapy in Australia* 12 (3): 48–55.

Giri, Ananta Kumar. 2002. *Building in the Margins of Shacks: The Vision and Projects of Habitat for Humanity.* Himayatnagar, Hyderabad: Orient Longman.

Givoni, Michal. 2011. "Beyond the Humanitarian/Political Divide: Witnessing and the Making of Humanitarian Ethics." *Journal of Human Rights* (10): 55–75.

Goldhammer, Jesse. 2005. *The Headless Republic: Sacrificial Violence in Modern French Thought.* Ithaca, NY: Cornell University Press.

Good, Mary-Jo Delvecchio, Sandra Hyde, Sarah Pinto, and Byron Good, eds. 2008. *Postcolonial Disorders.* Berkeley: University of California Press.

Gramsci, Antonio. 1971. *Selections from the Prison Notebooks.* New York: International Publishers.

———.1994. *Letters from Prison.* Edited by F. Rosengarten. New York: Columbia University Press.

Greene, Jeremy. 2011. "Making Medicines Essential: The Emergent Centrality of Pharmaceuticals in Global Health." *BioSocieties* 6 (1): 10–33.

Groenewold, Julia, and Eve Porter. 1997. *World in Crisis: The Politics of Survival at the End of the Twentieth Century.* London: Routledge.

Guibert, Emmanuel, Didier Lefèvre, and Frédéric Lemercier. 2009. *The Photographer.* New York: First Second.

Guillemoles, Alain. 2002. *Bernard Kouchner: La biographie.* Paris: Bayard.

Guly, Henry. 2005. *A History of Accident and Emergency Medicine: 1948–2004.* New York: Palgrave Macmillan.

Gutman, Roy, and David Rieff, eds. 1999. *Crimes of War: What the Public Should Know.* New York: W. W. Norton.

Haller, John. 1992. *Farmcarts to Fords: A History of the Military Ambulance, 1790–1925.* Carbondale: Southern Illinois University Press.

Hamlin, Christopher. 2009. *Cholera: The Biography.* Oxford: Oxford University Press.

Hammond, Laura. 2008. "The Power of Holding Humanitarianism Hostage and the Myth of Protective Principles." In *Humanitarianism in Question: Politics, Power, Ethics,* edited by M. Barnett and T. Weiss. Ithaca, NY: Cornell University Press, 172–195.

Hannerz, Ulf. 2004. *Foreign News: Exploring the World of Foreign Correspondents.* Chicago: University of Chicago Press.

Haraway, Donna. 1997. *Modest_Witness@Second_Millennium. FemaleMan©_Meets_Onco Mouse™: Feminism and Technoscience.* New York: Routledge.

Hardiman, David, ed. 2006. *Healing Bodies, Saving Souls: Medical Missions in Asia and Africa.* Amsterdam: Rodopi.

Harrell-Bond, B. E. 1986. *Imposing Aid: Emergency Assistance to Refugees.* Oxford: Oxford University Press.

Haskell, Thomas. 1985a. "Capitalism and the Origins of Humanitarian Sensibility, Part 1." *American Historical Review* 90 (2): 339–361.

————. 1985b. "Capitalism and the Origins of Humanitarian Sensibility, Part 2." *American Historical Review* 90 (3): 547–556.

Headrick, Daniel. 1981. *The Tools of Empire: Technology and European Imperialism in the Nineteenth Century.* Oxford: Oxford University Press.

Headrick, Rita. 1994. *Colonialism, Health and Illness in French Equatorial Africa, 1885–1935.* Edited by D. Headrick. Atlanta: African Studies Association Press.

Hecht, Gabrielle, ed. 2011. *Entangled Geographies: Empire and Technopolitics in the Global Cold War.* Cambridge, MA: MIT Press.

Hochschild, Adam. 2005. *Bury the Chains: Prophets and Rebels in the Fight to Free an Empire's Slaves.* Boston: Houghton Mifflin.

Hoffman, Susannah M., and Anthony Oliver-Smith, eds. 2002. *Catastrophe and Culture: The Anthropology of Disaster.* Santa Fe, NM: School for Advanced Research Press.

Homsy, J., E. Katabira, D. Kabatesi, F. Mubiru, L. Kwamya, C. Tusaba, S. Kasolo, D. Mwebe, L. Ssentamu, M. Okello, and R. King. 1999. "Evaluating Herbal Medicine for the Management of Herpes Zoster in Human Immunodeficiency Virus-Infected Patients in Kampala, Uganda." *Journal of Alternative and Complementary Medicine* 5 (6): 553–565.

Hoppe, Kirk A. 2003. *Lords of the Fly: Sleeping Sickness Control in British East Africa, 1900–1960.* Westport, CT: Praeger.

Hubert, Henri, and Marcel Mauss. 1964 [1898]. *Sacrifice: Its Nature and Functions.* Chicago: University of Chicago Press.

Hunt, Lynn. 2007. *Inventing Human Rights: A History.* New York: Norton.

Hutchinson, John F. 1996. *Champions of Charity: War and the Rise of the Red Cross.* Boulder, CO: Westview Press.

————. 1997. "Civilian Ambulances and Lifesaving Societies: The European Experience, 1870–1914." In *Accidents in History: Injuries, Fatalities and Social Relations,* edited by R. Cooter and B. Luckin. Amsterdam: Rodopi, 158–178.

Hyde, Sandra Teresa. 2007. *Eating Spring Rice: The Cultural Politics of AIDS in Southwest China.* Berkeley: University of California Press.

Hyndman, Jennifer. 2000. *Managing Displacement: Refugees and the Politics of Humanitarianism.* Minneapolis: University of Minnesota Press.

ICRC (International Committee of the Red Cross). 2000. *International Red Cross and Red Crescent Museum.* Geneva: ICRC.

————. 2004. *Logistics Field Manual.* Geneva: ICRC.

Ignatieff, Michael. 1984. *The Needs of Strangers.* London: Chatto and Windus.

Iliffe, John. 2002. *East African Doctors: A History of the Modern Profession.* Kampala: Fountain Publishers.

Irwin, Alec, Joyce Millen, Jim Kim, John Gershman, Brooke G. Schoepf, and Paul Farmer. 2002. "Suffering, Moral Claims and Scholarly Responsibility: A Response to Leslie Butt." *Medical Anthropology* 21 (1): 25–30.

Isaac, Ephraim. 1993. "Humanitarianism across Religions and Cultures." In *Humanitarianism across Borders: Sustaining Civilians in Times of War,* edited by T. Weiss and L. Minear. Boulder, CO: Lynne Rienner, 13–22.

Iserson, Kenneth, and John Moskop. 2007. "Triage in Medicine, Part I: Concept, History, and Types." *Annals of Emergency Medicine* 49 (3): 275–281.

James, Erica Caple. 2010. *Democratic Insecurities: Violence, Trauma and Intervention in Haiti.* Berkeley: University of California Press.

Jansson, Kurt, Michael Harris, and Angela Penrose. 1990. *The Ethiopia Famine.* London: Zed Books.

JRCIRC (Joint Relief Commission of the International Red Cross). 1944. *Materia Medica Minimalis.* Geneva: International Committee of the Red Cross and League of Red Cross Societies.

———. 1948. *Report of the Joint Relief Commission of the International Red Cross.* Geneva: International Committee of the Red Cross and League of Red Cross Societies.

Kaatrud, David, Ramina Samii, and Luk N. Van Wassenhove. 2003. "UN Joint Logistics Center: A Coordinated Response to Common Humanitarian Logistics Concerns." *Forced Migration Review* 18: 11–14.

Kasozi, A. B. K. 1999. *The Social Origins of Violence in Uganda.* Kampala: Fountain Publishers.

Keck, Margaret E., and Kathryn Sikkink. 1998. *Activists beyond Borders: Advocacy Networks in International Politics.* Ithaca, NY: Cornell University Press.

Kelly, Ann H. 2010. "Will He Be There? Mediating Malaria, Immobilizing Science." *Journal of Cultural Economy* 4 (1): 65–79.

Kidder, Tracy. 2003. *Mountains beyond Mountains: The Quest of Dr. Paul Farmer, a Man Who Would Cure the World.* New York: Random House.

Kirk, John M., and H. Michael Erisman. 2009. *Cuban Medical Internationalism: Origins, Evolution, and Goals.* New York: Palgrave MacMillan.

Klaits, Frederick. 2010. *Death in a Church of Life: Moral Passion during Botswana's Time of AIDS.* Berkeley: University of California Press.

Kleinman, Arthur, and Joan Kleinman. 1997. "The Appeal of Experience; The Dismay of Images: Cultural Appropriations of Suffering in Our Times." In *Social Suffering*, edited by Veena Das, Arthur Kleinman, and Margaret Lock. Berkeley: University of California Press, 1–23.

Knutsson, Karl-Eric. 1985. "Preparedness for Disaster Operations." In *Crisis in Uganda: The Breakdown of Health Services*, edited by C. Dodge and P. Wiebe. Oxford: Pergamon Press, 183–189.

Koselleck, Reinhardt. 1988 (1959). *Critique and Crisis: Elightenment and the Pathogenesis of Modern Society.* Cambridge, MA: MIT Press.

———. 2002. *The Practice of Conceptual History: Timing History, Spacing Concepts.* Stanford, CA: Stanford University Press.

———. 2006. "Crisis." *Journal of the History of Ideas* 67 (2): 358–400.

Kouchner, Bernard. 1985. "Un vrai samouraï." In *Michel Foucault: Une histoire de la vérité.* Paris: Syros, 85–89.

———. 1991. *Le malheur des autres.* Paris: Editions Odile Jacob.

Krause, Elliott. 1996. *Death of the Guilds: Professions, States and the Advance of Capitalism, 1930–Present.* New Haven: Yale University Press.

Kurzman, Charles, and Lynn Owens. 2002. "The Sociology of Intellectuals." *Annual Review of Sociology* 28: 63–90.

Lachenal, Guillaume, and Bertrand Taithe. 2009. "Une généalogie missionnaire et coloniale de l'humanitaire: Le cas Aujoulat au Cameroun, 1935–1973." *Le mouvement social* (227): 45–63.

Lakoff, Andrew. 2007. "Preparing for the Next Emergency." *Public Culture* 19 (2): 247–271.

———, ed. 2010a. *Disaster and the Politics of Intervention.* New York: Columbia University and Social Science Research Council.

———. 2010b. "Two Regimes of Global Health." *Humanity: An International Journal of Human Rights, Humanitarianism, and Development* 1 (1): 59–79.

Lakoff, Andrew, and Stephen J. Collier, eds. 2008. *Biosecurity Interventions: Global Health and Security in Question.* New York: Columbia University Press.

Laqueur, Thomas. 2009. "Mourning, Pity, and the Work of Narrative." In *Humanitarianism and Suffering: The Mobilization of Empathy,* edited by R. Wilson and R. Brown. Cambridge: Cambridge University Press, 31–57.

Latour, Bruno. 1987. *Science in Action: How to Follow Scientists and Engineers through Society.* Cambridge, MA: Harvard University Press.

———. 1999. *Pandora's Hope: Essays on the Reality of Science Studies.* Cambridge, MA: Harvard University Press.

———. 2004. "Why Has Critique Run Out of Steam? From Matters of Fact to Matters of Concern." *Critical Inquiry* 30 (2): 225–248.

Lemkin, Raphaël. 2002 [1944]. "Genocide." In *Genocide: An Anthropological Reader,* edited by A. L. Hinton. Malden, MA: Blackwell, 27–42.

Leopold, Mark. 2005. *Inside West Nile: Violence, History and Representation on an African Frontier.* Santa Fe, NM: School for Advanced Research Press.

Lévi-Strauss, Claude. 1966. *The Savage Mind.* Chicago: University of Chicago Press.

Lindqvist, Sven. 2001. *A History of Bombing.* New York: New Press.

Lippert, Randy. 2004. "Sanctuary Practices, Rationalities and Sovereignties." *Alternatives* 29: 535–555.

Lynn, John A., ed. 1993. *Feeding Mars: Logistics in Western Warfare from the Middle Ages to the Present.* Boulder, CO: Westview Press.

Lyons, Maryinez. 1992. *The Colonial Disease: A Social History of Sleeping Sickness in Northern Zaire, 1900–1940.* Cambridge: Cambridge University Press.

Magone, Claire, Michaël Neuman, and Fabrice Weissman. 2011. *Humanitarian Negotiations Revealed: The MSF Experience.* New York: Columbia University Press.

Malkki, Liisa. 1995. *Purity and Exile: Violence, Memory, and National Cosmology among Hutu Refugees in Tanzania.* Chicago: University of Chicago Press.

———. 1996. "Speechless Emissaries: Refugees, Humanitarianism, and Dehistoricization." *Cultural Anthropology* 11 (3): 377–404.

Mamdani, Mahmood. 1996. *Citizen and Subject: Contemporary Africa and the Legacy of Late Colonialism.* Princeton, NJ: Princeton University Press.

Maskalyk, James. 2009. *Six Months in Sudan: A Young Doctor in a War-Torn Village.* New York: Spiegel and Grau.

Mauss, Marcel. 1990 [1925]. *The Gift: Forms and Functions of Exchange in Archaic Societies.* New York: W. W. Norton.

Mazrui, Ali A. 1991. "Dr. Schweitzer's Racism." *Transition* 53: 96–102.

Mbembe, Achille, and Janet L. Roitman. 1995. "Figures of the Subject in Times of Crisis." *Public Culture* 7 (2): 323–352.

McFalls, Lawrence. 2010. "Benevolent Dictatorship: The Formal Logic of Humanitarian Government." In *Contemporary States of Emergency: The Politics of Military and Humanitarian Interventions,* edited by D. Fassin and M. Pandolfi. New York: Zone Books, 317–333.

Mei, Z., L. M. Grummer-Strawn, M. de Onis, and R. Yip. 1997. "The Development of a MUAC-for-Height Reference, Including a Comparison to Other Nutritional Status Screening Indicators." *Bulletin of the World Health Organization* 75 (4): 333–341.

Mertz, Elizabeth, and Andria Timmer. 2010. "Introduction: Getting It Done: Ethnographic Perspectives on NGOs." *PoLAR: The Political and Legal Anthropology Review* 33 (2): 171–177.

Miles, Steven. 2004. *The Hippocratic Oath and the Ethics of Medicine.* Oxford: Oxford University Press.

Mol, Annemarie. 2008. *The Logic of Care: Health and the Problem of Patient Choice.* New York: Routledge.

Moorehead, Caroline. 1998. *Dunant's Dream: War, Switzerland and the History of the Red Cross.* London: HarperCollins.

Moskop, John, and Kenneth Iserson. 2007. "Triage in Medicine, Part II: Underlying Values and Principles." *Annals of Emergency Medicine* 49 (3): 282–287.

Mosse, David, ed. 2011. *Adventures in Aidland: The Anthropology of Professionals in International Development.* Oxford: Berghahn Books.

Moyn, Samuel. 2006. "Empathy in History, Empathizing with Humanity." *History and Theory* 45 (3): 397–415.

———. 2010. *The Last Utopia: Human Rights in History.* Cambridge, MA: Harvard University Press.

MSF (Médecins Sans Frontières), ed. 1992. *Populations in Danger.* Edited by F. Jean. London: John Libbey.

———. 1997. *Refugee Health: An Approach to Emergency Situations.* London: Macmillan.

———. 1999. *Rapid Health Assessment of Refugee or Displaced Populations.* Paris: Médecins Sans Frontières / Epicentre.

———. 2002. *R.D. Congo: Silence, on meurt: Témoignages.* Paris: L'Harmattan.

———, ed. 2005. *My Sweet La Mancha.* Geneva: Médecins Sans Frontières International.

MSF-H (Médecins Sans Frontières Holland). 2002. *"The War Was Following Me": Ten Years of Conflict, Violence and Chaos in the Eastern DRC.* Amsterdam: MSF-Holland, Humanitarian Affairs Department.

Neff, Stephen. 2000. *The Rights and Duties of Neutrals: A General History.* Manchester: Manchester University Press.

Nelson, Diane. 2009. *Reckoning: The Ends of War in Guatemala.* Durham, NC: Duke University Press.

Nguyen, Vinh-Kim. 2010. *The Republic of Therapy: Triage and Sovereignty in West Africa's Time of AIDS.* Durham, NC: Duke University Press.

Nietzsche, Friedrich Wilhelm, and Walter Arnold Kaufmann. 1967 [1887/1888]. *"On the Genealogy of Morals" and "Ecce Homo."* New York: Vintage Books.

Nordstrom, Carolyn. 2004. *Shadows of War: Violence, Power, and International Profiteering in the Twenty-First Century.* Berkeley: University of California Press.

Nurok, Michael. 2003. "Elements of the Medical Emergency's Epistemological Alignment: 18th-20th-Century Perspectives." *Social Studies of Science* 33 (4): 563–579.

Nutton, Vivian. 1993. "Beyond the Hippocratic Oath." In *Doctors and Ethics: The Earlier Historical Setting of Professional Ethics,* edited by A. Wear, J. Geyer-Kordesch, and R. French. Amsterdam: Rodopi, 10–37.

Ong, Aihwa. 2006. *Neoliberalism as Exception: Mutations in Citizenship and Sovereignty.* Durham, NC: Duke University Press.

Orbinski, James. 2008. *An Imperfect Offering: Humanitarian Action for the Twenty-First Century.* New York: Walker.

Packard, Randall M. 2007. *The Making of a Tropical Disease: A Short History of Malaria.* Baltimore, MD: Johns Hopkins University Press.

Pandolfi, Mariella. 2000. "Une souveraineté mouvante et supracoloniale." *Multitudes* (3 [Nov.]), http://multitudes.samizdat.net/article.php3?id_article=182.

———. 2003. "Contract of Mutual Indifference: Governance and the Humanitarian Apparatus in Contemporary Albania and Kosovo." *Indiana Journal of Global Legal Studies* 10: 369–381.

Payet, Marc. 1996. *Logs: Les hommes-orchestres de l'humanitaire.* Paris: Éditions Alternatives.

Petryna, Adriana, Andrew Lakoff, and Arthur Kleinman. 2006. *Global Pharmaceuticals: Ethics, Markets, Practices.* Durham, NC: Duke University Press.

Pfeifer, Michael. 2004. *Rough Justice: Lynching and American Society, 1874–1947.* Urbana: University of Illinois Press.

Porter, Roy. 1997. "Accidents in the Eighteenth Century." In *Accidents in History: Injuries, Fatalities and Social Relations,* edited by R. Cooter and B. Luckin. Amsterdam: Rodopi, 90–106.

Power, Samantha. 2002. *A Problem from Hell: America and the Age of Genocide.* New York: Basic Books.

Proctor, Robert. 1992. "Nazi Doctors, Racial Medicine and Human Experimentation." In *The Nazi Doctors and the Nuremberg Code: Human Rights and Human Experimentation,* edited by G. Annas and M. Grodin. New York: Oxford University Press, 17–31.

Pupavac, Vanessa. 2010. "Between Compassion and Conservatism: A Genealogy of Humanitarian Sensibility." In *Contemporary States of Emergency: The Politics of Military and Humanitarian Interventions,* edited by D. Fassin and M. Pandolfi. New York: Zone Books, 129–149.

Rabben, Linda. 2011. *Give Refuge to the Stranger: The Past, Present and Future of Sanctuary.* Walnut Creek, CA: Left Coast Press.

Rabinow, Paul. 1999. *French DNA: Trouble in Purgatory.* Chicago: University of Chicago Press.

———. 2003. *Anthropos Today: Reflections on Modern Equipment.* Princeton, NJ: Princeton University Press.

Rabinow, Paul, George Marcus, James Faubion, and Tobias Rees. 2008. *Designs for an Anthropology of the Contemporary.* Durham, NC: Duke University Press.

Rabinow, Paul, and Nikolas Rose. 2006. "Biopower Today." *BioSocieties* 1: 195–217.

Rackley, Edward B. 2001. *Bearing Witness: Strategies and Risks: A Reference Tool for MSF Field Workers.* Brussels: Centre de Recherche, MSF-Belgium.

———. 2002. "Solidarity and the Limits of Humanitarianism: A Critique of Humanitarian Reason." PhD diss., New School University.

Rademacher, Anne, and Raj Patel. 2002. "Retelling Worlds of Poverty: Reflections on Transforming Participatory Research for a Global Narrative." In *Knowing Poverty: Critical Reflections on Participatory Research and Policy,* edited by K. Brock and R. McGee. London: Earthscan Publications, 166–188.

Rancière, Jacques. 2004. "Who Is the Subject of the Rights of Man?" *South Atlantic Quarterly* 103 (2/3): 297–310.

Rankin, Johanna. 2005. "A New Frontier for Humanitarianism? Médecins Sans Frontières Responds to Neglected Diseases." Honors thesis, University of North Carolina at Chapel Hill.

Rawson, Elizabeth. 1969. *The Spartan Tradition in European Thought.* Oxford: Claredon Press.

Ray, Gene. 2004. "Reading the Lisbon Earthquake: Adorno, Lyotard and the Contemporary Sublime." *Yale Journal of Criticism* 17 (1): 1–18.

Redfield, Marc. 1996. *Phantom Formations: Aesthetic Ideology and the Bildungsroman.* Ithaca, NY: Cornell University Press.

Redfield, Peter. 2005. "Doctors, Borders and Life in Crisis." *Cultural Anthropology* 20 (3): 328–361.

Rees, Tobias, and Carlo Caduff. n.d. "What Was Biopower? And What Form(s)—If Any— Has It Assumed or Does It Assume Today?" Unpublished manuscript prepared for "Biopower Today" Workshop, University of Zurich, June 9–11, 2011.

Rice, Andrew. 2009. *The Teeth May Smile but the Heart Does Not Forget: Murder and Memory in Uganda.* New York: Metropolitan Books.

Rieff, David. 2002. *A Bed for the Night: Humanitarianism in Crisis.* New York: Simon and Schuster.

Riles, Annelise. 2000. *The Network Inside Out.* Ann Arbor: University of Michigan Press.

Robbins, Bruce. 1999. *Feeling Global: Internationalism in Distress.* New York: New York University Press.

Robertson, David, Richard Bedell, James Lavery, and Ross Upshur. 2002. "What Kind of Evidence Do We Need to Justify Humanitarian Medical Aid?" *Lancet* 360 (July 27): 330–333.

Robins, Steven. 2009. "Humanitarian Aid beyond Bare Survival: Social Movement Responses to Xenophobic Violence in South Africa." *American Ethnologist* 36 (4): 637–650.

———. 2010. *From Revolution to Rights in South Africa: Social Movements, NGOs and Popular Politics after Apartheid.* Oxford: James Currey.

Ross, Kristin. 2002. *May '68 and Its Afterlives.* Chicago: University of Chicago Press.

Rottenburg, Richard. 2009. *Far-Fetched Facts: A Parable of Development Aid.* Cambridge, MA: MIT Press.

Rousseau, Jean-Jacques. 2000 [1756]. "Letter to Voltaire on Optimism, 18 August 1756." In *"Candide" and Related Texts,* edited by D. Wooten. Indianapolis: Hackett, 108–122.

Scheper-Hughes, Nancy. 1993. *Death without Weeping: The Violence of Everyday Life in Brazil.* Berkeley: University of California Press.

Schmitt, Carl. 1985 [1922]. *Political Theology: Four Chapters on the Concept of Sovereignty.* Cambridge, MA: MIT Press.

Schrift, Alan, ed. 1997. *The Logic of the Gift: Toward an Ethic of Generosity.* New York: Routledge.

Schweitzer, Albert. 2003. *The African Sermons.* Edited by S. Melamed. Syracuse, NY: Syracuse University Press.

———. 2005. *Essential Writings.* Edited by J. Brabazon. Maryknoll, NY: Orbis Books.

———. 2009 [1933]. *Out of My Life and Thought.* Baltimore, MD: Johns Hopkins University Press.

Scott, David, and Charles Hirschkind. 2006. *Powers of the Secular Modern: Talal Asad and His Interlocutors.* Stanford, CA: Stanford University Press.

Seftel, Adam, ed. 1994. *Uganda: The Bloodstained Pearl of Africa and Its Struggle for Peace, from the Pages of "Drum."* Nairobi: JRA Bailey.

Setel, Philip. 1999. *A Plague of Paradoxes: AIDS, Culture, and Demography in Northern Tanzania.* Chicago: University of Chicago Press.

Shapin, Steven. 1994. *A Social History of Truth: Civility and Science in Seventeenth-Century England.* Chicago: University of Chicago Press.

Shaw, Rosalind, Lars Waldorf, and Pierre Hazan, eds. 2010. *Localizing Transitional Justice: Interventions and Priorities after Mass Violence.* Stanford, CA: Stanford University Press.

Shevchenko, Olga, and Renée C. Fox. 2008. "'Nationals' and 'Expatriates': Challenges of Fulfilling 'sans frontières' ('without Borders') Ideals in International Humanitarian Action." *Health and Human Rights* 10 (1), www.hhrjournal.org/index.php/hhr/article/view/21/112.

Siméant, Johanna. 2005. "What Is Going Global? The Internationalization of French NGOs 'without Borders.'" *Review of International Political Economy* 12 (5): 851–883.

Slaughter, Joseph. 2007. *Human Rights, Inc.: The World Novel, Narrative Form, and International Law.* New York: Fordham University Press.

———. 2009. "Humanitarian Reading." In *Humanitarianism and Suffering: The Mobilization of Empathy,* edited by R. Wilson and R. Brown. Cambridge: Cambridge University Press, 88–107.

Slim, Hugo. 1997. "Doing the Right Thing: Relief Agencies, Moral Dilemmas and Moral Responsibility in Political Emergencies and War." *Disasters* 21 (3): 244–257.

Slovic, Paul. 2007. "'If I Look at the Mass I Will Never Act': Psychic Numbing and Genocide." *Judgment and Decision Making* 2 (2 [Apr.]): 79–95.

Smith, Adam. 1976 [1759]. *The Theory of Moral Sentiments.* Oxford: Claredon Press.

Sontag, Susan. 2003. *Regarding the Pain of Others.* New York: Picador.

Soussan, Judith. 2008. "MSF and Protection: Pending or Closed?" In *Les cahiers du CRASH.* Paris: Fondation Médecins Sans Frontières.

Spivak, Gayatri. 1988. "Can the Subaltern Speak?" In *Marxism and the Interpretation of Culture,* edited by C. Nelson and L. Grossberg. Chicago: University of Illinois Press, 271–313.

Starn, Randolph. 1971. "Historians and 'Crisis.'" *Past and Present* (52 [Aug.]): 3–22.

———. 2005. "Crisis." In *New Dictionary of the History of Ideas.* Vol. 2. Edited by M.C. Horowitz. New York: Charles Scribner's Sons / Thompson Gale, 500–501.

Steinberg, Jonny. 2008. *Sizwe's Test: A Young Man's Journey through Africa's AIDS Epidemic.* New York: Simon and Schuster.

Stirrat, Jock. 2006. "Competitive Humanitarianism: Relief and the Tsunami in Sri Lanka." *Anthropology Today* 22 (5): 11–16.

Stirrat, R. L. 2008. "Mercenaries, Missionaries and Misfits: Representations of Development Personnel." *Critique of Anthropology* 28 (4): 406–425.

Taithe, Bertrand. 1998. "The Red Cross Flag in the Franco-Prussian War: Civilians, Humanitarians and War in the 'Modern Age.'" In *War, Medicine and Modernity,* edited by R. Cooter, M. Harrison, and S. Sturdy. Phoenix Mill, UK: Sutton, 22–47.

———. 2004. "Reinventing (French) Universalism: Religion, Humanitarianism and the 'French Doctors.'" *Modern and Contemporary France* 12 (2): 147–158.

Tanguy, Joëlle. 1999. "The Médecins Sans Frontières Experience." In *Framework for Survival: Health, Human Rights and Humanitarian Assistance in Conflicts and Disasters,* edited by K. M. Cahill. New York: Routledge, 226–244.

Tanguy, Joëlle, and Fiona Terry. 1999. "On Humanitarian Responsibility." Adapted from "Humanitarian Responsibility and Committed Action: Response to 'Principles, Politics, and Humanitarian Action.'" *Ethics & International Affairs* 13 March (1999), 29–34.

Terry, Fiona. 2002. *Condemned to Repeat? The Paradox of Humanitarian Action.* Ithaca, NY: Cornell University Press.

Thompson, E. P. 1971. "The Moral Economy of the English Crowd in the Eighteenth Century." *Past and Present* 50 (1): 76–136.

Ticktin, Miriam. 2011a. *Casualties of Care: Immigration and the Politics of Humanitarianism in France.* Berkeley: University of California Press.

———. 2011b. "The Gendered Human of Humanitarianism: Medicalising and Politicising Sexual Violence." *Gender & History* 23 (2): 250–265.

Tilley, Helen. 2004. "Ecologies of Complexity: Tropical Environments, African Trypanosomiasis, and the Science of Disease Control Strategies in British Colonial Africa, 1900–1940." *Osiris* 19: 21–38.

Tronto, Joan. 1993. *Moral Boundaries: A Political Argument for an Ethic of Care.* New York: Routledge.

Tsing, Anna Lowenhaupt. 2005. *Friction: An Ethnography of Gobal Connection.* Princeton, NJ: Princeton University Press.

Vallaeys, Anne. 2004. *Médecins sans frontières: La biographie.* Paris: Fayard.

Van Herp, Michel, Véronique Parqué, Edward B. Rackley, and Nathan Ford. 2003. "Mortality, Violence and Lack of Access to Healthcare in the Democratic Republic of Congo." *Disasters* 27 (2): 141–153.

Vaughn, Megan. 1991. *Curing Their Ills: Colonial Power and African Illness.* Stanford, CA: Stanford University Press.

Vidal, Claudine, and Jacques Pinel. 2011. "MSF 'Satellites': A Strategy Underlying Different Medical Practices." In *Medical Innovations in Humanitarian Situations: The Work of Médecins Sans Frontières,* edited by J.-H. Bradol and C. Vidal. New York: Médecins Sans Frontières USA / Doctors Without Borders, 22–38.

Voltaire. 1991. *Candide.* Translated and edited by R. Adams. New York: W. W. Norton.

Waters, Ken. 2004. "Influencing the Message: The Role of Catholic Missionaries in Media Coverage of the Nigerian Civil War." *Catholic Historical Review* 90 (4 [Oct.]): 697–718.

Weber, Olivier. 1995. *French Doctors: L'épopée des hommes et des femmes qui ont inventé la médecine humanitaire.* Paris: Editions Robert Laffont.

Weiss, Thomas. 1999. "Principles, Politics and Humanitarian Action." *Ethics and International Affairs* 13: 1–22.

Weissman, Fabrice, ed. 2004. *In the Shadow of "Just Wars": Violence, Politics and Humanitarian Action.* Ithaca, NY: Médecins Sans Frontières / Cornell University Press.

———. 2011. "Silence Heals . . . From the Cold War to the War on Terror, MSF Speaks Out: A Brief History." In *Humanitarian Negotiations Revealed: The MSF Experience,* edited by C. Magone, M. Neuman, and F. Weissman. New York: Columbia University Press, 177–198.

Well, Melissa. 1985. "The Relief Operation in Karamoja: What Was Learned and What Needs Improvement." In *Crisis in Uganda: The Breakdown of Health Services,* edited by C. Dodge and P. Wiebe. Oxford: Pergamon Press, 177–182.

Wendland, Claire. 2010. *A Heart for the Work: Journeys through an African Medical School.* Chicago: University of Chicago Press.

Westad, Odd Arne. 2007. *The Global Cold War: Third World Interventions and the Making of Our Times.* Cambridge: Cambridge University Press.

Wilson, Richard, and Richard Brown, eds. 2009. *Humanitarianism and Suffering: The Mobilization of Empathy.* Cambridge: Cambridge University Press.

Zelizer, Viviana. 1994 (1985). *Pricing the Priceless Child: The Changing Social Value of Children.* Princeton, NJ: Princeton University Press.

Zink, Brian. 2006. *Anyone, Anywhere, Anytime: A History of Emergency Medicine.* Philadelphia, PA: Mosby Elsevier.

INDEX

Abbé Pierre, 255n61

Access Campaign, 27, 99, 106, 116, 117, 201–3, 241, 245

Action Against Hunger (ACF), 227

Action Aid, 24

Adorno, Theodor, 235

advocacy work, MSF's, 29, 64, 66, 96, 190, 201, 202, 219, 230, 261n13; and moral witness, 99, 105, 106, 108, 110, 115, 116, 261n13

Afghanistan: MSF's activity in, 28, 38, 61, 76, 103, 114, 142, 143, 157, 161, 162–63; Soviet invasion of, 76, 103; U.S. invasion of, 105, 259n47

Agamben, Giorgio, 19–20, 21, 251n20, 263n43

AIDS, MSF's work relating to, 13, 14, 27, 28, 64, 106, 203–4, 230, 245, 272n2; in South Africa, 181, 246–47; in Uganda, 87–88, 179–83, 184, 187–201, 215, 216, 221, 226, 227. See also antiretroviral (ARV) drugs

Algerian war, 51, 52, 53, 100

Allen, Tim, 215

ambulances, 25, 33, 71, 75

Amin, Idi, 29, 37, 205–6, 211, 212, 213, 214

Amnesty International, 12

amputation, patients' resistance to, 158–59

Angola, MSF's activity in, 28, 87, 157–58

anthropology, 3–4, 5–6; and Agamben's work, 19, 251n20; and sacrifice, 41, 164, 266–67n20; and secularism, 43

anticolonialism, 34, 51, 149, 239, 246

anti-communism, 62, 76, 103 255n67, 256n86

antiretroviral (ARV) drugs, 28, 87, 179, 181–82, 184, 187–88, 190–91, 194–97, 199–200, 216, 230, 234, 246–47, 269n19

Arendt, Hannah, 16, 19, 44, 253n15

Aristotle, 16

Armenia, earthquake in, 225

Aron, Raymond, 60

Asad, Talal, 43

Australia, MSF section in, 71

authenticity, medical, 30–32

Bangladesh, 83

Barthes, Roland, 60

Bateson, Gregory, 150, 151

Belgium, MSF section in, 27, 61–62, 64, 81, 83, 96, 112, 143, 181, 185, 222, 256n86, 257n89; témoignage practiced by, 103, 107–8, 113

Benjamin, Walter, 19

Bérès, Jacques, 54, 58, 62

Bernier, Philippe, 55, 56, 58, 65

Biafra, conflict in, 52–53; MSF founded in context of, 12, 19, 38, 53, 54, 56, 57, 58, 61, 102; Red Cross's relief efforts in, 38, 52, 53, 54

bildungsroman, 2, 4, 231, 241, 249n2, 264n70

biopolitics, minimal, 20–21, 31, 156, 170, 178

biopower, Foucault's concept of, 18, 21

bios, 16

biosecurity, 87

boat people, 60, 76, 252n34